Endocrinology of Pregnancy

Endocrinology of Pregnancy

Edited by

Fritz Fuchs, M.D., Dr. Med., F.A.C.O.G.

Professor of Obstetrics and Gynecology,
Cornell University Medical College; and
Obstetrician and Gynecologist-in-Chief,
The New York Hospital, New York City

AND

Arnold Klopper, M.D., Ph.D., F.R.C.O.G.

Reader in Obstetrics and Gynaecology,
University of Aberdeen, Aberdeen, Scotland

BY 17 AUTHORS

WITH 102 ILLUSTRATIONS

MEDICAL DEPARTMENT
Harper & Row, Publishers
New York, Evanston, and London

 Printed in the United States of America. For information address Medical Department, Harper & Row, Publishers, Inc., 49 East 33rd Street, New York, N.Y. 10016.

First Edition

LIBRARY OF CONGRESS CATALOG CARD NUMBER: 72-114592

Contents

List of Authors

CARL G. BELING, M.D., Med. Dr.
Associate Professor of Endocrinology in Obstetrics and Gynecology, Cornell University Medical College, New York City

RUDI BORTH, D.Sc.
Associate Professor, Department of Obstetrics and Gynecology, The University of Toronto Faculty of Medicine, Toronto, Ontario, Canada

ROBERTO CALDEYRO-BARCIA, M.D.
Professor of Physiopathology, Faculty of Medicine, University of the Republic; and Director of the Latin American Center of Perinatology and Human Development, Montevideo, Uruguay

JUAN A. COCH, Ph.D.
Associate Professor of Physical Chemistry, School of Chemistry, University of the Republic, Montevideo, Uruguay

ANNA-RIITTA FUCHS, M.Sc.
Research Associate, The Population Council, The Rockefeller University, New York City

FRITZ FUCHS, M.D., Dr. Med., F.A.C.O.G.
Given Foundation Professor of Obstetrics and Gynecology, Cornell University Medical College; and Obstetrician and Gynecologist-in-Chief, The New York Hospital, New York City

EUGENE D. FURTH, M.D.
Associate Professor of Medicine, Division of Endocrinology and Metabolism, Albany Medical College of Union University, Albany, New York

HORTENSE M. GANDY, M.D.
Associate Professor of Endocrinology in Obstetrics and Gynecology, Cornell University Medical College, New York City

ERLIO GURPIDE, Ph.D.

Professor of Biochemistry and Professor of Obstetrics and Gynecology, Departments of Biochemistry and Obstetrics and Gynecology, University of Minnesota Health Sciences Center, Minneapolis

JOHN B. JOSIMOVICH, M.D.

Associate Professor of Obstetrics and Gynecology, Magee-Womens Hospital, The University of Pittsburgh School of Medicine, Pittsburgh, Pennsylvania

ARNOLD KLOPPER, M.D., Dr. Med., F.R.C.O.G.

Reader in Obstetrics and Gynaecology, University of Aberdeen, Aberdeen, Scotland

STIG MELANDER, M.D., Med. Dr.

Associate Professor of Obstetrics and Gynecology, University of Uppsala, Uppsala, Sweden

PATRICK J. MULROW, M.D.

Professor of Medicine, Yale University School of Medicine, New Haven, Connecticut

ANTHONY S. PAGLIARA, M.D.

Post-doctorial Research Fellow in Metabolism and Endocrinology, Washington University, St. Louis; and Instructor in Pediatrics, St. Louis Children's Hospital, St. Louis, Missouri

RALPH E. PETERSON, M.D.

Professor of Medicine, Cornell University Medical College, New York City

SAMUEL SOLOMON, Ph.D.

Professor, Departments of Biochemistry and Experimental Medicine, McGill University and the University Clinic, Royal Victoria Hospital, Montreal, Quebec, Canada

WILLIAM N. SPELLACY, M.D.

Associate Professor of Obstetrics and Gynecology, Department of Obstetrics and Gynecology, University of Miami School of Medicine, Miami, Florida

Preface

This book began with the first Cornell Postgraduate Course on the Endocrinology of Pregnancy held in New York in the autumn of 1966. The course was such a success that as many as possible of the members of the original faculty were reassembled in San Juan two years later to give the course again. As there appeared to be some need for a book of this kind, we persuaded our colleagues to prepare their material in a form suitable for publication and later to update their writings.

The book is intended to provide the obstetrician and endocrinologist with a comprehensive review of the endocrinology of human pregnancy and labor. The book does not purport to be a record of the two Cornell courses on the endocrinology of pregnancy. Our collaborators have reviewed their fields in more detail and in a different manner from what is possible in a verbal presentation. In addition, we have tried to cover aspects of the endocrinology of pregnancy not considered at the meetings by inviting additional contributors.

The scope of the book is not limited to those hormones which are assumed to be directly involved in the maintenance of pregnancy and the initiation of labor. All endocrine systems in the mother undergo specific changes during pregnancy, and knowledge of these changes is important for the evaluation of each system. We are fully aware that some subjects have not been covered in this book. No mention has been made of calcitonin, which is important to calcium homeostasis and probably plays a role in the mechanism providing the fetus with the inorganic substance in greatest demand. Nor has the recent demonstration of thyroid-stimulating hormone activity of placental origin been considered; with chorionic gonadotrophin and placental lactogen, we now have three placental hormones which are closely related to anterior pituitary hormones. Perhaps we shall find placental counterparts to all trophic hormones.

The term "feto-placental unit" has been helpful for our understanding of the interdependence of the fetal endocrine glands and the placenta with regard to certain steroid hormones. Although the fetus and placenta may be considered a functional unit in many respects, the term should be reserved for this unique complementary function with regard to steroid synthesis and metabolism, unless a more descriptive term could be devised.

We owe a special word of gratitude to our publishers, the Medical Department of Harper & Row, who have done a truly professional job coping with an Afrikaner-Scottish and Danish-American editorial partnership. The contributors represent more countries than revealed by their present affiliations, and we reflect with satisfaction that such a mixture is in some sense representative of our polyglot scientific community. As editors we would like to acknowledge and thank not only the authors, but also their collaborators, assistants, and secretaries, as well as our own, for their valuable contributions to this endeavor.

There are many writings on various aspects of the endocrinology of pregnancy, but, so far as we are aware, none in English which puts them within a single cover. By doing so, we hope the book will fill a need.

Fritz Fuchs
Arnold Klopper

Endocrinology of Pregnancy

Chapter One

Dynamics of Hormone Production and Metabolism

Erlio Gurpide and Hortense M. Gandy

The concentration (c) of a hormone in blood is usually considered the best index of availability of hormone to tissues and is a most useful parameter in distinguishing normal and pathological hormonal environments.[66] The total concentration of hormones can now be measured with such new techniques as double isotope dilution procedures,[6, 19, 42] radioimmunoassays,[5, 12, 13, 25, 28, 34, 43, 45, 46] and competitive binding methods.[27] However, the concentration of free hormone (hormone not bound to protein) may correlate better with evidence of biological activity than does the total concentration. This is true for cortisol[33] and thyroxin.[29] Ultrafiltration,[7] equilibrium dialysis,[9] electrophoresis,[10] and gel filtration[11] are used in measurement of free hormone in body fluids.

However, other dynamic parameters must be considered in the evaluation of hormone activity. One of these is the rate of glandular secretion of the hormone, usually expressed in milligrams or micrograms per day. The secretion rate of a hormone by a specific endocrine gland can be calculated from the arteriovenous difference in hormone concentration, provided organ blood flow is known. Since direct sampling of organ blood and measurement of blood flow are not practical clinical pro-

Supported in part by U.S.P.H.S. Research Grant AMO7328.

cedures, it is desirable to establish a relationship between blood concentration and rate of secretion of a hormone. This relationship appears to be a simple proportionality in a wide range of physiological conditions for such hormones as progesterone[22] and placental lactogen in pregnant women,[18] testosterone in men,[36,39] chorionic gonadotropin,[26,31,47] pituitary gonadotropins,[8,20] thyroxin,[29] and aldosterone.[41] For many other hormones the situation is complicated by the formation of circulating hormone by peripheral metabolic conversion of other secreted compounds. Circulating testosterone and androstenedione are interconverted;[3,30,39] both are precursors of estradiol and estrone, which are themselves interconverted peripherally.[2] In these cases, c may not be proportional to the secretory rate.

The concept of production rate (PR) of a circulating hormone was introduced to describe the rate at which the hormone enters the circulation de novo, irrespective of its origin. By definition, therefore, production rate equals the secretory rate of the hormone plus the fractions of the rates of secretion of other compounds which are converted peripherally into the circulating hormone. In the absence of metabolic conversions as sources for the circulating hormone, the hormone production rate in blood is identical to its secretory rate.

At physiological levels, the concentration of a hormone in peripheral blood is proportional to its blood production rate. The proportionality factor is referred to as the metabolic clearance rate (MCR, in liter/day) of the circulating hormone, i.e., $MCR = PR/c$. Tait *et al.*[38,41] named this factor and provided insight about its significance. By utilizing this formula, if the metabolic clearance rate of a circulating hormone is known, its production rate can be calculated from its concentration in the blood. As mentioned earlier, the production rate may equal the secretory rate for some hormones but not for all. For instance, the production rate of circulating estradiol in women results from ovarian secretion of estradiol, estrone, and androstenedione, as well as adrenal secretion of androstenedione. Thus, studies on estrogen production must include several dynamic parameters to define what fraction of the circulating hormone is contributed by gland secretion and what fraction by peripheral interconversion. Study of secretory and production rates has been facilitated by use of radioisotopically labeled hormones or hormone precursors.

LABELED HORMONES AS TRACERS

A tracer of a hormone has attached to its molecule a label or "tag" that permits the metabolic fate of the hormone to be followed; a tracer should behave identically to the endogenous compound in all metabolic reactions. The molecule may be labeled by introducing isotopic atoms into it, e.g., deuterium (a heavy hydrogen atom), ^{18}O (an oxygen atom with an atomic weight 2 units heavier than the common species ^{16}O), and ^{13}C. The ratio of labeled to unlabeled molecules can be measured in a mass spectrometer.

However, radioactive isotopes are more commonly used for labeling. These atoms are also heavier than the common species but are unstable, emitting measurable radiation as they disintegrate. Carbon-14 and tritium (^{3}H), radioactive isotopes of carbon and hydrogen, are used to label steroids. The list of tritium- and ^{14}C-labeled steroids available commercially is impressive. The ^{14}C is usually present at C-4 and tritium is usually attached to C-7. The numbering system for steroids is illustrated in Figure 1-1, which shows the structure of cholesterol. The number of ^{14}C and ^{3}H atoms present in a sample is usually measured with a liquid scintillation counter. In these systems, the energy of the β radiation emitted as a result of the disintegration of these radioisotopes is converted into light by organic compounds, called "phosphors," dissolved in an appropriate solvent. This light is detected by photoelectric cells. Tritium and ^{14}C can be measured simultaneously in the same solution because the energy of the electrons derived from the latter is about ten times greater than that derived from the former.

The unit of radioactivity commonly used in tracer experiments with hormones is the microcurie, which corresponds to 2.22×10^{6} dpm (atoms disintegrating per minute). Only a fraction of these disintegrations are

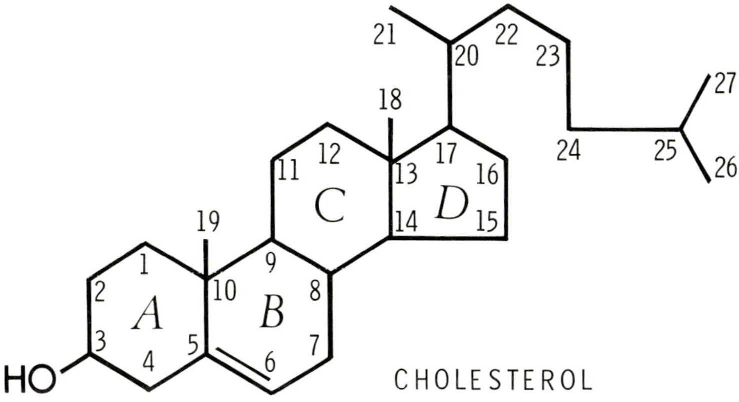

Fig. 1-1. Structural formula of cholesterol illustrating the typical cyclopentane phenantrene nucleus of the steroids (rings A,B,C, and D), the angular methyl groups (C-18, C-19), and the side chain attached to C-17.

counted; the efficiency of the counting depends on the isotope, the scintillation counter, and the counting conditions employed. Therefore, the amount of radioactivity is usually expressed in counts per minute (cpm). The specific activity of a compound is the amount of radioactivity per unit of weight, e.g., dpm/micromole or cpm/microgram.

A common procedure for labeling protein hormones consists of iodinating with ^{131}I or ^{125}I. Since only a few atoms of iodine attach to the protein molecule, the behavior of labeled and the unsubstituted molecules is very similar. In contrast to ^{3}H and ^{14}C, the radioactive iodine atoms emit gamma rays which are measured with NaI crystal scintillation counters. The amount of radioactivity is also expressed as cpm. Thyroid hormones are available labeled with ^{3}H, ^{14}C, or radioactive iodine.

Radioactive labeled hormones administered intravenously reflect only the metabolic fate of the hormone released into circulation. For instance, if labeled progesterone is injected intravenously, practically no labeled cortisol is formed, although cortisol is made in the adrenals from cholesterol via progesterone. Lack of formation of labeled cortisol indicates that circulating progesterone is not utilized by the adrenal for cortisol synthesis.

CALCULATION OF PR AND MCR FROM TRACER EXPERIMENTS

It is possible to calculate production rates (PR) and metabolic clearance rates (MCR) from tracer experiments.[14,23,39,41] The box in Figure 1-2 represents the circulating hormone under study. The hormone enters the pool de novo at a rate which, by definition, is the rate of production of the hormone in blood. The compound leaves the circulation irreversibly at a rate v, which equals the production rate if the system is at the steady state. Some of the hormone returns to circulation, at a rate w, from other tissues or by reversible metabolic reactions. This scheme does not impose a limitation on the number of spaces in which the hormone may be distributed in the organism, nor does it establish any restriction on the multiplicity of metabolic pathways, reversible and irreversible, in which the hormone may be involved. On the other hand, it implies a rapid mixing of the hormone in circulation, or at least an identical fate for tracer and endogenous circulating hormone.

Trace Infused at a Constant Rate

If the labeled hormone is infused at a constant rate (P, in cpm/min), a steady state in the specific activity (constant specific activity = a^*) of

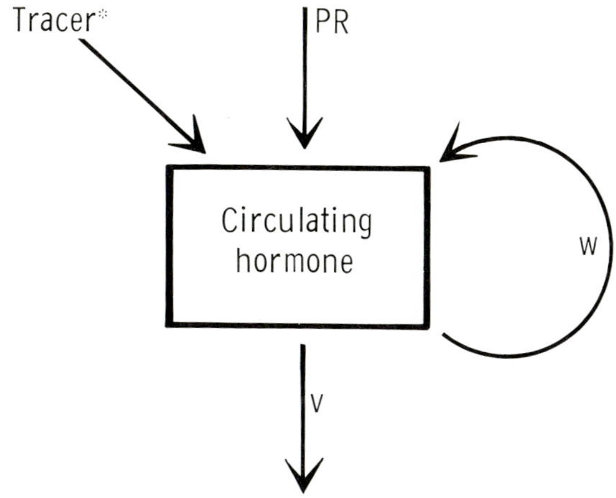

Fig. 1-2. Schematic representation of the rates of entry and removal of a circulating hormone. *PR* = production rate of hormone; *v* = rate at which hormone irreversibly leaves circulation; *w* = rate at which hormone returns to circulation.

the hormone in blood will eventually be reached. At such an isotopic steady state, the same amount of radioactive hormone enters and leaves the pool. Therefore,

$$P + wa^* = (v + w)a^*$$

If the term wa^* is cancelled from both sides of the equation, it follows that $v = \frac{P}{a^*}$ at the steady state, and since v equals the production rate (PR),

$$PR = v = \frac{P}{a^*} \qquad \text{(Equation 1)}$$

and, furthermore,

$$MCR = \frac{PR}{c} = \frac{P}{c^*} \qquad \text{(Equation 2)}$$

The concentration of the hormone (c, in μg/ml) is obtained from a blood sample taken before the infusion is started. After administration of the tracers at a constant rate, another blood sample is taken to determine the concentration of the tracer (c^*, in cpm/ml). The constant specific activity is calculated from these samples, since $a^* = c^*/c$. Achievement of the isotopic steady state is verified by taking several samples at different intervals and showing that c^* remains constant.

Tracer Injected as a Single Dose

Instead of using a continuous infusion technique, the tracer may be administered in a single injection and the changes in the specific activities (Sp. act.) of the hormone in plasma may be measured as a function of time. The specific activities are plotted against time and the areas of the resulting curves, extrapolated to zero time and negligibly low values of specific activities, are measured. The equivalence between single injection and constant infusion experimental designs[16] is shown by the following equality:

$$\left[\frac{\text{Area under Sp. act. curve}}{\text{Dose injected (cpm)}}\right]_{\substack{\text{single}\\\text{injection}}} = \left[\frac{\text{Sp. act. at steady state}}{\text{Infusion rate (cpm/min)}}\right]_{\substack{\text{constant}\\\text{infusion}}}$$

Therefore, Equations 1 and 2 are equivalent to

$$\text{PR} = \text{v} = \frac{\text{Dose injected}}{\text{Area under Sp. act. curve}} \qquad \text{(Equation 3)}$$

and

$$\text{MCR} = \frac{\text{Dose injected}}{\text{Area under tracer concentration curve}} \qquad \text{(Equation 4)}$$

CALCULATION OF RATES OF INTERCONVERSION OF CIRCULATING HORMONES

The use of tracers also permits the calculation of rates of interconversion of circulating hormones.[23,40] Supply and removal of two hormones in blood are illustrated in Figure 1-3. The symbol v_{AB} indicates the rate (μg/hr) of conversion of circulating compound A to circulating compound B, regardless of pathways or sites where such conversions occur. The symbol v_A denotes the rate at which A is removed irreversibly from circulation without being converted into circulating B. The rate at which A enters the circulation de novo excluding any contribution from circulating B is represented by the symbol Q_A. The rate, w_A, refers to the re-entry of A into circulation by all paths, except through circulating B. The remaining symbols represent the corresponding rates for conversion of compound B.

Two Tracers Infused Simultaneously at a Constant Rate

If a tracer of compound A labeled with tritium is mixed with a tracer of compound B labeled with ^{14}C, and the mixture is infused intra-

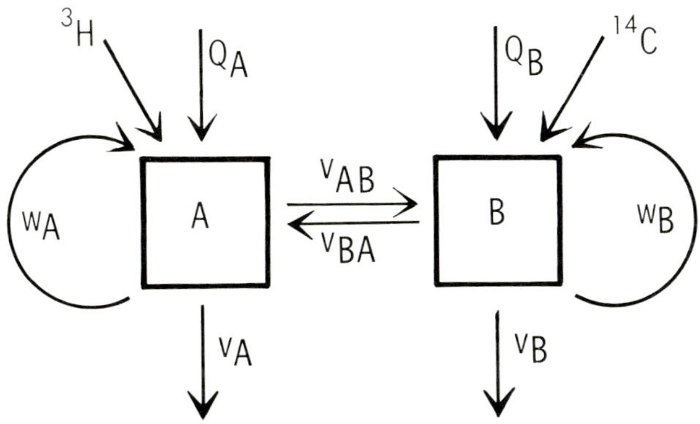

Fig. 1-3. Schematic representation of interconversion of two circulating hormones. v_{AB} = rate of conversion of compound A to compound B; v_A = rate at which A is removed irreversibly from circulation without being converted to B; Q_A = rate at which A enters circulation de novo without contribution from B; w_A = re-entry of A into circulation by all paths except through B. (Remaining symbols represent corresponding rates for conversion of compound B.)

venously at a constant rate, an isotopic steady state will eventually be reached for both circulating compounds. The Q and the v values shown in Figure 1-3 can be calculated from the six steady-state equations cited in Table 1-1. The steady-state equations express the identity of the rates of entry into, and exit from, circulation for labeled and unlabeled compounds A and B. The rates w_A and w_B are not shown in these equations since, by definition, they indicate re-entry, without losses or gains, at the steady state.

TABLE 1–1

STEADY-STATE EQUATIONS APPLICABLE TO INFUSION OF TRACERS AT CONSTANT RATE

	Compound A	Compound B
^{3}H	$P_A^{3H} + v_{BA}a_B^{3H} = (v_A + v_{AB})a_A^{3H}$	$v_{AB}a_A^{3H} = (v_B + v_{BA})a_B^{3H}$
^{14}C	$v_{BA}a_B^{14C} = (v_A + v_{AB})a_A^{14C}$	$P_B^{14C} + v_{AB}a_A^{14C} = (v_B + v_{BA})a_B^{14C}$
Endogenous	$Q_A + v_{BA} = v_A + v_{AB}$	$Q_B + v_{AB} = v_B + v_{BA}$

The solution of these equations is quite simple and yields the formulas shown in Table 1-2. It is important to emphasize that these calculations are valid regardless of the complexity of metabolic pathways and of the number of spaces of distribution of the compound under study.

TABLE 1-2

FORMULAS FOR CALCULATION OF RATES OF SECRETION AND INTERCONVERSION OF CIRCULATING HORMONES FROM TRACER DATA

$$Q_A = P_A^{3H} \times \frac{a_B^{14C} - a_A^{14C}}{a_A^{3H}\, a_B^{14C} - a_B^{3H}\, a_A^{14C}}; \quad v_{AB} = P_B^{14C} \times \frac{a_B^{3H}}{a_A^{3H}\, a_B^{14C} - a_B^{3H}\, a_A^{14C}}$$

$$Q_B = P_B^{14C} \times \frac{a_A^{3H} - a_B^{3H}}{a_A^{3H}\, a_B^{14C} - a_B^{3H}\, a_A^{14C}}; \quad v_{BA} = P_A^{3H} \times \frac{a_A^{14C}}{a_A^{3H}\, a_B^{14C} - a_B^{3H}\, a_A^{14C}}$$

Two parameters can now be introduced. One describes the fraction of the circulating compound (e.g., A) which is derived from the other. More precisely,[23]

$$\Delta_{BA} = \frac{v_{BA}}{(v_{BA} + Q_B)} = \frac{a_A{}^{14C}}{a_B{}^{14C}}$$

The other describes the fraction of the circulating compound (e.g., A) which is converted into the other. Specifically,[23]

$$\rho_{AB} = \frac{v_{AB}}{v_{AB} + v_A} = \frac{\left(\dfrac{{}^3H}{{}^{14}C}\right)_B}{\left(\dfrac{{}^3H}{{}^{14}C}\right)_{\text{infused}}}$$

The fraction ρ_{AB} also represents that part of Q_A which is converted into circulating B "for the first time," that is, excluding the part of the transfer from A to B which corresponds to recycled material.

The contributions of metabolic sources to the hormone in blood can be estimated from the data obtained from the two-tracer experiments described above. If testosterone and androstenedione are substituted for compounds A and B, respectively, in Figure 1-3, $\frac{\rho_{BA} Q_B}{PR_A}$ equals the contribution of secreted androstenedione to circulating testosterone. The symbol Q_A then corresponds to the rate of glandular secretion of testosterone, since the contribution of other possible metabolic precursors of the circulating hormone, such as dehydroisoandrosterone and androstenediol as well as their respective sulfates, might be negligible.

The model in Figure 1-2 applies not only to pairs of circulating compounds but also to the same compounds in two different spaces, as in fetal and maternal circulations. The application of this experimental design to study of fetal-maternal hormone transfers, production of hormones by the fetus, and supply of placental hormones to the fetus and mother have been discussed by Gurpide and Vande Wiele.[17]

Two Tracers Injected Simultaneously as a Single Dose

If the mixture of tracers is administered intravenously as a single injection, the formulas for calculating Q and v values from the experimental data can be obtained from the formulas in Table 1-2 merely by replacing infusion rates (P's) by the amounts of radioactivity injected and by replacing the specific activities at the steady state by areas under the specific activity curves.

CALCULATION OF SECRETORY RATES USING URINARY METABOLITES

Parameters of secretion and metabolism of hormones can also be estimated from specific activities of urinary metabolites.[14, 37, 39] If there is a metabolite entirely derived from one secreted hormone, calculation of the rate of secretion of the hormone is straightforward, provided the assumption is made that the fate of the intravenously injected tracer is identical with the fate of the secreted compound. This assumption is reasonable, since both tracer and secreted hormone are immediately transported to a common place—the right heart. The specific activity of the metabolite (e.g., $\bar{a}_I$ for metabolite I) isolated from pooled urine collected for an adequate period of time following the injection of the tracer is, by definition, equal to the ratio of labeled and unlabeled material. Thus,

$$\bar{a}_I = \frac{\text{amount of radioactivity appearing as I}}{\text{amount of I excreted}} = \frac{fR}{fQt}$$

where R is the dose injected (cpm), Q is the secretory rate (mg/day), t is the number of days taken to excrete all the labeled metabolite, and f is the fraction of the dose injected appearing as I (equal to the ratio of the rate of urinary excretion of I and to the rate of secretion of the hormone). Then,

$$Q = \frac{R}{\bar{a}_I t}$$

This expression appears to be applicable to the measurement of the rate of secretion of aldosterone, since this hormone seems to be the sole secreted precursor of urinary tetrahydroaldosterone glucuronide.[21]

However, urinary metabolites of steroid hormones are usually derived from more than one secreted precursor.[44] Although the above equation is not applicable for such instances, similar formulas can be derived. Consider that two urinary metabolites (I and II) are common products of two secreted precursors (A and B) but do not derive from any other secreted hormone. If a mixture of ^{3}H-A and ^{14}C-B is injected, then, by the same reasoning indicated above, it follows that[15]

$$\bar{a}_I^{3H} = \frac{f_{AI} R_A^{3H}}{(f_{AI}Q_A + f_{BI}Q_B)\,t} = \frac{R_A^{3H}}{\left[Q_A + \left(\frac{f_{BI}}{f_{AI}}\right) Q_B\right] t}$$

and

$$\bar{a}_{II}^{14C} = \frac{f_{BII} R_B^{14C}}{(f_{AII}Q_A + f_{BII}Q_B)\,t} = \frac{R_B^{14C}}{\left[\left(\frac{f_{AII}}{f_{BII}}\right) Q_A + Q_B\right] t}$$

where f's are the fractions of the injected doses excreted with each of the metabolites. The ratios $\frac{f_{AI}}{f_{BI}}$ and $\frac{f_{AII}}{f_{BII}}$ are given by the isotope ratios in the metabolite, i.e.,

$$\frac{f_{BI}}{f_{AI}} = \frac{\left(\frac{^3H}{^{14}C}\right)_{\text{injected}}}{\left(\frac{^3H}{^{14}C}\right)_I} \quad \text{and} \quad \frac{f_{AII}}{f_{BII}} = \frac{\left(\frac{^3H}{^{14}C}\right)_{II}}{\left(\frac{^3H}{^{14}C}\right)_{\text{injected}}}$$

Solving Q_A and Q_B in the equations above, expressions very similar to those shown in Table 1-2 are obtained:

$$Q_A = \frac{R_A^{3H}}{t} \times \frac{\bar{a}_{II}^{14C} - \bar{a}_I^{14C}}{\bar{a}_I^{3H}\bar{a}_{II}^{14C} - \bar{a}_{II}^{3H}\bar{a}_I^{14C}}, \quad Q_B = \frac{R_B^{14C}}{t} \times \frac{\bar{a}_I^{3H} - \bar{a}_{II}^{3H}}{\bar{a}_I^{3H}\bar{a}_{II}^{14C} - \bar{a}_{II}^{3H}\bar{a}_I^{14C}}$$

It is evident from these equations that the specific activities of the two urinary metabolities must be different with respect to at least one of the isotopes. However, it must be emphasized again that it is not required that one metabolite be exclusively derived from either A or B. These formulas have been used to estimate the rates of secretion of dehydroisoandrosterone and its sulfate.[44]

The multiplicity of precursors of urinary metabolites makes it imperative to evaluate carefully each particular situation before calculating rates of secretion by this method. For example, urinary pregnanediol, which was supposed to be a metabolite that reflected the secretion of progesterone, was found to be also derived from secreted pregnenolone or pregnenelone sulfate.[1] Testosterone glucuronide in urine is derived not only from secreted testosterone but also from secreted androstenedione, dehydroisoandrosterone and its sulfate.[44] Thus, to measure the secretion rate of testosterone by isotopic methods involving urinary metabolites, tracers of all of the precursors listed above would have to be administered and the specific activities of four urinary metabolites measured. Although these calculations are theoretically possible, the results of such studies would be imprecise owing to expected accumulation of experimental errors.

CURVE ANALYSIS

All tracer data used in the formulas given in the preceding sections were either constant values obtained during infusion of the tracers or areas under specific activity or concentration curves obtained following a single injection of the labeled hormone. If the shape of the curve is analyzed, further information about the system may be obtained. A typical curve of disappearance of a tracer from blood can be described by the sum of exponential terms, usually less than four. Since the number of terms is two for most of the experimental curves, we shall consider the function,

$$c^* = Ae^{-\alpha t} + Be^{-\beta t} \qquad \text{(Equation 3)}$$

to describe the concentration of the tracer in blood; c^* shall be expressed as the per cent of the injected dose/liter of blood. The values of A, B, α and β can easily be obtained by the "peel-off" graphic method[32] or by using suitable computer programs.[4] From these values, the following parameters can be estimated without resorting to the use of models.

Volume of Fast Initial Distribution of the Hormone

At the moment of injection ($t = 0$), the tracer distributes in a volume (V) such that, at a uniform concentration, $c^*_0 = \frac{100}{V}$. But, since $e^0 = 1$, it follows from Equation 3 that $c^*_0 = A + B$. Then,

$$V = \frac{100}{(A + B)}$$

Therefore, the hormonal content of the space of fast initial distribution is

$$M = Vc$$

Rate Constant of Total Removal of the Hormone from the Space of Fast Initial Distribution

Since at the time of injection ($t = 0$), there is no re-entry of the tracer into circulation, the rate of change of concentration of the tracer is simply given by the processes of removal, i.e., $\left(\frac{dc^*}{dt}\right)_0 = -k_{total}c^*_0$. The value of $\left(\frac{dc^*}{dt}\right)_0$ results from differentiating Equation 3 and evaluating the resulting equation for $t = 0$. Then, $k_{total} = \frac{A\alpha + B\beta}{(A + B)}$.

The rate at which the hormone leaves the circulation then equals $r_{total} = k_{total}M$. It is then possible to estimate what fraction of the hormone leaving the pool is lost irreversibly:

$$\phi = \frac{\text{rate of irreversible removal}}{\text{rate of total removal}} = \frac{PR}{r_{total}} = \frac{MCR}{k_{total}V}$$

The rate w in Figure 1-1 ($w = r_{total} - v$) as well as the rates w_A and w_B in Figure 1-3 (e.g., $w_A = r_{A, total} - v_{AB} - v_A$) can be calculated in this manner.

These calculations do not depend upon models. Other procedures currently used to interpret tracer data are based on models consisting of as many pools as exponential terms are necessary to describe the experimental curve. However, such procedures are essentially arbitrary and require a more extensive justification than is usually provided.[24, 35]

The clinical significance of measurement of production rates and rates of peripheral interconversion of hormones are discussed in the chapters that follow.

REFERENCES

1. Arcos, M., Gurpide, E., Vande Wiele, R. L., and Lieberman, S. Precursors of urinary pregnanediol and their influence on the determination of the secretory rate of progesterone. *J. Clin. Endocr. 24:*237, 1964.
2. Baird, D., Horton, R., Longcope, C., and Tait, J. F. Steroid prehormones. *Perspect. Biol. Med. 11:*384, 1968.
3. Bardin, C. W., and Lipsett, M. B. Testosterone and androstenedione blood production rates in normal women and women with idiopathic hirsutism or polycystic ovaries. *J. Clin. Invest. 46:*891, 1967.
4. Berman, M. "Compartmental Analysis In Kinetics." In *Computers in Biomedical Research,* R. W. Stacy and B. D. Waxman (Eds.), Academic Press, New York, 1965, Vol. II, p. 173.
5. Berson, S. A., and Yalow, R. S. Radioimmunoassay of ACTH in plasma. *J. Clin. Invest. 47:*2725, 1968.
6. Bojesen, E., and Degn, H. A double isotope derivative method for the determination of aldosterone in peripheral plasma. *Acta Endocr. (Kobenhavn) 37:*541, 1961.

7. Chen, P. S., Jr., Mills, I. H., and Bartter, F. C. A simple ultrafiltration method for determining non-protein bound steroids. *4th Int. Biochem. Congr.*, Vienna, p. 119, 1958.

8. Coble, Y. D., Jr., Kohler, P. O., Cargille, C. M., and Ross, G. T. Production rates and metabolic clearance rates of human follicle-stimulating hormone in premenopausal and postmenopausal women. *J. Clin. Invest. 48:*359, 1969.

9. Daughaday, W. H. Binding of corticosteroids by plasma proteins. III. The binding of corticosteroid and related hormones by human plasma and plasma protein fractions as measured by equilibrium dialysis. *J. Clin. Invest. 37:*511, 1958.

10. Daughaday, W. H. Binding of corticosteroid binding globulin. *J. Clin. Invest. 37:*519, 1958.

11. DeMoor, P., Heirwegh, K., Heremans, J. F., and Declerck-Raskin, M. Protein binding of corticoids studied by gel filtration. *J. Clin. Invest. 41:*816, 1962.

12. Demura, H., West, C. D., Nugent, C. A., Nakagawa, K., and Tyler, F. H. A sensitive radioimmunoassay for plasma ACTH levels. *J. Clin. Endocr. 26:*1297, 1966.

13. Glick, S. M., Kumaresan, P., Kagan, A., and Wheeler, M. Radioimmunoassay of oxytoxin. *Excerpta Med. Int. Congr. Sr. 161:*81, 1968.

14. Gurpide, E., MacDonald, P. C., Chapdelaine, A., Vande Wiele, R. L., and Lieberman, S. Studies on the secretion and interconversion of the androgens. II. Methods of estimation of rates of secretion and of metabolism from specific activities of urinary metabolites. *J. Clin. Endocr. 25:*1537, 1965.

15. Gurpide, E., and Mann, J. Estimation of secretory rates of hormones from the specific activities of metabolites which have multiple secreted precursors. *Bull. Math. Biophys. 27:*389, 1965.

16. Gurpide, E., Mann, J., and Lieberman, S. Analysis of open systems of multiple pools by administration of tracer at a constant rate or as a single dose as illustrated by problems involving steroid hormones. *J. Clin. Endocr. 23:*1155, 1963.

17. Gurpide, E., and Vande Wiele, R. L. "Estimation of Rates of Production and Transfer of Hormones in Pregnancy." In *Diagnosis and Treatment of Fetal Disorders,* K. Adamson (Ed.), Springer-Verlag, New York, 1969, p. 113.

18. Kaplan, S. L., Gurpide, E., Sciarra, J. J., and Grumbach, M. M. Metabolic clearance rate and production rate of chorionic growth hormone—prolactin in late pregnancy. *J. Clin. Endocr. 28:*1450, 1968.

19. Kliman, B., and Peterson, R. Double isotope derivative assay of aldosterone in biological extracts. *J. Biol. Chem. 235:*1639, 1960.

20. Kohler, P. O., Ross, G. T., and Odell, W. D. Metabolic clearance and production rates of human luteinizing hormone in pre- and postmenopausal women. *J. Clin. Invest. 47:*38, 1968.

21. Laragh, J. H., Ulick, S., Januszewicz, V., Deming, Q. B., Kelly, W., and

LIEBERMAN, S. Aldosterone secretion and primary and malignant hypertension. *J. Clin. Invest. 39:*1091, 1960.

22. LITTLE, B., TAIT, J. E., TAIT, S. A. S., and ERLENMEYER, F. Progesterone clearance in non pregnant and pregnant subjects. *Excerpta Med. Int. Sr. 111:*150, 1966.
23. MANN, J., and GURPIDE, E. Generalized rates of transfer in open systems of pools in the steady state. *J. Clin. Endocr. 26:*1346, 1966.
24. MANN, J., and GURPIDE, E. Interpretation of tracer data: significance of the number of terms in specific activity functions. *Biophys. J. 9:*810, 1969.
25. MIDGLEY, A. R., JR. Radioimmunoassay: a method for human chorionic gonadotropin and human luteinizing hormone. *Endocrinology 79:*10, 1966.
26. MIDGLEY, A. R. JR., and JAFFE, R. B. Regulation of human gonadotropins: II. Disappearance of human chorionic gonadotropin following delivery. *J. Clin. Endocr. 28:*1712, 1968.
27. MURPHY, B. E. Some studies of the protein-binding of steroids and their application to the routine micro and ultra-micro measurement of various steroids in body fluids by competitive protein-binding radioassay. *J. Clin. Endocr. 27:*973, 1967.
28. ODELL, W. D., ROSS, G., and RAYFORD, P. L. Radioimmunoassay for human luteinizing hormone. *Metabolism 15:*287, 1966.
29. OPPENHEIMER, J. H. Role of plasma proteins in the binding, distribution and metabolism of the thyroid hormones. *New Eng. J. Med. 278:*1153, 1968.
30. RIVAROLA, M., SAEZ, A., MEYER, J. M., JENKINS, and MIGEON, C. J. Metabolic clearance rate and blood production rate of testosterone and androst-4-ene-3, 17-dione under basal conditions, ACTH and HCG stimulation. *J. Clin. Endocr. 26:*1208, 1966.
31. RIZKALLAH, T., GURPIDE, E., and VANDE WIELE, R. L. Metabolism of HCG in man. *J. Clin. Endocr. 29:*92, 1969.
32. ROBERTSON, J. S. Theory and use of tracers in determining transfer rates in biological systems. *Physiol. Rev. 37:*133, 1957.
33. SANDBERG, A. A., ROSENTHAL, H., SCHNEIDER, S. L., and SLAUNWHITE, W. R., JR. "Interactions and Their Role in the Transport and Metabolism of Steroids." In *Steroid Dynamics,* G. Pincus, T. Nakao, and J. F. Tait (Eds.), Academic Press, New York, 1966, p. 1.
34. SAXENA, B. B., DEMURA, H., GANDY, H. M., and PETERSON, R. E. Radioimmunoassay of human follicle stimulating and luteinizing hormones in plasma. *J. Clin. Endocr. 28:*519, 1968.
35. SHARNEY, L., WASSERMAN, L. R., and GEVIRTZ, N. R. Representation of certain mammillary n-pool systems by two-pool models. *Amer. J. Med. Electronics 3:*249, 1964.
36. SOUTHERN, A. L., GORDON, G. G., and TOCHIMOTO, S. Further study of factors affecting the metabolic clearance of testosterone in man. *J. Clin. Endocr. 28:*1105, 1968.
37. TAIT, J. F. Review the use of isotopic steroids for the measurement of production rates *in vivo. J. Clin. Endocr. 23:*1285, 1963.
38. TAIT, J. F., and BURSTEIN, S. *"In Vivo* Studies of Steroid Dynamics in

Man." In *The Hormones,* G. Pincus, K. V. Thimann and E. B. Astwood (Eds.), Academic Press, New York, 1964, Vol. 5, p. 441.

39. TAIT, J. F., and HORTON, R. "The *In Vivo* Estimation of Blood Production and Interconversion Rates of Androstenedione and Testosterone and the Calculation of Their Secretion Rates." In *Steroid Dynamics,* G. Pincus, T. Nakao, and J. F. Tait (Eds.), Academic Press, New York, 1966, p. 393.
40. TAIT, J. F., and HORTON, R. Androstenedione production and interconversion rates measured in peripheral blood and studies on the possible site of its conversion to testosterone. *J. Clin. Invest. 45:*301, 1966.
41. TAIT, J. F., LITTLE, B., TAIT, S. A. S., and FLOOD, C. The metabolic clearance rate of aldosterone in pregnant and non pregnant subjects estimated by both single injection and constant infusion methods. *J. Clin. Invest. 41:*2093, 1962.
42. TAIT, S. A. S., and TAIT, J. F. "Assay of Aldosterone and Metabolites." In *Methods of Hormone Research,* R. I. Dorfman (Ed.), Academic Press, New York, 1962, Vol. 1, p. 265.
43. UTIGER, R. D. Radioimmunoassay of thyrotropin. *J. Clin. Invest. 44:*1277, 1965.
44. VANDE WIELE, R. L., MACDONALD, P. C., GURPIDE, E., and LIEBERMAN, S. Studies on the secretion and interconversion of the androgens. *Recent Progr. Hormone Res. 19:*275, 1963.
45. YALOW, R. S., and BERSON, S. A. Immunoassay of endogenous plasma insulin in man. *J. Clin. Invest. 39:*1157, 1960.
46. YALOW, R. S., GLICK, S. M., and BERSON, S. A. Radioimmunoassay of human plasma ACTH. *J. Clin. Endocr. 24:*1219, 1964.
47. YEN, S. S. C., LLERENA, O., LITTLE, B., and PEARSON, O. H. Disappearance rates of endogenous luteinizing hormone and chorionic gonadotropin in man. *J. Clin. Endocr. 28:*1763, 1968.

Chapter Two

Chorionic Gonadotrophin

Rudi Borth

Traditionally, reviews on human chorionic gonadotrophin (HCG) begin by quoting Aschheim and Zondek's epochal discovery in 1927,[3] that the blood and urine of pregnant women contain a hormone, then thought to originate in the anterior pituitary gland, which in immature female mice produces ovarian follicular growth and corpus luteum formation and, as a secondary effect, vaginal estrus. But the HCG story may be traced farther back to Aschner, who in 1913 described ovarian hyperemia, corpus luteum formation, and estrus in virgin guinea pigs injected with placental extracts.[4] He stated that the agent was soluble in water and destroyed by heat, and suggested its therapeutic use in amenorrhea and sterility. One may trace the story even farther back to Halban who, in 1905[39], from a masterly analysis of clinical observations, arrived at statements such as the following (my translation) : "Only the fertilized egg can be the cause triggering the changes in the maternal organism. Also, the occurrence of the corpus luteum verum must be understood as a reaction to the egg. . . . There is nothing else left . . . but to put the source of the active substances in the placenta." The marked ovarian and other changes seen in hydatidiform mole "may well be attributed to a particularly increased secretion of specific substances from the overgrown chorionic epithelium. . . . The active pregnancy substances are an effect of the placenta, or of the trophoblast and the chorionic epithelium."

To postulate that the placenta is an endocrine gland is one thing, to obtain direct experimental evidence of this is quite another. The traditional systematic approach in endocrinological studies includes the production of deficiency symptoms by removal of the gland, and the alleviation or disappearance of such symptoms following the administration of glandular extracts and purified fractions. But the chorionic villi secure the development of the fetus not only by influencing the maternal organism through endocrine agents produced in the feto-placental unit, but also by feeding the fetus from the maternal circulation. Obviously, it is impossible to remove the feto-placental unit as a source of internal secretion and at the same time keep it intact in all other respects. In spite of this intrinsic difficulty, a respectable store of knowledge on HCG and the other placental hormones has accumulated over the last 40 years. Much of this is due to the fortunate fact that these hormones produce their well-known effects in nonpregnant rodents.

In this chapter, those established facts which can be found in textbooks and reviews, and which can still be considered as true, will be dealt with rather briefly. Prominence will be given to some aspects which appear less familiar or more problematic. Following the usage of the World Health Organization, and in agreement with the convincing arguments advanced by Corner,[24] Russell and Wilhelmi,[55] and others, the spelling gonadotrophin is preferred to gonadotropin.

CHEMISTRY

It is a truism that a compound must be obtained in a chemically pure state before its composition and structure can be elucidated. Has pure HCG been prepared and used in such studies? The evidence on this point seems somewhat conflicting. A substance is supposed to be homogeneous or pure if further attempts at fractionation fail to produce any changes in its physical, chemical, and biological properties. However, it should not be overlooked that the procedures used in such attempts may by themselves cause a certain small degree of destruction, that is, chemical change.

In any case, it is unsatisfactory to note that different preparations of similar biological activity per unit weight were found to be homogeneous by some authors, and to contain more than one protein by others.[41, 67, 69] Recent evidence has established the existence of various components differing from each other in potency and sialic acid content.[42]

On the other hand, not too much should be made of the fact that the highest activities reported are not exactly the same. Some of the differences are well within the error of bioassay, others can easily be attributed to the now well-established fact that relative potencies of standard and unknown preparations may vary with the end point used if the two preparations differ in composition. The model of the *analytical* or *dilution assay*—which we have to use in bioassay and which we take, wishfully, for granted—is only an approximation; reality, not only in the gonadotrophin field, is sometimes noticeably different.[32,35]

Despite these limitations, and unless one wishes to adopt the rather extreme hypothesis that all the chemical data obtained so far refer to carrier proteins "contaminated" with a chemically undetectable small amount of the hormone, it seems now fairly likely that urinary HCG is a group of glycoproteins containing about 8–15 percent each of hexoses, hexosamines, and sialic acids. The biological activity of some components is of the order of 12–20 IU per μg, and the molecular weight (determined by methods as different as ultracentrifugation[38] and radiation inactivation[54]) is in the order of 30,000. A dimer may exist.[42] By way of comparison, the molecular weights of a few other compounds are as follows: progesterone, 314; thyroxin, 777; oxytocin, 1007; ACTH, 10,000; human growth hormone, 27,000; serum albumin, 69,000; fibrinogen, 400,000.

SITE OF PRODUCTION

The evidence leaves no doubt now that the placenta is the source of HCG in pregnancy.[29] HCG can be detected in tissues and body fluids only if chorionic tissue is also present, even in the absence of a living fetus or of the hypophysis.[8] Tissue culture and perfusion studies have shown that placental tissue can produce HCG in vitro.

The cellular site of production within the placenta remains uncertain. Histological and histochemical evidence from both in vivo and in vitro material seems inconclusive and, according to different authors, points to different cell types as the source of HCG.[29] The method of localization based on "staining" with fluorescent antibody has been applied to the problem[64] and may well be expected to solve it, provided that the difficulty of establishing specificity, common to all immunochemical methods, can be overcome (see discussion later in chapter).

Is the placenta the only source of gonadotrophic activity during pregnancy, or does the hypophysis contribute? This is a question of fact, not of ideology: the observation that the hypophysis is not required to maintain pregnancy[8] does not answer it. The question still arises mainly because FSH activity has been consistently found by some investigators (though not by all) in placental extracts and in urine from pregnant women.[29] If it is accepted that the protein HCG has some intrinsic follicle-stimulating activity,[1] the conflicting findings may perhaps be attributed to differences in dosage. It is difficult, however, to see how this explanation could apply to the claim that HCG and FSH can be extracted separately by benzoic acid and by kaolin used in sequence,[25] or to the observation that, of two different groups of antigens found in normal pregnancy urine reacting with antisera to HCG and to HMG, respectively, the HMG antigen could not be identified in one urinary extract obtained from a pregnant patient after hypophysectomy.[36] This may be, however, an isolated observation. Experiments showing differential inhibition of the biphasic-mouse-uterine-weight-response to HCG preparations by antisera to HCG and to HMG[43] are of great interest regarding sites of activity in protein mixtures, but they do not (and were not meant to) provide conclusive information on the origin of these proteins.

In spite of the new serological evidence brought forward, the view expressed in 1961 by Diczfalusy and Troen that a separate "FSH is not produced by the placenta, nor, with the possible exception of early stages of gestation, by the pituitary"[29] may well turn out to be the correct one in the end.

CONTROL OF SECRETION AND SECRETION RATES

Clear evidence regarding the factors which regulate the release or production of HCG is lacking. One may say, of course, that the production parallels the functional state of the trophoblast. But such a statement is little more than a tautology, and it fails to account for the decrease in secretion occurring after the third month of gestation.

For the time being, the only way to estimate approximately the rate at which HCG enters the maternal circulation is to divide the excretion rate in pregnancy urine by the percentage of HCG recovered in urine after delivery or following its injection into nonpregnant humans. This calculation yields figures of the order of 500,000–1,000,000 IU/day in the third month of gestation, and about 80,000–120,000 IU/day in late pregnancy.[29] It should be clear that these cannot be more than rough approximations; as such, they are nevertheless useful in physiological and therapeutic considerations.

For the future, isotope dilution comes to mind as the method of choice for the determination of secretion and production rates. But even if labeled HCG were available and its administration authorized, the intricacies involved in a multicompartment model (mother, placenta, fetus) make the collection of reliable data difficult and complicate their interpretation.

The implication that labeled HCG is not yet available calls for a short comment. Labeling, in a narrow sense, means replacing an atom of the molecule by its radioactive isotope. The preparations currently used in radioimmunological assays (see later) are protein mixtures containing, not the labeled hormone, but iodinated derivatives labeled with, for instance, iodine-125.

METABOLISM

The renal clearance of HCG is about 1 ml/minute or less; low values in this range are typical of proteins in general. By way of comparison, the creatinine clearance is about 100 ml/minute; the renal plasma flow is about 600 ml/minute.[30] The clearance remains fairly constant throughout pregnancy.[46,47] From data obtained in the immediate postpartum period (i.e., in the absence of placental production and, hypothetical, utilization), it has been demonstrated convincingly that only about 6–8 per cent of the circulating HCG is excreted in the urine in biologically active form; over 90 per cent must be assumed to be inactivated in the body.[44,56] The recovery from urine is much higher when known amounts of HCG are administered to nonpregnant individuals.[2]

These are the meager facts. Nothing seems to be known yet on the biosynthesis of HCG or on its inactive metabolites. Obviously, the latter would be of great clinical interest. Are they small fragments of the hormone molecule, perhaps even amino acids and hexoses which may re-enter metabolic cycles? Is activation achieved by partial breakdown of the main structure or by minor chemical changes not affecting the molecular size? These are interesting questions and the answers, as yet unknown, have important implications for clinical research, diagnosis, and therapy.

ASSAYS

Bioassay

The methods available for bioassay and the requirements in design and evaluation have been discussed frequently[2,9,11,15,28,32,35,46,47] and will not be reconsidered here in any detail. It is now common knowledge that assay results obtained under different conditions, in different laboratories, or by using different end points can only be compared in a meaningful way when: (1) a standard has been used, (2) the results are expressed in international units, (3) the precision has been estimated, and (4) the validity of the assumptions underlying the method of evaluation has been checked. Computers have greatly facilitated the routine use of correct statistical methods.[50]

Even so, many problems remain. Otherwise inert contaminants present in the standard or unknown preparations may affect the relative potency in different ways depending on the end point used.[13] Many bioassay procedures are costly and tedious. Their precision is considerably lower than that of techniques not affected by the biological variation in test animals. Colonies and strains of the animals may differ so much as to render the use of certain end points impossible in some places. In spite of these shortcomings, bioassays will remain an indispensable tool for the estimation of a protein hormone as long as its presence in a mixture can be ascertained only by means of its biological activity. This is certainly still true for HCG.

In many respects bioassays will become obsolete once it is demonstrated either that the hormone itself can be measured in a mixture without the use of a biological end point, or that some representative metabolites can be so measured. With the development of immunochemical methods, this moment is approaching rapidly. Widespread premature and uncritical use of these promising new methods, however, will do more harm than good.

Immunochemical Assay

Competent reviews on the immunochemical assay of HCG and other protein hormones have been published,[7,22,34,48] and no attempt will be made here to summarize this information. It is, however, emphasized that the nonspecialized user of immunochemical assay methods should read these texts.

These methods are superior to biological methods in many ways, particularly with regard to precision and practicability. Specificity, however, remains a problem, regardless of whether the end point used is hemolysis indicating the absence of complement fixation,[18] inhibition of the agglutination of antigen-coated erythrocytes[66] or latex particles,[37] or isotope dilution of antibody-bound antigen.[33,52,68] The nature of the problem, however, is different for each end point. It is essential to understand these differences, but the technical details involved are beyond the scope of this chapter.

For the method based on agglutination inhibition, complete kits including reagents, test tubes, etc., are available commercially. Most manufacturers set the sensitivity of their kits at 0.8–8 IU-eq/ml. The high speed of the slide tests is sometimes an advantage in pregnancy diagnosis. Assays, on the other hand, require serial dilutions, and for this purpose test tubes may be more practical. The precision of the assays is limited by the dilution factor employed. If two two-fold dilution series are used (the concentration points of one series being midway between the points of the other) the effective dilution factor is $\sqrt{2} = 1.41$, and the standard deviation of results from replicate assays will be of the order of 20 per cent.[5] If the end point is of the quantal or all-or-none type (presence or absence of agglutination), the serial spacing of concentrations cannot be made much closer without impairing the readability of the end point. Most variants of the technique are not suitable for the graded-response type of assay.

The complement fixation test has been adapted for the graded-response type of assay by measuring the degree of hemolysis colorimetrically rather than just noting the presence or absence of the reaction.[18] The sensitivity can be adjusted to 0.5–5 IU-eq/ml. The standard deviation of results from replicate assays is of the order of 3–5 per cent.

Radioimmunoassays require expensive equipment for counting the radioactive label, as well as special equipment or reagents for separating free from antibody-bound antigen. Small amounts of highly purified hormone must be available for labeling, that is, iodination with iodine-125 (the isotope now used most widely), and the experimental conditions for this chemical reaction are critical. The reward for mastering these requirements (which are obviously more demanding than those for other methods of immunoassay) is the thousand times higher sensitivity of radioimmunoassays as compared to the other systems discussed. The working range is of the order of 1–10 mIU-eq/ml (immunochemical equivalents of international milliunits of HCG per milliliter). The standard deviation of replicates is 3–5 per cent.

The special techniques which are used by immunologists to test and characterize a serological system have been widely employed to provide evidence on the specificity of immunochemical assay procedures for HCG.[20,34] Such evidence, though important and convincing in its own context, is necessarily incomplete since the molecular sites of antigenicity and biological activity are not the same, and the latter may be destroyed without loss of the former. This difference in sites has been demonstrated by immunological and biological methods,[41,66] as well as by radiation inactivation.[54] Terms such as "biologically inactivated HCG preparations," although sometimes used in describing this situation, are confusing and meaningless since "HCG without biological activity" is not HCG (just as progesterone after its chemical conversion to biologically inactive steroids cannot be called "inactive progesterone").

There is no doubt that HCG is *included* in the group of proteins measured by the immunochemical assay systems now available. If any such system measures *only* or *mainly* HCG, the results should agree with those obtained by bioassay of the same specimens (bearing in mind, however, the possible variation between different biological methods). Such comparisons have been reported by various authors with results ranging from almost perfect to complete absence of correlation.[6,12,48] Moreover, the ratio of the two values may differ from unity and vary considerably between samples, and even according to week of gestation.[66] Some of the variation found in these comparative studies must certainly be attributed to the assay error which is, of course, greater for the biological end points than for the immunochemical in vitro procedures. But once this is taken into account, a difference in specificity is the only explanation for major discrepancies in the results obtained by the two techniques, when such discrepancies exist.

A lack of specificity in terms of the hormone itself would become an asset if this could be attributed to the presence of biologically inactive metabolites and decomposition products of HCG. In wishful anticipation, this interpretation is often taken for granted without much evidence. Studies designed to test whether the immunochemical methods measure biologically inactive metabolites of HCG as well as the original hormone would be of great interest. It was reported recently that some HCG components which differed in chemical and biological properties were immunochemically identical.[57]

In the absence of sufficient evidence on specificity, it is well to remember that immunochemical assays in a given serological system do not give measurements in international units of HCG, but in immunochemical equivalents of these in terms of the standard preparation used. To avoid semantic as well as factual confusion, results should be reported in careful terminology reflecting this fact. The World Health Organization Expert Committee on Biological Standardization, in its 20th and 21st reports, has suggested distinguishing between "IU" and "IU (immunoassay)." According to another recent proposal, the required distinction could be achieved by calling biological units "bions," and immunochemical units "imms."[10]

While the high accuracy of the serological pregnancy tests is well established, it should not be overlooked that, in addition to HCG, the presence of other urinary antigens related to pregnancy may often have contributed to the highly satisfactory performance reported for these methods.

Chemical Assay

Despite repeated claims to the contrary in the older literature, no chemical method exists for the assay of HCG in body fluids. Attempts have been made to base such a method on the colorimetric estimation of the carbohydrate moiety of the hormone molecule. Assuming that HCG has a specific activity of only 15,000 IU/mg and a carbohydrate content of as much as 30 per cent, 1 IU would correspond to 20 ng of carbohydrate. It follows that colorimetric estimation does not seem to be a practical proposition.

CONCENTRATION IN TISSUES AND BODY FLUIDS

The facts concerning the concentration of HCG in tissues and body fluids have been summarized in many books and reviews,[17,29,47] and they are so well established that they need not be repeated here in any detail. As a hormone produced in the placenta and transported in the blood, HCG permeates most maternal tissues and is also excreted in the urine. The levels in tissue, blood, and urine run parallel throughout pregnancy, and it is customary to describe these curves as reaching a sharp peak between the 7th and 12th weeks, followed by an equally steep drop to levels which remain fairly constant from about the 15th week onwards until term. A much smaller rise may occur during the last trimester.

The magnitude of the changes in the first trimester is perhaps overemphasized if they are plotted on an arithmetic scale. For general biological and biochemical reasons, a logarithmic scale reflecting relative changes rather than differences seems to be more appropriate.[14,19,21,26] The drop in HCG levels is to about one-fifth or one-tenth of the peak value; a change of this magnitude is not exceptional in endocrine secretion.

The subject of HCG levels in placental disorders is outside the scope of this chapter. It should, however, be emphasized that, although different authors may agree about the qualitative changes associated with various clinical conditions, the actual values reported in normal as well as disturbed pregnancies may differ according to the assay methods used.[6,29] Clinical interpretation of individual assay results obtained in one laboratory should not be based on reference points reported by another.

The results of immunochemical assays of placental antigens often differ from those of bioassays of HCG, and the latter may also differ from each other depending on the end point used.[6,47] Nevertheless, the general shape of excretion and concentration curves (see Fig. 2-1), as well as the changes associated with various clinical conditions,[19,21,26,31,49,53,65,66] are very similar, and there remains little doubt that the antigen levels determined by the current immunochemical assay systems for HCG reflect placental function to about the same degree as do HCG levels determined by bioassay.

The concentration in urine varies throughout the day and also inversely with fluid volume; therefore, as a clinical parameter the 24-hour excretion rate seems preferable to the concentration in random samples or even morning urine.[5]

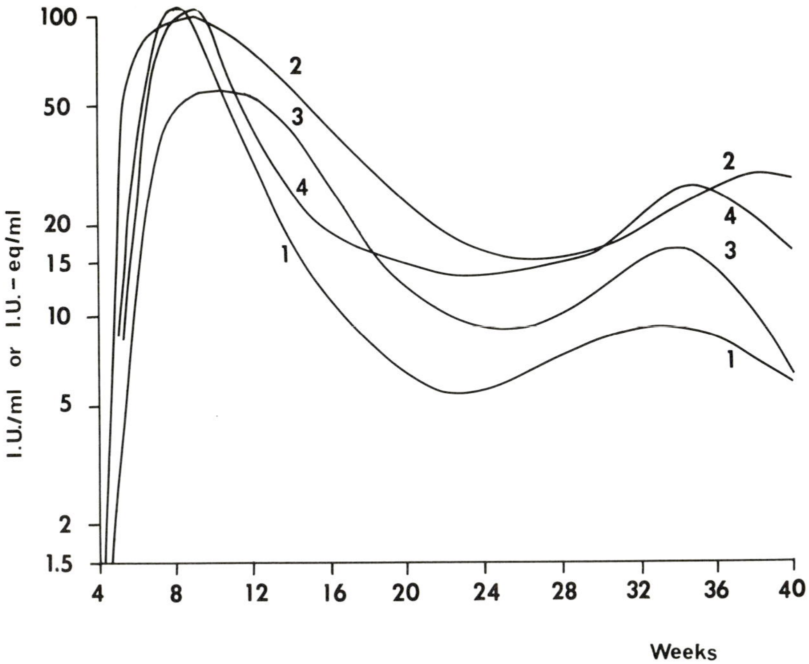

Fig. 2-1. Mean serum levels of chorionic gonadotrophin in normal pregnancy. The curves are based on results reported by various authors using different bioassay and immunoassay methods. Curve 1: uterine weight increase in rats;[45] Curve 2: ovarian hyperemia in rats (Borth and Menzi, unpublished); Curve 3: complement fixation;[19] Curve 4: hemagglutination inhibition.[51]

PLACENTAL TRANSFER AND FETO-MATERNAL RELATIONSHIP

HCG concentrations in fetal tissues are much lower than in maternal tissues.[29] In the amniotic fluid of early pregnancy, the concentration is very variable and, on the average, about one-tenth of that found in maternal serum.[16] From the distribution pattern of HCG it has been suggested that some of the hormone released from the chorion into the maternal blood seeps through the membranes into the fetal system.[23] It is also a possibility that rapid inactivation in the fetus helps to keep the concentration at a low level.[29]

PHYSIOLOGICAL ROLE IN PREGNANCY

Various theories have been advanced on the function of HCG.[29] According to the oldest and most widely taught concept, HCG keeps the corpus luteum functional until the steroids required for the development of the conceptus are produced in sufficient amounts by the feto-placental unit. This theory is in accordance with the known pharmacological effects of HCG and with the secretion peak in early pregnancy. It fails to attribute a role to the still considerable amounts produced later, and it is not easily reconciled with the uneventful continuation of pregnancy after early removal of the corpus luteum by operation.

Various authors have suggested a role for HCG in the stimulation of the fetal adrenal cortex, in the stimulation of the maternal adrenal gland, in placental estrogen synthesis, or in a placental feedback mechanism integrated with steroid metabolism. There is so far no conclusive or even strong evidence in support of any of these views.

A series of experimental papers published several years ago has resulted in an interesting attempt to link HCG (or a glycoprotein with similar properties) with the phenomenon of inhibition of uterine motility.[27, 58–63] These investigations may be summarized as follows: Therapeutic interruption of pregnancy can be done by intra-amniotic injection of hypertonic saline (10% NaCl). For various reasons, uterine or placental or fetal trauma, direct effect of the sodium chloride, and a drop in placental progesterone secretion can all be eliminated as the most likely cause of the onset of labor resulting from this clinical procedure. On the other hand, the observations made are compatible with the hypothesis that a functional anatomical lesion of the epithelium of the fetal membranes and the removal of an inhibitor of uterine motility are the determining factors.

The amniotic fluid of women with a normal pregnancy inhibited uterine motility in guinea pigs, rats, and rabbits, in vitro as well as in vivo. Amniotic fluid obtained during spontaneous abortion or delivery did not produce this effect.

The contractions induced in a pregnant woman by the intra-amniotic hypertonic saline were inhibited when the latter was removed and replaced by amniotic fluid from a normally pregnant woman; replacement by physiological saline had no such inhibitory effect.

The medium from chorionic tissue culture contained the motility-inhibiting factor as well as HCG. The presence of the latter was evidenced by the production of ovarian hyperemia in immature rats. A purified fraction, obtained from pregnancy urine and containing less nitrogen and more carbohydrate than those reported[38] for HCG, inhibited uterine motility in vitro at a concentration of 50 ng/ml; like HCG, it produced ovarian hyperemia at doses of 10–25 ng per rat. Purified commercial HCG preparations inhibited contractions of the rat uterus in vitro as well as in vivo and in pregnant animals. Negative results may occur in vitro or on intraperitoneal (instead of intramuscular) injection if crude or denatured preparations are used, since these may be toxic or oxytocic whereas amniotic fluid and suitably purified fractions are not.

These investigations have had to be discontinued; attention is called to them in the hope that it may stimulate further work.

It seems appropriate to conclude this section with a quotation. "The pharmacological action of HCG in different animal species, or in the human male and nonpregnant female—in instances in which the hormone normally does not occur—is relatively well understood. However, its physiological actions on the mother, on the fetus, and on the placenta are still obscure."[29]

CONCLUSIONS

It would be a thankless task to summarize this selective and condensed chapter. However, it may be useful to emphasize some of the points made.

1. HCG is produced by the trophoblast.
2. HCG is probably a glycoprotein with a molecular weight of approximately 30,000.
3. Immunochemical methods of assay are on the way to replace methods of bioassay for HCG; in promoting this development, attention should be paid to the problem of specificity.
4. The concentration of HCG in maternal tissues and body fluids is much higher than in the fetal compartment.
5. Most of the endogenous HCG is inactivated in the organism, but the pathways and the products of its metabolism are not known.
6. Many pharmacological effects of HCG preparations have been studied, but the physiological role of HCG in pregnancy is not known.

REFERENCES

1. Albert, A., and Derner, I. Studies on the biologic characterization of human gonadotropins. VI. Nature and number of gonadotropins in human pregnancy urine. *J. Clin. Endoc. 20:*1225, 1960.
2. Apostolakis, M., and Voigt, K.-D. *Gonadotropine.* Thieme, Stuttgart, 1965.
3. Aschheim, S., and Zondek, B. Hypophysenvorderlappenhormon und Ovarialhormon im Harn von Schwangeren. *Klin. Wschr. 6:*1322, 1927.

4. ASCHNER, B. Ueber brunstartige Erscheinungen (Hyperämie und Hämorrhagie am weiblichen Genitale) nach subkutaner Injektion von Ovarial- oder Placentarextrakt. *Arch. Gynaek. 99:*534, 1913.
5. BAECHLER, C., BORTH, R., and MENZI, A. Immunoassay of human chorionic gonadotrophin: diurnal variation in urinary antigen excretion. *Acta Endocr.* (Kobenhavn) *52:*199, 1966.
6. BELL, E. T., and LORAINE, J. A. (Eds.) *Recent Research on Gonadotrophic Hormones.* Livingstone, Edinburgh, 1967.
7. BERSON, S. A., and YALOW, R. S. "Immunoassay of Protein Hormones." In *The Hormones,* G. Pincus, K. V. Thimann, and E. B. Astwood (Eds.), Academic Press, New York, 1964, vol. IV, p. 557.
8. BETTENDORF, G., BRECKWOLDT, M., KNÖRR, and STEGNER, H.-E. Gravidität nach Hypophysektomie und Behandlung mit hypophysärem Humangonadotropin. *Deutsch. Med. Wschr. 89:*1952, 1964.
9. BORTH, R. Simplified mathematics for multiple bioassays. *Acta Endocr.* (Kobenhavn) *35:*454, 1960.
10. BORTH, R. A terminology for units of biological and immunochemical activity. *Acta Endocr.* (Kobenhavn) *60:*1, 1969.
11. BORTH, R., Diczfalusy, E., and Heinrichs, H. D. Grundlagen der statistischen Auswertung biologischer Bestimmungen. *Arch. Gynaek. 188:*497, 1957.
12. BORTH, R., FERIN, M., and MENZI, A. Comparison of bioassay and immunoassay of human chorionic gonadotrophin in urine. *Acta Endocr.* (Kobenhavn) *50:*335, 1965.
13. BORTH, R., LINDER, A., and LUNENFELD, B. Relative potency of human pituitary gonadotrophin preparations from urine in different types of bioassay. *Acta Endocr.* (Kobenhavn) *31:*192, 1959.
14. BORTH, R., LUNENFELD, B., STAMM, O., and DE WATTEVILLE, H. Gonadotrophin and steroid excretion in a case of twin pregnancy. *Acta Obstet. Gynec. Scand. 38:*417, 1959.
15. BORTH, R., LUNENFELD, B., and DE WATTEVILLE, H. Le dosage des gonadotrophines, méthode et intérêt clinique. *Bull. Soc. Roy. Belg. Gynec. Obstet. 27:*639, 1957.
16. BORTH, R., MENZI, A., and MIKAMO, K. Concentration of HCG in amniotic fluid in early pregnancy. In *Recent Research on Gonadothrophic Hormones,* E. T. Bell and J. A. Loraine (Eds.), Livingstone, Edinburgh and London, 1967, p. 87.
17. BORTH R., and DE WATTEVILLE, H. Hormone assays in obstetrics and gynecology. *Vitamins Hormones (N.Y.) 10:*141, 1952.
18. BRODY, S. Immunoassay of human chorionic gonadotrophin. Methodological and statistical aspects of a graded-response procedure based on complement fixation. *Acta Endocr.* (Kobenhavn) *52:*113, 1966.
19. BRODY, S., and CARLSTRÖM, G. Immuno-assay of human chorionic gonadotrophin in normal and pathologic pregnancy. *J. Clin. Endocr. 22:*564, 1962.
20. BRODY, S., and CARLSTRÖM, G. The problem of specificity in serologic deter-

mination of human chorionic gonadotrophin. *Acta Endocr.* (Kobenhavn) *42*:485, 1963.

21. Brody, S., and Carlström, G. Human chorionic gonadotrophin in abnormal pregnancy. Serum and urinary findings using various immunoassay techniques. *Acta Obstet. Gynec. Scand. 44*:32, 1965.
22. Brody, S., and Carlström, G. Problems associated with the quantitative immunoassay of human chorionic gonadotropin. *Ciba Found. Study Group No. 22*:70, 1965.
23. Bruner, J. A. Distribution of chorionic gonadotropin in mother and fetus at various stages of pregnancy. *J. Clin. Endocr. 11*:360, 1951.
24. Corner, G. W., Sr. -tropic versus -trophic in the terminology of the pituitary hormones. *Endocrinology 33*:405, 1943.
25. Crooke, A. C., and Butt, W. R. The excretion of follicle stimulating hormone by pregnant women. *J. Obstet. Gynaec. Brit. Emp. 66*:297, 1959.
26. Danielsson, M. Urinary excretion of human chorionic gonadotropin during prolonged pregnancy and labor. *Amer. J. Obstet. Gynec. 91*:895, 1965.
27. Dessarzin, D., and Stamm, O. Action inhibitrice des gonadotrophines choriales sur l'utérus. *Gynaecologia* (Basel) *154*:272, 1962.
28. Diczfalusy, E., and Heinrichs, H. D. Gonadotropine and ihre Bestimmung. *Arch. Gynaek. 187*:556, 1956.
29. Diczfalusy, E., and Troen, P. Endocrine functions of the human placenta. *Vitamins Hormones* (*N.Y.*) *19*:229, 1961.
30. Diem, K. (Ed.) *Scientific Tables.* Documenta Geigy, Basel, 1962, 6th edition, p. 545.
31. Enein, M. A. A., and Sharman, A. Immuno-assay of human chorionic gonadotrophin in threatened abortion. *J. Obstet. Gynaec. Brit. Comm. 74*:583, 1967.
32. Finney, D. J. *Statistical Method in Biological Assay,* Ed. 2, Griffin, London, 1964.
33. Franchimont, P. Dosage radio-immonologique des gonadotrophines folliculostimulante et lutéinisante. *J. Labelled Compounds 2*:303, 1966.
34. Franchimont, P. *Le dosage des hormones hypophysaires somatotrope et gonadotropes et son application en clinique. Thèse d'agrégation.* Arscia, Brussels, 1966.
35. Gaddum, J. H. Bioassays and mathematics. *Pharmacol. Rev. 5*:87, 1953.
36. Goss, D. A., and Lewis, J. Immunologic studies of the origin of follicle-stimulating substances in pregnancy urine extracts. *J. Clin. Endocr. 23*:986, 1963.
37. Goss, D. A., and Taymor, M. L. A rapid immunologic method for the semiquantitative determination of human chorionic gonadotropin in urine. *Fertil. Steril. 16*:151, 1965.
38. Got, R. Récentes acquisitions sur la gonadotropine choriale humaine. *Path. Biol.* (Paris) *8*:1583, 1960.
39. Halban, J. Die innere Secretion von Ovarium und Placenta und ihre Bedeutung für die Function der Milchdrüse. *Arch. Gynaek. 75*:353, 1905.

40. Hamashige, S., and Arquilla, E. R. Immunologic and biologic study of human chorionic gonadotropin. *J. Clin. Invest. 43:*1163, 1964.
41. van Hell, H., Goverde, B. C., Schuurs, A. H. W. M., de Jager, E., Matthijsen, R., and Homan, J. D. H. Purification, characterization and immunochemical properties of human chorionic gonadotropin. *Nature* (London) *212:*261, 1966.
42. van Hell, H., Matthijsen, R., and Homan, J. D. H. Studies on human chorionic gonadotrophin. I. Purification and some physio-chemical properties. *Acta Endocr.* (Kobenhavn) *59:*89, 1968.
43. Isersky, C., Lunenfeld, B., and Shelesnyak, M. C. Immunologic studies on gonadotropins: II. Biological assessment of the antigenic nature of the follicle-stimulating principle in human chorionic gonadotropin preparations. *J. Clin. Endocr. 23:*54, 1963.
44. Johnson, C. E., Albert, A., and Wilson, R. B. Renal and extrarenal disposal of chorionic gonadotropin in the immediate postpartum period. *J. Clin. Endocr. 10:*371, 1950.
45. Jones, G. E. S., Delfs, E., and Stran, H. M. Chorionic gonadotropin and pregnanediol values in normal pregnancy. *Bull. Hopkins Hosp. 75:*359, 1944.
46. Loraine, J. A. Bioassay of pituitary and placental gonadotropins in relation to clinical problems in man. *Vitamins Hormones* (N.Y.) *14:*305, 1956.
47. Loraine, J. A., and Bell, E. T. *Hormone Assays and Their Clinical Application,* Ed. 2, Livingstone, Edinburgh, 1966.
48. Lunenfeld, B., and Eshkol, A. Immunology of human chorionic gonadotropin. *Vitamins Hormones* (N.Y.) *25:*137, 1967.
49. MacGregor, W. G., Gale, C. W., Simmons, E., and Knight, G. J. The urinary excretion of human chorionic gonadotrophin in normal and abnormal pregnancy. *J. Obstet. Gynaec. Brit. Comm. 73:*775, 1966.
50. McArthur, J. W., Ulfelder, H., and Finney, D. J. A flexible computer program for the composite analysis of symmetrical and asymmetricial biologic assays of parallel-line type. *J. Pharmacol. Exp. Ther. 153:*573, 1966.
51. McCarthy, C. Pennington, G. W., and Crawford, W. S. Chorionic gonadotrophin excretion in normal and abnormal pregnancy. *J. Obstet. Gynaec. Brit. Comm. 71:*86, 1964.
52. Midgley, A. R., Jr. Radioimmunoassay: A method for human chorionic gonadotropin and human luteinizing hormone. *Endocrinology 79:*10, 1966.
53. Mishell, D. R., and Davajan, V. Quantitative immunologic assay of human chorionic gonadotropin in normal and abnormal pregnancies. *Amer. J. Obstet. Gynec. 96:*231, 1966.
54. Paul, W. E., and Odell, W. D. Radiation inactivation of the immunological and biological activities of human chorionic gonadotropin. *Nature* (London) *203:*979, 1964.
55. Russell, J. A., and Wilhelmi, A. E. Terminology for the anterior pituitary hormones (correspondence). *Science 138:*725, 1962.
56. Salvatierra, V. Über den Gonadotropinstoffwechsel während der Schwangerschaft. *Arch. Gynaek. 184:*617, 1954.

57. SCHUURS, A. H. W. M., DE JAGER, E., and HOMAN, J. D. H. Studies on human chorionic gonadotrophin. III. Immunochemical characterisation. *Acta Endocr.* (Kobenhavn) *59:*120, 1968.

58. STAMM, O. Untersuchungen über uterusinhibierende Eigenschaften des Fruchtwassers. *Arch. Gynaek. 182:*663, 1953.

59. STAMM, O. Action inhibitrice de liquide amniotique de grossesse chez la femme en travail. *Bull. Fed. Gynec. Obstet. Franc. 9:*117, 1957.

60. STAMM, O. Effet inhibiteur des gonadotrophines choriales sur la motilité utérine. *Schweiz. Med. Wschr. 89:*383, 1959.

61. STAMM, O. Extraction et isolement d'une hormone placentaire à effet inhibiteur sur l'utérus. *Experientia 17:*506, 1961.

62. STAMM, O., MONNIER, J., and LOOS, U. Mise en evidence d'une hormone placentaire à effet inhibiteur sur l'utérus. *Bull. Soc. Chim. Biol.* (Paris) *43:*1347, 1961.

63. STAMM, O., and DE WATTEVILLE, H. Étude expérimentale sur le mécanisme d'avortement par hydramnios artificiel. *Gynec. Obstet.* (Paris) *53:*171, 1954.

64. THIEDE, H. A., and CHOATE, J. W. Chorionic gonadotropin localization in the human placenta by immunofluorescent staining. 2. Demonstration of HCG in the trophoblast and amnion epithelium of immature and mature placentas. *Obstet. Gynec. 22:*433, 1963.

65. WÉRY, P. Estimation quantitative de l'hormone gonadotrope chorionique par une technique immunologique. *Bull. Soc. Roy. Belg. Gynec. Obstet. 35:*403, 1965.

66. WIDE, L. An immunological method for the assay of human chorionic gonadotrophin. *Acta Endocr.* (*Suppl.*) *70:*1, 1962.

67. WILDE, C. E., and BAGSHAWE, K. D. The purification of chorionic gonadotropin (and the discussion following this paper). *Ciba Found. Study Group No. 22:*46, 1965.

68. WILDE, C. E., ORR, A. H., and BAGSHAWE, K. D. A radioimmunoassay for human chorionic gonadotrophin. *Nature* (London) *205:*191, 1965.

69. YODER, J. M., ADAMS, E. C., JR., CHAMBLISS, K. W., and LOUGHMAN, B. E. Antigens of human chorionic gonadotropin preparations. I. Fractionation of pregnancy urine human chorionic gonadotropin and isolation of one of its specific antigens. *J. Clin. Endocr. 27:*509, 1967.

Chapter Three

Estrogens

Carl G. Beling

During the last few years there has been an increasing interest in the functional role of estrogens during pregnancy, and several groups of investigators have been engaged in the study of steroidogenic problems. The concept of the fetus and the placenta as a functional metabolic unit introduced by Diczfalusy some 10 years ago has proved most rewarding in the general understanding of steroid metabolic processes during pregnancy.[23,25,26] Before this concept, interest was predominantly focused on the endocrinology of the placenta; the active role of the fetus was not realized. Recent studies have clarified the biosynthetic pathways for a number of steroid metabolites in the fetoplacental unit, and it has been shown that the estrogen metabolic functions during pregnancy are delicately balanced between the fetus and the placenta.

The endocrine function of the placenta and the fetoplacental unit has been reviewed a number of times in recent years.[23,24,35,38,48,50,62,87] In the following chapter an attempt has been made to describe the present concept of the metabolism of the estrogens during pregnancy. Even though new data in this field tend to add to the complexity of the already established metabolic pathways, our concept of synthesis and deactivation of the estrogens are continuously being confirmed and further extended by different groups of investigators.

The functional role of estrogens during pregnancy is incompletely understood at the present time. It is generally believed that they are necessary for the maintenance of pregnancy, but their specific action on the uterus and the growing fetus is not known. It may be difficult to resolve questions related to the functional role of the estrogens without experiments in which estrone and estradiol or their precursors are administered during pregnancy. Because of the danger to the fetus such studies can not be performed in the human and experimental models have to be used. Subhuman primates may serve this purpose. Merkatz and Beling have shown that the pregnant baboon is an experimental model with great promise for the future because of its well defined excretion pattern of the major steroids of pregnancy.[68] Higher mammals may also provide useful information. A recent study in our laboratory has shown that injection of a small amount of estradiol to pregnant dogs during the last trimester of gestation results in characteristic changes in the fetuses.[43] These findings indicate that a proper balance in the synthesis of different estrogens of pregnancy is important for a normal fetal growth and development.

Only part of our present knowledge of estrogens during pregnancy has been directly applied to clinical problems. The determination of urinary estriol in various forms of pathological pregnancy is of particular interest in this respect. Data accumulated over the last few years have shown that, used with adequate restraint, such studies are of great value to determine the viability of the fetus in high-risk pregnancies. On the other hand, it is questionable whether the many studies of estriol excretion in pathological pregnancies have resulted in a better understanding of the functional role of the estrogens. Studies of estrogen metabolites other than estriol may prove to be more useful for the understanding of estrogen metabolism in pathological pregnancies.

CHEMISTRY

More than twenty different estrogens have been demonstrated in the urine of pregnant women. They are all phenolic steroids with an aromatic A ring and 18 carbon atoms. The chemical configuration of the three classical estrogens, estrone (E1), estradiol (E2), and estriol (E3) is shown in Figure 3-1. In spite of differences in the chemical structure, the estrogens are closely related to androgens, progestagens, and corticosteroids. In fact, progestagens and androgens serve as precursors for the formation of estrogens. The metabolic pathways for the synthesis and metabolism of the three main estrogens will be discussed in some detail because of their importance for the understanding of the physiological role of the estrogens during pregnancy. The structural formulas of the steroids involved and the major metabolic pathways in the steroid synthesis during pregnancy are shown in Figure 3-2.

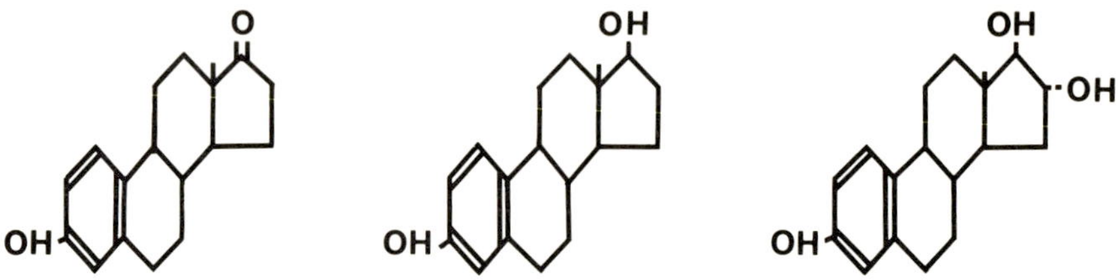

Estrone (E1) **Estradiol (E2)** **Estriol (E3)**

Fig. 3-1. The chemical structure of estrone, estradiol, and estriol.

ESTROGEN METABOLISM IN THE FETOPLACENTAL UNIT

The different experimental approaches used in studying estrogen synthesis in the fetus and the placenta are summarized in Table 3-1. Incubation experiments with placental and fetal tissue have been of great significance for our understanding of the endocrinology of pregnancy, and many conversions of estrogens have been demonstrated for the first time in such in vitro assays. On the basis of incubation experiments, Ryan, Villee, Migeon, and other investigators made the first outlines of estrogen synthesis in the placenta and the fetus, and their pioneer work has had a great impact on the development of the research in this field.

Placental perfusion studies have by and large confirmed and further extended the findings from in vitro assays. Perfusion of previable fetuses, carried out at the 18th to 20th week of gestation, has clarified the steroid metabolism in different fetal organs and has further demonstrated the extensive sulphate conjugation which takes place in the fetus. The feto-placental unit has been studied by different approaches including chemi-

TABLE 3-1
EXPERIMENTAL APPROACHES IN STUDYING THE STEROID PATHWAYS DURING PREGNANCY

In vitro studies	Incubation of placental tissue Incubation of fetal tissue
Perfusion studies	Perfusion of the placenta after its removal from the uterine wall Perfusion of placenta in situ Perfusion of previable fetuses
Studies of the intact feto-placental unit	Chemical determination of steroids on the fetal or maternal side Injection of labeled steroids on the fetal or maternal side

cal determination of estrogen metabolites and estrogen precursors in the umbilical artery and vein. On the basis of such determinations the fetal production of estriol precursor has been estimated and metabolic pathways for the formation of estriol have been outlined. Studies of the feto-placental unit also have been performed by administration of labeled steroids to the fetus and to the mother. Even though some difficulties have been encountered in the interpretation of the data because of the complex compartmentalization during pregnancy, the results from experiments with labeled steroids have clarified a number of estrogen pathways in the feto-placental unit.

Estrogen Precursors

All steroids, including progesterone and estrogens, can be made from acetate[55] and cholesterol[101] and the fetus as well as the placenta is ultimately dependent on the supply of precursor substances from the maternal side for the synthesis of steroids. Available evidence suggests that pregnenolone is the predominant precursor of progesterone and estrogens during pregnancy. Conversion of pregnenolone to progesterone has been demonstrated by Vande Wiele and Jailer[101] in placental incubation experiments and by Solomon *et al.*[98] and Pion, Conrad, and Wolf[76] in placental perfusion experiments.

The placenta is not capable of converting pregnenolone or progesterone to estrogens. This lack of enzyme systems for the formation of phenolic steroids was demonstrated by Jaffe *et al.* in experiments involving perfusion of placentas with labeled pregnenolone[47] and by Morato, Lemus, and Gual in placental incubation experiments.[72] Placental incubation with progesterone[58,63] and perfusion of the placenta with 17α-OH-progesterone[58] has also demonstrated the absence of aromatizing enzymes in placental tissue. Jaffe *et al.* found that both the fetus and the placenta contained no radioactive estrogens following injection of labeled progesterone into the umbilical vein.[47]

Fetal Conjugation

As shown in Figure 3-2, the fetus is actively involved in the formation of all three classical estrogens even though estrone and estradiol are synthesized by pathways quite different from those utilized for estriol. Pregnenolone, which serves as the precursor to all three estrogens, is transferred from the placenta to the fetus where it is conjugated to pregnenolone sulphate. The efficient sulphate conjugation of all the estrogens and estrogen precursors reaching the fetus has been strongly emphasized by Diczfalusy and his group.[23,25,26] This concept was further pursued by Emerman *et al.* who demonstrated in perfusion experiments with previable fetuses that the steroid molecule is also metabolized in conjugated form by the fetus (Table 3-2).[30] Similar results indicating that the fetal liver is the site of this metabolism of estrogens conjugated by the fetus were obtained by Schwers, Eriksson, and Diczfalusy.[90] The findings are in agreement with the tissue incubation studies of Wengle which showed a high sulphurylating capacity in the fetal liver.[108]

DHAS and Other Intermediates

As shown in Figure 3-2, pregnenolone is first converted to 17α-OH-pregnenolone and then to dehydroisoandrosterone sulphate (DHAS). DHAS is formed predominantly in the fetal adrenals and is of particular interest because of its multiple precursor role for the synthesis of the placental estrogens. The amount of DHAS produced by the fetal adrenals was estimated by Simmer *et al.* to be approximately 75 mg per 24 hours at term.[95] It seems that during pregnancy enough DHAS is formed by the fetus to serve as precursor to the large amounts of estrogens excreted in the maternal urine.

DHAS is utilized as a precursor for the synthesis of estrone and estradiol. Production-rate studies of Siiteri and MacDonald have shown that precursor-DHAS for the formation of estradiol during pregnancy is supplied in approximately equal amounts from the maternal and fetal side.[94] DHAS is further metabolized in the placenta to estrone and estradiol by pathways involving the formation of androstenedione and testosterone[2, 9, 41, 42, 44, 46, 48, 77, 84] as illustrated in Figure 3-2. The importance of this "neutral" pathway for formation of estrogens has been demonstrated by Meyer,[69] Ryan,[85] Baggett *et al.*,[2] Gual *et al.*,[1] and other investigators. The synthesis from DHAS via androstenedione to estrone and via testosterone to estradiol was outlined on the basis of placental perfusion experiments by Bolté *et al.*[9, 10] (Table 3-3). However, intermediate metabolites other than androstenedione and testosterone are also involved in the synthesis of estrone and estradiol. Longchampt *et al.*[59] and Wilcox and Engel[109] showed in placental incubation experiments and Cedard, Varangot, and Yannotti[18] showed in placental perfusion studies that 19-hydroxylation of androstenedione and testosterone is a necessary step preceding the formation of estrone and estradiol. These experiments also showed conclusively that no estriol is formed from DHA by the placenta, which confirms earlier findings that no 16-hydroxylating enzymes are present in human placental tissue.

Protective Fetal Mechanisms

Even though precursor DHAS is produced by the fetal adrenals, the fetus does not possess enzyme systems to convert DHAS to androgens.

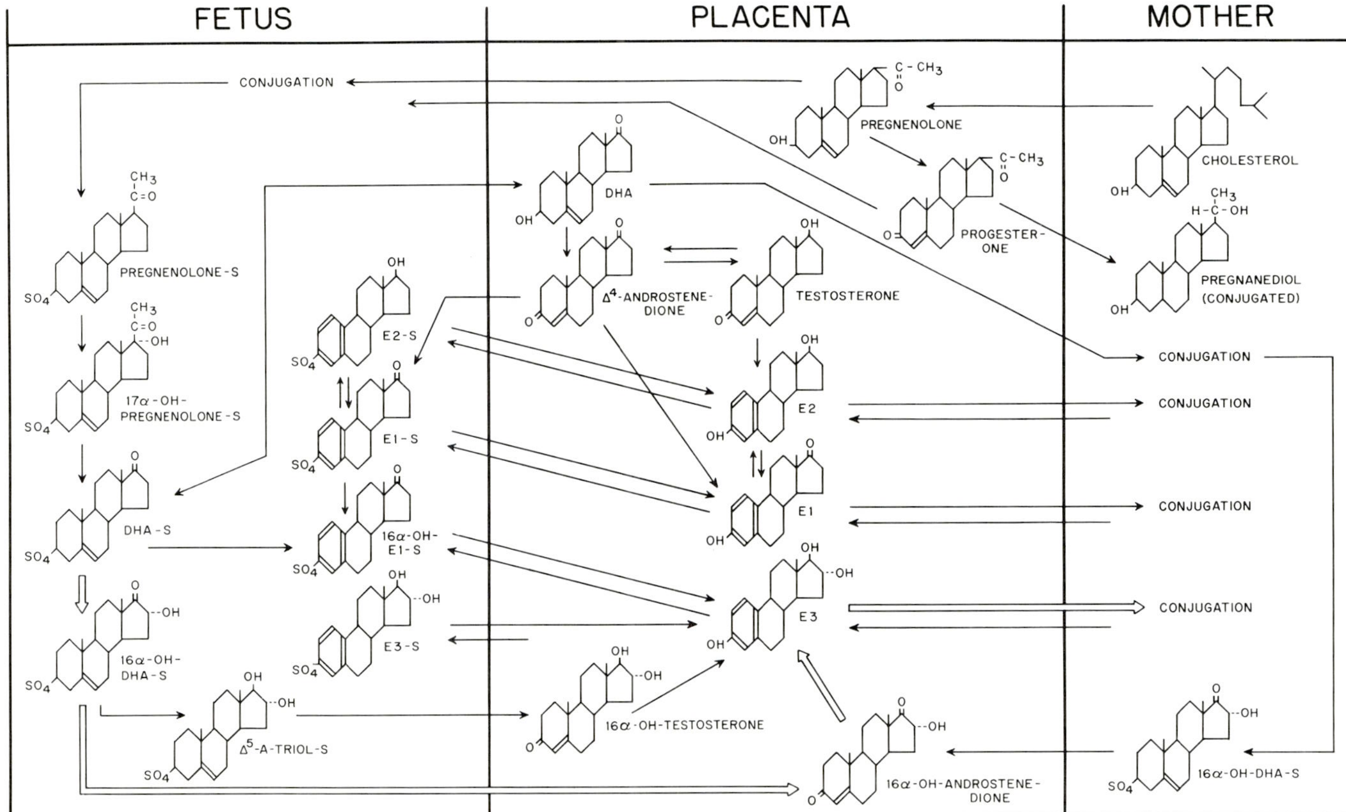

Fig. 3-2. Estrogen metabolism in the fetoplacental unit. E1 = estrone, E2 = estradiol, E3 = estriol, DHA = dehydroisoandrosterone, Δ^5-triol = androst-5-ene-3β, 16α, 17β-triol, S = sulphate conjugation.

TABLE 3-2

FETAL ESTROGEN METABOLISM: INCUBATION OF FETAL ORGANS AND FETAL PERFUSION STUDIES*

Type of study	Findings	Interpretation	Authors
Incubation of fetal adrenal slices and homogenate with progesterone-C^{14}	17-OH-progesterone and 16α-OH-progesterone and 16α, 17 dihydroxy progesterone formed	Fetal adrenal capable of 16-hydroxylation	Villee *et al.*, 1961[103, 104]
Sulphatase activity measured in various fetal organs	No steroid sulphatase present in kidneys, adrenals, pancreas, or the spleen; E1-S but not DHAS split by the fetal liver	No sulphatase activity in fetal organs (except for the fetal liver)	Pulkkinen, 1961[78]
Perfusion of previable fetuses with E1-C^{14}	Estrogen sulphates but no glucuronides formed; E1 converted to E2 but not to E3	The fetus is capable of forming steroid sulphates	Levitz, Condon, and Dancis, 1961[55]
Perfusion of previable fetuses with E2 and E3	Conjugated estrogens formed in the liver, lungs, intestine, and adrenals; E1-S, E2-S, and E3-S identified	Sulfate conjugation predominant in the fetus	Diczfalusy *et al.*, 1961[25, 26]
Incubation of fetal liver tissue slices with E1 and E2	E1 and E2 converted to E3; E2 converted to E3 and 16-epi-E3; E3-glucuronide found in the liver	16-hydroxylation carried out by the fetal liver, but the over-all fetal estrogen metabolism is not extensive	Engel, Baggett, and Halla, 1962[31]
Perfusion of previable fetuses with E3-C^{14}	Estrogens in the fetus mostly conjugated as sulphates; small amounts of E3-16-glucuronide was found in the fetal liver	Predominantly sulphate conjugation in the fetus	Mikhail, Wiqvist, and Diczfalusy, 1963[71]

Perfusion of previable fetuses with E2-C^{14}	E1-S and E2-S identified in fetal tissue following perfusion	Extensive sulphurylation in the fetus; E3 not a major metabolite of E2 in the fetus	Haynes *et al.*, 1964[44]
Investigation of the sulphurylating capacity of fetal adrenals	Sulphurylation of DHA and various androstane and estrane derivatives	High sulphurylating capacity of the fetal adrenals	Wengle, 1964[108]
Perfusion of previable fetuses with T-H^3, DHA-H^3, and A-C^{14}	No estrogens formed from DHA; A and T converted to E1 and E2, respectively	DHA not converted to A and T by the fetus; fetal A probably of placental origin	Mancuso *et al.*, 1965[66]
Perfusion of previable fetuses with E1-H^3, E2-C^{14}, and E1-S-C^{14}	Isolation of 15α-OH-E2 from the fetal liver	Fetus may protect itself against estrogen action by forming 15α-OH-E2, which is biologically relatively inactive	Schwers *et al.*, 1965[91]
Perfusion of previable fetuses with E1-H^3 and E1-S-C^{14}	E1-S not hydrolyzed by the fetus; 15α-OH-E2 and E3 found in the fetal liver	15- and 16-hydroxylation take place exclusively in the fetal liver	Schwers *et al.*, 1965[92]
Perfusion of previable fetuses with E1-S-H^3	E1-S-H^3 and small amounts of E2-S-H^3 and E3-S-H^3 found in the fetal liver	Metabolism of E1-S in conjugated form in the fetus	Emerman *et al.*, 1965[30]
Perfusion of previable fetuses with DHA-C^{14} and DHAS-H^3	DHA sulphurylated by the fetus; perfused DHAS not hydrolyzed by the fetus; DHAS and Δ^5-triol present in fetal tissue	16-hydroxylation takes place predominantly in the fetal liver	Bolté, Wiqvist, and Diczfalusy, 1966[13]
Perfusion of previable fetuses with T-H^3 and A-C^{14}	A converted to T and T converted to A	Reductive metabolism of A and T in the fetus discussed	Benegiano *et al.*, 1968[7]
Perfusion of previable fetuses with T-H^3 and A-C^{14}	E2 and 15α-OH-E2 found in the fetal liver	Aromatization takes place in the fetal liver	Mancuso *et al.*, 1968[65]

* El = estrone, E2 = estradiol, E3 = estriol, A = androstenedione, T = testosterone, DHA = dehydroisoandrosterone, 5-triol = androst-5-ene-3β,16α,17β-triol, S = sulphate conjugation, C^{14} and H^3 = carbon and tritium labeling, respectively.

TABLE 3-3

PLACENTAL ESTROGEN METABOLISM: INCUBATION AND PERFUSION STUDIES*

Type of study	Findings	Interpretation	Authors
Incubation of (dog) placental microsomal fraction with A and 19-OH-A	Conversion to E1 by the placenta	Conversion of A and 19-OH-A to E1 by the placenta	Meyer, 1955[69]
Incubation of placental microsomal fraction with Δ^5-triol	Estriol formation by the placenta	Conversion of Δ^5-triol to E3 by the placenta	Ryan, 1958[83]
Incubation of placental microsomal fraction with A	Formation of E1 and T by the placenta; no E3 found	Conversion of A to E1, but not to E3 by the placenta	Ryan, 1958[84]
Incubation of placental microsomal fraction with T-C^{14}	E1 and E2 formed, but no E3	Conversion of T to E1 and E2 but no conversion to E3	Baggett *et al.*, 1959[2]
Incubation of placental microsomal fraction with 16-OH-A, 16α-OH-T and Δ^5-triol	Formation of E3	Pathways suggested in the placenta: 16α-OH-A $\longrightarrow$ 16α-OH-E1 $\longrightarrow$ E3, and Δ5-triol $\longrightarrow$ 16α-OH-T $\longrightarrow$ E3	Ryan, 1959[85]
In situ placental perfusion with maternal blood	E1, E2 and E3 excretion in the maternal urine was maintained by placental perfusion	Circulation through the placenta favors placenta estrogen production	Cassmer, 1959[16]
Incubation of placental microsomal fraction with 16-OH-E1	16-oxo-E2 and E3 formed by the placenta	Pathway suggested: 16-oxo-E1 $\longrightarrow$ 16α-OH-E1 $\longrightarrow$ E3. No conversion 16-oxo-E2 to E3	Ryan, 1960[86]
Placental tissue incubation with progesterone	Conversion to 17α-OH-progesterone	Conversion of progesterone to 17α-OH-progesterone by the placenta	Little and Shaw, 1960[57]

Incubation of placental microsomal fraction with A-C^{14}	19-OH-A as well as E1 found in the incubate	19-OH-A suggested as an intermediate in the synthesis of placental estrogens	Lonchampt *et al.*, 1960[59]
Term placenta homogenates incubated with steroid sulphates	Steroid sulphatase present in the placenta	Steroid sulphatase present in the placenta	Pulkkinen, 1961[78]
Incubation of placental microsomal fraction with T-C^{14} and A	Formation of E1 and E2 from both T and A	T and A converted to E1 and E2 by the placenta	Gual *et al.*, 1962[41]
In vitro placental perfusion with 16α-OH-E1	Conversion to E3	16-hydroxylation precedes aromatization; pathway: 16α-OH-E1 ⟶ E3	Cedard, Varangot, and Yannotti, 1962[17]
Incubation of placental microsomal fraction with A-C^{14} and 19-OH-A	A converted to E1 and E2; 19-OH-A converted to E1; and E2; specific activity studies	19-OH-A is not an obligatory intermediate for formation of E1 and E2 from A	Hollander, 1962[46]
Placental incubation with labeled acetate	No estrogens formed	No estrogens formed from acetate by the placenta	Levitz, Emerman, and Dancis, 1962[55]
Determination of sulphatase activity in term placenta (and in fetal blood and tissue)	Sulphatase present in the placenta (but not in fetal blood or tissue)	Sulphatase present in the placenta	Warren and Timberlake, 1962[106]
Incubation of placental microsomal fraction with progesterone	Formation of 16α-OH-progesterone and A in low yield	Very low 16-hydroxylating capacity in the placenta	Little, Shaw, and Purdy, 1963[58]
In vitro placental perfusion with 19-OH-A, A, T and DHA, and 17α-OH-progesterone	No estrogen formed from 17α-OH-progesterone; no E3 formed from DHA; E1 and E2 formed from 19-OH-A, A, and T	C-19 steroids aromatized by the placenta; no 16-hydroxylation in the placenta	Cedard, Varangot, and Yannotti, 1963[18]

* E1 = estrone, E2 = estradiol, E3 = estriol, A = androstenedione, T = testosterone, DHA = dehydroisoandrosterone, 5-triol = androst-5-ene-3β,16α,17β-triol, S = sulphate conjugation, C^{14} and H^3 = carbon and tritium labeling, respectively.

(*continued*)

TABLE 3-3 (*continued*)*

Type of study	Findings	Interpretation	Authors
Incubation of placental homogenate with progesterone-C^{14} and 17α-OH-progesterone	A formed in low yield; 17α-OH-progesterone gave a similarly low yield of A	Since A is formed from progesterone, progesterone is considered an estrogen precursor	Warren and Cheatum, 1964[105]
Incubation of placental microsomal fraction for 1 hour with 16α-OH-DHA	Low values for Δ^5-triol; 16α-OH-DHA converted to E3; tentative formation of 16α-OH-A from 16α-OH-DHA	16-hydroxylation is involved in the major pathway of formation of E3	Magendantz and Ryan, 1964[63]
In situ placental perfusion with DHA-C^{14}, DHAS-H^3 and labeled A, T, and E2	DHA, A, and T converted to E1 and E2; DHAS aromatized more slowly; no E3 in the perfusate	Placental barrier limits the passage of androgens to the maternal side	Bolté *et al.*, 1964[10]
In situ placental perfusion with T-C^{14}-H^3	T converted to E1, E2, A, and T; T converted to E2 without involving E1	T directly converted to E2, and E1 derived from A; E1-E2 equilibrium in the placenta favors E2	Bolté *et al.*, 1964[9]
Incubation of placental microsomal fraction with DHA-C^{14}, DHAS-H^3, A-C^{14} and pregnenalone-S-H^3	Higher yield of estrogens from DHAS than from DHA; pregnenolone-S not converted to estrogens	DHA and DHAS metabolized to E1 in two placental compartments or else DHAS metabolized in one compartment via 19-hydroxylation of A, DHA, or DHAS	Morato, Lemus, and Gual, 1965[72]
Incubation of placental microsomal fraction with A-C^{14}	19-OH-A appeared in the incubate before the estrogens were detectable; E1 and E2 formed after 10 min. of incubation	19-OH-A is an obligatory intermediate in the conversion of A to E1 or E2	Wilcox and Engel, 1965[109]

In situ placental perfusion with pregnenolone-H^3	No E1, E2, or E3 found in the placenta or perfusate	No conversion of pregnenolone to estrogens by the placenta	Jaffe *et al.*, 1965[47]
In situ placental perfusion with pregnenolone-H^3-S	Labeled progesterone found in the placenta	Placental conversion of pregnenolone-S to progesterone	Pion, Conrad, and Wolf, 1966[76]
In situ placental perfusion with 16α-OH-DHA-H^3, 16α-OH-C^{14}, and 16α-OH-T-H^3	16α-OH-DHA converted to 16α-OH-A and E3, but not to 16α-OH-T; 16α-OH-T and 16α-OH-A converted to E3, but not to E1 and E2	Pathways suggested in the placenta: Δ^5-triol $\longrightarrow$ 16α-OH-T $\longrightarrow$ E3, and 16α-OH-DHA $\longrightarrow$ 16α-OH-A $\longrightarrow$ E3	Dell'Acqua *et al.*, 1967[21]
In situ placental perfusion (umbilical artery) with DHA-C^{14} and DHAS-H^3	Higher contribution of DHAS to A than to DHA and E1	DHA and DHAS metabolized in two different placental compartments; small amounts of A and T transferred to the fetus from the placenta	Lamb *et al.*, 1967[53]
In situ placental perfusion with 16-oxo-Δ^5-triol-C^{14}	Conversion to E3 and 16-epi-E3	Pathways suggested in the placenta: 16-oxo-Δ^5-triol $\longrightarrow$ 16-oxo-T $\longrightarrow$ 16-oxo-E2 $\longrightarrow$ E3 and 16-epi-E3	Reynholds *et al.*, 1968[79]

* El = estrone, E2 = estradiol, E3 = estriol, A = androstenedione, T = testosterone, DHA = dehydroisoandrosterone, 5-triol = androst-5-ene-3β,16α,17β-triol, S = sulphate conjugation, C^{14} and H^3 = carbon and tritium labeling, respectively.

This was shown conclusively by Mancuso *et al.* in fetal perfusion experiments.[66] The lack of these enzyme systems may serve the purpose of providing the fetus with a relatively androgen-free milieu. Another mechanism acting in the direction of protecting the fetus from the influence of androgens produced in the placenta is the efficient conversion of androgens to estrone and estradiol in the placenta. This conversion, which functions as a "placental metabolic barrier," was carefully studied by Bolté *et al.*[12]

No placental barrier exists to prevent the transfer of estrone and estradiol from the placenta to the fetus; this is of interest considering the fact that the production rate of estrone and estradiol is relatively high at the end of pregnancy. Siiteri and MacDonald estimated the average estradiol production to be 15 mg per day,[93,94] and it appears, therefore, that the fetus, at least by the end of pregnancy, would be exposed to relatively large amounts of estradiol. It is evident, however, that the fetus is in possession of various mechanisms to protect itself against biologically active estrogens. Schwers *et al.* showed that the fetal liver is capable of metabolizing estradiol to estriol and to 15α-OH-estradiol, both of which are estrogens of low biological activity.[92] It is noteworthy that 15-hydroxylation of estradiol results in a reduction of its uterotropic activity to less than $\frac{1}{1000}$. Also the 16-hydroxylating enzymes in the fetal liver may be involved in protecting the fetus against estradiol exposure. Thus, an efficient 16-hydroxylation of fetal DHAS favors the formation of estriol and makes less DHAS available for conversion to estrone and estradiol.

Estriol

Estriol is quantitatively the most important estrogen during pregnancy, and large amounts of estriol are excreted in the maternal urine, particularly during the last trimester of pregnancy. The aromatization of estriol takes place in the placenta. The principal precursor is DHAS produced in the fetal adrenals and 16-hydroxylized in the fetal liver.[90] As shown by Ryan, the further metabolism involves conversion of 16α-OH-DHA to estriol via 16α-OH-androstenedione and conversions of androstenetriol to estriol via 16α-OH-testosterone (Fig. 3-2).[85]

A great deal of evidence exists in support of the present concept of estriol synthesis. Production-rate studies by Simmer *et al.*[95] and studies of the arteriovenous difference of circulating DHAS in the fetal umbilical cord by Colas, Heinrichs, and Tatum[19] have shown that the fetal adrenals indeed have a large capacity to synthesize DHAS. The studies of Frandsen and Stakeman are significant in this respect. They observed that pregnancies with anencephalic fetuses with atrophic adrenal cortexes were associated with significantly low estrogen excretion.[37] Siiteri and Mac-

Donald showed that most of the estriol produced during normal pregnancy is derived from the fetal DHAS and that the maternal contribution of DHAS for formation of estriol is minimal during pregnancy.[94] The contribution of maternal DHAS to the estriol pool was calculated to be less than 10 per cent. Bolté *et al.* showed that maternal DHA and DHAS serve as precursors to placental estriol via 16-hydroxylated intermediates formed in the fetal liver.[11] The DHAS from the maternal side is metabolized differently from the DHAS from the fetal side and more estrone and estradiol in relation to estriol is formed from maternal DHAS than from fetal DHAS[12] (Table 3-4). This characteristic metabolism of DHAS has been confirmed in cases of anencephaly[40,87] and also in cases of hydatiform mole,[93] where DHAS is supplied exclusively from the maternal side. The ratio of estriol to estrone and estradiol is somewhat higher in cases of anencephaly than in the mole, but it is still much lower than in normal pregnancy. Since maternal DHAS in normal pregnancy passes through the placenta on its way to the fetus, it is likely to be exposed to the placental enzymes and be partly converted to androstenedione and testosterone and subsequently to estrone and estradiol by the placenta before it reaches the 16-hydroxylating enzymes in the fetal liver. This may explain why maternal DHAS in normal pregnancy (as well as in cases of anencephaly) is converted to estriol to a much less extent than the fetal DHAS. The absence of the 16-hydroxylating capacity of the fetal liver may explain the low production of estriol in relation to estrone and estradiol from maternal DHAS in cases of hydatiform mole.

Studies in Pregnant Dogs

Recent studies in our laboratory in which pregnant dogs have been used as experimental models have shown that the placental production of estradiol and the amount of estradiol to which the fetus is exposed during pregnancy is important for the growth and development of the fetus.[43] In a study involving 14 pregnant dogs, it was shown that administration of a small amount of estradiol (45–60 μg of estradiol-17β per kilogram of body weight) to the pregnant bitches during the last three weeks of gestation resulted in significant developmental changes in the pups. At six weeks of age the pups showed retarded skeletal growth, delayed ossification, poor development of the subcutaneous connective tissue, and enlarged inguinal rings. These changes were interpreted to be an effect of exogeneous estradiol entering the fetuses in utero, as evidenced by the finding that similar developmental changes could be produced in pups of untreated bitches by injection of a small amount of estradiol directly to the pups during the first six weeks of life. The fact that administration of estradiol during pregnancy can cause these

TABLE 3-4

ESTROGEN METABOLISM IN THE INTACT FETOPLACENTAL UNIT*

Type of study	Findings	Interpretation	Authors
Oral administration of deuterio cholesterol in 8th month of pregnancy	Isolation of deuterio-pregnanediol glucuronide in the maternal urine	Pathway suggested: cholesterol ⟶ progesterone ⟶ pregnanediol-glucuronide	Bloch, 1945[8]
Determination of conjugated DHA in plasma of fetal cord blood and maternal blood	Higher DHA(S) values in umbilical cord plasma (average 36.7 μg/100 ml) than in maternal plasma (18.1 μg/100 ml)	DHA produced by the fetal adrenals	Migeon, Keller, and Holmstrom, 1955[70]
Intravenous infusion of 100 mg E3 during pregnancy	Small increase in the conjugated E3 fraction in the fetal liver	Very little E3 from the maternal side reaches the fetus	Diczfalusy *et al.*, 1961[23, 25, 26]
Isolation from the placenta	Isolation of 16α-OH-T from the placenta (35 μg per kg)	Relatively high concentration of 16α-OH-T in the placenta	Neher and Stark, 1961[74]
E2-H^3 administrated intravenously to pregnant women	E1, E2, and E3 isolated from maternal urine; E2 secretory-rate studies	Various mathematical models for E2 metabolism during pregnancy discussed	Gurpide *et al.*, 1962[42]
E2-C^{14} administered intravenously during pregnancy	Labeled E1, E2, and E3 secreted in urine; specific activity of E3 lower than that of E1 and E2	Higher secretory rate for E3 than for E1 and E2; a precursor of E3 from sources other than E2 suggested	Fishman *et al.*, 1962[33]
Intravenous administration of DHAS-H^3, A-C^{14}, and T-C^{14} during pregnancy	Higher E3 conversion from DHAS than from A or T	Preferably neutral pathway for maternal DHAS into E3; pathway DHAS ⟶ 16, 17-di-OH-Δ^5-one suggested	Baulieu and Dray, 1963[3]

Simultaneous intravenous administration of DHAS-H^3 and E2-C^{14}	Higher specific activity in urinary E3 following administration of DHAS than following injection E2	Placental E3 derived via a pathway which does not involve E1 or E2	Siiteri and MacDonald, 1963[93]
E3 injected into umbilical cord; analysis of placental and fetal tissues	E3-3-S found in fetal tissue; small amounts of E3-3-glucuronide in fetal liver; free E3 in the placenta	Placental E3 sulphurylated by the fetus; E3-3-S from fetal side hydrolyzed by the placenta	Mikhail, Wiqvist, and Diczfalusy, 1963[71]
E3-C^{14} administered in 20th week of pregnancy; after 30 min. of circulation fetuses removed surgically	Less than 0.5% of the radioactivity found in amniotic fluid, fetus, and placenta; in maternal blood 40% of E3 in free form, in urine glucuronide form	Conjugation procedure in mother relatively slow; E3 not metabolized to other estrogens	Wilson, Eriksson, and Diczfalusy, 1964[110]
DHAS-H^3 administered at term and four days after delivery	36–55% of the radioactivity recovered in urinary phenolic fraction at term; after delivery only 0.5% found in phenolic fraction	DHAS hydrolyzed and subsequently aromatized by the placenta	Warren and Timberlake, 1964[107]
Injection of DHA-C^{14} and DHAS-H^3 simultaneously into the uterine artery; fetal tissue and placenta analyzed 12–15 min. after injection	More DHA metabolized to placental E1 and E2 than to DHAS; E3 incompletely identified	DHA and DHAS serve as direct precursors to placental E1 and E2, and as indirect precursors to placental E3 via a fetal metabolite	Bolté *et al.*, 1964[11]
Simultaneous administration of DHAS-C^{14} and DHAS-H^3 to umbilical and maternal antecubital vein respectively; maternal urine collected for 6 days	DHAS (administered on the maternal side) converted to phenolic steroids only to a small extent	Both maternal and fetal DHAS serve as estrogen precursors, but maternal DHAS is aromatized much more slowly	Bolté *et al.*, 1964[12]

* El = estrone, E2 = estradiol, E3 = estriol, A = androstenedione, T = testosterone, DHA = dehydroisoandrosterone, 5-triol = androst-5-ene-3β,16α,17β-triol, S = sulphate conjugation, C^{14} and H^3 = carbon and tritium labeling, respectively.

(*continued*)

TABLE 3-4 (*continued*)*

Type of study	Findings	Interpretation	Authors
Determination of conjugated DHA and 16α-OH-DHA in plasma after solvolysis	Higher DHA values in arterial plasma (81 μg/100 ml) than in vein plasma (68 μg/100 ml); lower values in maternal plasma (32 μg/100 ml); corresponding values for 16α-OH-DHA: 147, 114, and 7 μg/100 ml	16α-OH-DHA of fetal origin reaches the placenta where estriol is synthesized	Colás, Heinrichs, and Tatum, 1964[19]
Determination of DHAS in fetal umbilical blood plasma and in maternal vein plasma	Identification of DHAS; higher values in umbilical arterial plasma (162 μg/100 ml) than in fetal vein (130 μg/100 ml); lowest in maternal vein (100 μg/100 ml); fetal production rate of DHA estimated at 75 mg per 24 hours	Uptake of fetal DHAS (75 mg per 24 hours) in the placenta; different pathways of estrogen synthesis suggested	Simmer *et al.*, 1964[95]
Isolation of 16α-OH-DHAS; determination of Δ^5-steroids following solvolysis of pooled umbilical (arterial and venous) plasma	Following solvolysis an average of 80 μg 16α-OH-DHA per 50 ml cord plasma (arterovenous difference not significant)	Major pathway of estriol synthesis: DHA ⟶ 16α-OH-DHA ⟶ 16α-OH-A ⟶ E3. Alternative pathway: DHA ⟶ 16α-OH-DHA ⟶ Δ^5-triol ⟶ 16α-OH-T ⟶ E3	Magendantz and Ryan, 1964[63]
Isolation from umbilical cord blood (placentas at delivery)	Isolation of pregnenolone-S and 17α-OH-pregnenolone-S from cord blood	Δ^5-3β OH-steroids are produced in the fetal adrenals	Eberlein, 1964[28]

Injection of E2-C^{14} into fetal umbilical vein	90% of the fetal estrogens in conjugated form: E1-S and E2-S, no conjugated E3; no conjugated estrogens found in the placenta	Rapid transfer of E2 to maternal side; E3 not a major and instantaneously formed fetal metabolite of E2	Haynes *et al.*, 1964[44]
E1-H^3 and E2-C^{14} injected simultaneously into fetal umbilical cord at midpregnancy	Predominantly conjugated estrogens in the fetus (92%); very little conjugated estrogen (14%) found in the placenta	E1 to E2 interaction takes place in fetal liver, probably in conjugated form	Schwers, Eriksson, and Diczfalusy, 1965[90]
Progesterone-C^{14} injected into fetal umbilical vein	Both placental and fetal tissue free of estrogens	Progesterone not a precursor of placental estrogens	Jaffe *et al.*, 1965[47]
Injection of E2-H^3 and DHAS-C^{14} into women pregnant with anencephalic fetuses	Placental estrogens found in the urine derived from DHAS circulating in the maternal plasma	In cases of anencephaly, maternal DHAS is utilized by the placenta for estrogen synthesis	MacDonald and Siiteri, 1965[61]
Injection of DHAS-H^3 and E1-S-C^{14} into umbilical cord	E3 mainly derived from DHAS and to a lesser extent from E1-S; more DHAS converted to E3 than to E1 or E2	Fetal DHAS metabolized to E3 preferably via neutral pathway	Kirschner, Wiqvist, and Diczfalusy, 1966[49]
Injection of Δ^5-triol-H^3 into the fetal umbilical cord	Labeled Δ^5-triol, 16α-OH-T, and E3 found in the placenta; only Δ^5-triol found in the fetus	Δ^5-triol converted into 16α-OH-T by the placenta; no transfer of 16α-OH-T to the fetus	Dell'Acqua *et al.*, 1967[22]

* El = estrone, E2 = estradiol, E3 = estriol, A = androstenedione, T = testosterone, DHA = dehydroisoandrosterone, 5-triol = androst-5-ene-3β,16α,17β-triol, S = sulphate conjugation, C^{14} and H^3 = carbon and tritium labeling, respectively.

changes in the offspring indicates that the balance between biologically more active and less active estrogens during pregnancy is of great significance. It may well be that the study of estradiol and estrone production will prove to be more fruitful for the understanding of the role of the estrogens during pregnancy than the study of the amount of estriol produced under normal and pathological conditions.

ESTROGEN ASSAYS

Various methods have been devised for the assay of the three main estrogens, individually or combined, in urine, blood, and other body fluids. The bioassays of estrogens in the urine have only historical interest. The chemical assays of estrogens in pregnancy urine can achieve a high degree of accuracy and reliability. Assays on blood, bile, amniotic fluid, etc., are more complicated and, apart from the assay on estriol in blood, have not yet proven of clinical value. Since estriol is excreted in milligram amounts in the urine, and since it is believed to reflect most closely the condition of the fetus, a great deal of work has been devoted to the development of simple, rapid, and yet reliable methods for assaying estriol. During the last few years a number of new methods have been described, but not all of them fulfill the basic criteria of precision, accuracy, sensitivity, and specificity.

From a chemical point of view the determination of estriol in normal pregnancy urine is not a complicated matter and does not necessarily have to involve elaborate chemical techniques. This is due mainly to the fact that relatively large amounts of estriol are present in normal pregnancy urine, particularly during the last trimester when the estriol tests are generally applied. The situation is different in patients with severe diabetes or toxemia. The estriol level of these patients is usually considerably lower than normal, and the urine specimens are often concentrated and heavily pigmented. A relatively extensive purification procedure is necessary in order to obtain accurate estriol values in the urine of such patients. It is our belief that estriol should not be measured in patients with toxemia or diabetes until it has been shown clearly that reliable values can be obtained in urine specimens from patients with other pathological conditions. A number of methods have been tested carefully in various clinical conditions and seem to fulfill the basic criteria of reliability. Among these are the colorimetric methods published by Eberlein *et al.*,[29] Taylor *et al.*,[99] Klopper and Wilson,[52] Greene and Touchstone,[40] Brown and Coyle,[15] Beling,[5] and Frandsen,[34] Oakey *et al.*,[75] and the gas chromatographic methods published by Wotiz and Martin,[111] Yousem,[112] and Schindler and Herrmann.[88]

In our study of pathological pregnancies, the method of Beling[5] has been used for urinary assays of estriol. This method is based on gel filtration on Sephadex, enzyme hydrolysis of the purified estriol conjugates, and further purification in a benzene-petroleum ether:water partition. The capacity is 20–25 urine samples per day, and the reports can be delivered 20 hours after the urine has been collected. Even though this represents a considerable delay in regard to the condition of the fetus, the estriol values have proven to be of value in clinical situations. The gel filtration method measures specifically estriol-16-glucuronide, which constitutes approximately 80 per cent of the total conjugated estriol in late pregnancy urine.

The estriol level during the second half of pregnancy is of particular interest from the clinical point of view, and most of the work has been concentrated, therefore, on the determination of urinary estriol during this period (Table 3-5). The estriol level during the first trimester is relatively low and quantitative determination requires a refined chemical technique involving column chromatography and the formation of derivatives. The methods, therefore, tend to be relatively time-consuming. Estriol assays have not been used much for diagnostic purposes during the first trimester of pregnancy, even though low values (5–10 μg estriol per 24 hours) have proven to be useful in the diagnosis of intrauterine fetal death.[5]

The determination of estrone and estradiol in pregnancy urine also involves extensive chemical techniques, and the available methods are

TABLE 3–5
URINARY ESTRIOL LEVELS
REPORTED BY DIFFERENT INVESTIGATORS

Weeks of gestation	Mean estriol values (μg/24 hours)	Range of values (μg/24 hours)	Authors
From 36th week to term	29.1	16.0–41.0	Brown, 1956[14]
From 36th week to term	19.8	14.9–31.2	Hobkirk and Nilsen, 1962[45]
From 37th week to term	24.2	8.0–52.0	Beling, 1963[5]
From 37th week to term	27.5	15.0–52.0	Govaertz-Videtsky, 1965[39]
From 37th week to term	27.2	12.2–36.6	Frandsen and Lundwall, 1966[36]
From 38th week to 41st week	24.0	12.0–40.0	McLeod *et al.*, 1967[67]
At term	17.0	7.0–27.0	Greene and Touchstone, 1963[40]
At term	34.5	±9.3	Klopper and Billewicz, 1963[51]

not suitable for routine use. The levels of estrone and estradiol during normal pregnancy are well documented (Table 3-6). On the other hand, the excretion of these two estrogens in various forms of pathological pregnancy has not been systematically investigated.

Estrogen determination in blood or plasma offers certain advantages over urinary determination since changes in the placental estriol supposedly appear in the blood earlier than in the urine. Various assay methods for estriol have been suggested but none of them can be considered routine. Only very small amounts of estriol are present in the blood (Table 3-7). An extensive chemical work-up as well as a sensitive end point determination (such as gas chromatography and fluorimetry) is therefore necessary for the chemical determination. Of particular interest is the method of Nachtigall *et al.*,[73] which has enough capacity to be used in follow-up studies of pathological pregnancies. It should be pointed out, however, that a great deal of skill is required to handle this very delicate fluorimetric method.

ESTROGEN CONCENTRATIONS IN URINE AND BLOOD

Estriol levels during normal pregnancy have been studied by many workers in recent years, and there is a close agreement on the normal values. This is also evident from Table 3-5 where the estriol levels near term reported by different investigators are shown.

Klopper carried out a survey of nine publications of the past 10 years and found an over-all average of 10.1 mg at 28 weeks, 14.2 mg at 32 weeks, 19.8 mg at 36 weeks, and 26.0 mg at 40 weeks.[50] These values are in agreement with those found in our laboratory (Fig. 3-3).

The mean estriol excretion curve is characterized by relatively low values during the first trimester, increasing values after the 10th to 12th week, a leveling off after the 24th to 26th week, and a sharp rise during the last 3 to 4 weeks of pregnancy. After delivery there is a dramatic fall in the estriol values. The features of the estriol curve were analyzed carefully by Govaerts-Videtzky. She confirmed the lognormal distribution of estriol values during pregnancy and found that the increase of the logarithmic means fits well with a set of two regression lines with different slopes before and after the 24th week.[39] This leveling of the estriol curve at midpregnancy cannot be satisfactorily explained at the present time, even though one may speculate that it is caused by a change in fetal growth and development or by a change in fetal or placental estrogen metabolism.

The general shape of the estrone and estradiol curves is similar to the estriol curve, but the level of excretion is much lower (Table 3-6). The

TABLE 3–6

URINARY LEVELS OF ESTRONE AND ESTRADIOL REPORTED BY DIFFERENT INVESTIGATORS

Weeks of gestation	Mean values (μg/24 hours)		Range of values (μg/24 hours)	Authors
From 36th week to term	estrone	1.4	0.7–2.1	Brown, 1956[14]
	estradiol	0.5	0.3–0.9	
From 36th week to term	estrone	1.2	0.6–1.8	Hobkirk and Nilsen, 1962[45]
	estradiol	0.5	0.3–0.6	
From 37th week to term	estrone	1.4	0.5–4.0	Govaertz-Videtsky, 1965[39]
	estradiol	0.3	0.1–0.7	
From 37th week to term	estrone + estradiol	1.9	0.8–4.5	Frandsen and Lundwall, 1966[36]

TABLE 3–7

PLASMA AND BLOOD ESTRIOL LEVELS REPORTED BY DIFFERENT INVESTIGATORS

Fluid analyzed	Mean estriol values (μg/100 ml)	Range of values (μg/100 ml)	Authors
Pooled plasma from 36th week to term	16.4	12.2–20.4	Smith and Hagerman, 1965[97]
Plasma from 37th week to term	17.8	15.3–20.0	Aitken *et al.*, 1958[1]
Plasma from 37th week to term	11.4	3.9–27.0	Preedy and Aitken, 1961[77]
Plasma from 37th week to term	9.1	2.9–20.0	Roy and Macay, 1962[81]
Plasma at term	23.3	12.6–38.0	Smith and Arai, 1963[96]
Plasma at term	5.4	2.5–8.2	Roy and Harkness, 1963[82]
Plasma at term	15.3	9.9–19.6	Touchstone *et al.*, 1963[100]
Plasma at term	14.1	5.0–40.0	Schwers, 1965[89]
Plasma at term	27.0	9.3–56.0	Nachtigall *et al.*, 1966[73]
Blood at term	11.3	1.7–33.0	Varangot and Seeman, 1958[102]
Blood from 36th week to term	7.8	2.3–19.6	Roy and Brown, 1960[80]

increase in estrone and estradiol from the level at conception to the end of pregnancy is about a hundredfold. Thus, approximately 1.5 mg of estrone and 0.5 mg of estradiol is present in the urine at term.

The blood level of estriol varies a great deal during pregnancy, as

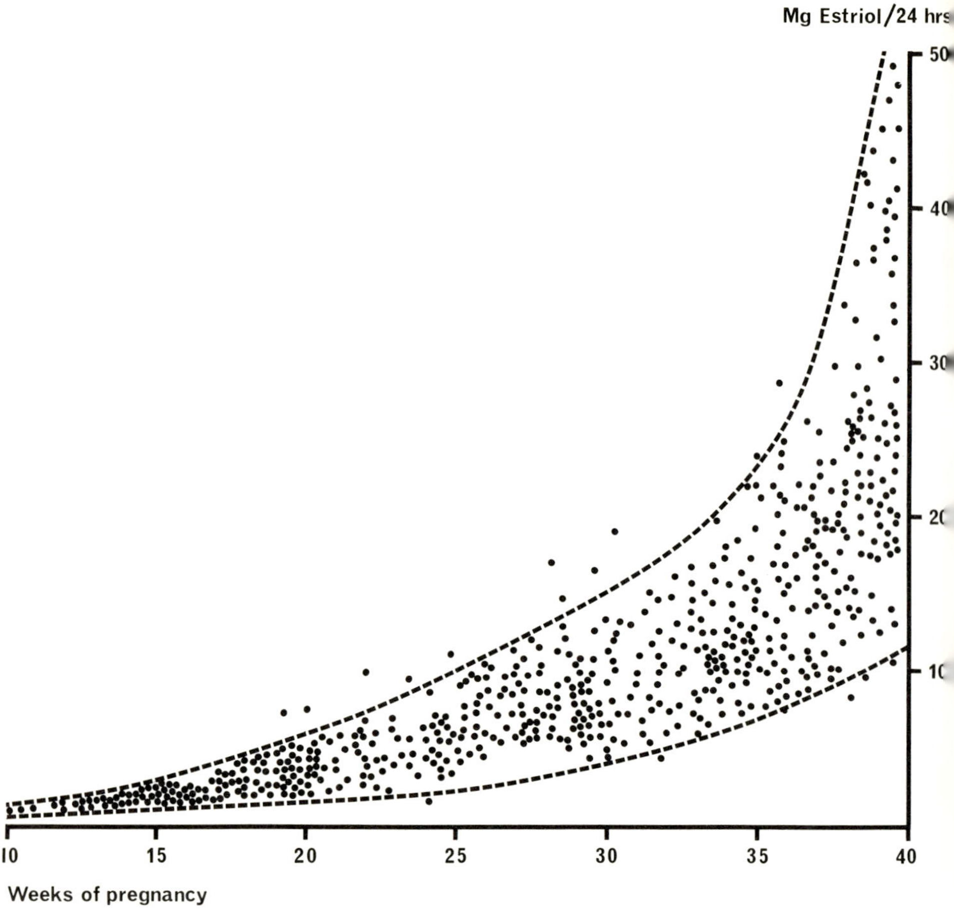

Fig. 3-3. Urinary excretion of estriol-16-glucuronide during pregnancy in 31 normal women. The upper and lower dashed lines are 95% confidence limits.

shown in Table 3-7. Values as low as 1.7–5.0 mg/100 ml have been reported by different investigators.[77, 80, 81, 82, 89, 102] It is difficult, therefore, to distinguish between low values and normal values in cases of pathological pregnancies. Whether or not this difficulty can be overcome by performing serial determinations of estriol in blood remains to be shown.

The estrogen content of amniotic fluid was investigated by Diczfalusy and Magnusson. They found 4.4 μg of estrone, 3.1 μg of estradiol, and 794 μg of estriol per 1000 ml at the end of pregnancy.[27] Schindler and Herrmann found a mean concentration of 979 μg of estriol in the amniotic fluid of 37 normal women at term.[88] It is of interest that even though the values in amniotic fluid were found to be distributed over a relatively wide range (19–3000 μg/liter), pathologically low values could be distinguished in cases of Rh disease.[88] Determination of estriol in amniotic fluid, therefore, may prove to be of definite diagnostic value in pathological pregnancies.

CLINICAL APPLICATION OF ESTROGEN ASSAYS

The estriol level is believed to reflect the intrauterine situation of the fetus, and depressed estriol values have been considered indicative of fetal distress. Even though estriol assays have proved to be of great value as a guide to the clinical management of the pregnant patient, the interpretation of the estriol values in various clinical conditions has not been agreed upon by different workers in the field. This discrepancy may be explained, in part, on the basis of our present income understanding of the mechanism involved in regulating the production of estriol in pathological pregnancies. It is well established that dramatically falling estriol values indicate impending fetal death, but it has not been fully clarified to what extent the estriol level is influenced by other factors such as the length of pregnancy, size of the fetus, presence of more than one fetus, disturbed feto-placental circulation, separation of the placenta from the uterine wall, disturbed fetal development, and malformation of the fetus. Thus, further work is required to demonstrate the nature and details of the mechanisms that almost certainly exist to regulate estriol production in normal and pathological pregnancies.

Even though estrogen biosynthesis during pregnancy has been explored in great detail in recent years, it has been difficult to find clinical applications for the new discoveries in the biochemical field. This is partly due to the difficulties involved in establishing experimental conditions for studying the mechanism of action of different estrogens in the fetus and the placenta without interfering with functions essential for the maintenance of pregnancy. The clinical research in this area, therefore, has been limited to studies of estrogen excretion products and the concentration of estrogens in different organs and in biological fluids such as blood and liquor amni. However, in spite of the obvious difficulties, a large body of information has accumulated describing the hormonal situation in a variety of pathological conditions during pregnancy. Particularly interesting in this regard are the studies of estriol excretion in cases of high-risk pregnancies.

Estriol Level and Weight of Newborn

The relationship between the urinary estriol level in normal pregnancy and the weight of the newborn has been studied by different investigators. Coyle and Brown,[20] Greene and Touchstone,[40] Frandsen,[35] and Lundwall and Stakemann[60] reported a positive correlation between the weight of the newborn and the estriol level at term. A positive correlation between the mean of the estriol values during the last five days prior to delivery was also reported by Beling.[5] Klopper and Billewicz, on the other hand, did not find that the estriol level was correlated to the weight of the newborn.[51]

Estriol determinations have been used in our laboratory to estimate the weight of the fetus. Single values are not considered reliable, but the mean excretion of estriol during at least three to five days seems to give a fairly good estimate of fetal weight at or near term. Whether or not the estriol level all through the pregnancy is correlated to the size of the fetus is not known at the present time. However, the finding that women carrying small babies show a continuously low estriol level, and those with larger fetuses show a high level, supports the idea that the estriol level reflects the size of the growing fetus all through the gestation. Also, clinical estimations of the size of the fetus and radiographic examinations tend to support the idea that at least during the last trimester the fetal size is correlated to the estriol level. However, direct evidence for the existence of such a correlation is difficult to produce, since estimates of the fetal weight are not reliable during the course of pregnancy.

Pathological Pregnancies

In pathological pregnancies estriol assays have been used either to evaluate impending fetal hazard (at the time when the fetus is mature enough to be delivered) or to evaluate the fetal condition at any time during pregnancy.

The frequency of the determinations varies depending on the reason for the estriol assay. Daily determinations are necessary in order to detect suddenly falling values. Since this situation occurs only during the last few weeks of pregnancy when the fetus is mature enough to be delivered, daily determinations are not essential before the 34th to 35th week. The use of a short and simple assay technique is absolutely necessary for these follow-up studies.

When estriol assays are used as a general control of fetal viability, daily determinations are not necessary. In our experience, estriol assays once or twice a week seem to be enough to provide information on the fetal viability and assurance that the fetus is not in immediate danger. Weekly assays have been used in cases of antepartum hemorrhage, habitual abortion, placenta previa, suspected intrauterine fetal death, and also to monitor diabetic and toxemic pregnancies before the 35th week.

A number of studies exist describing estriol levels in different clinical conditions. In diabetic pregnancies, estriol assays have been studied predominantly as a guide to the optimum time for termination of the pregnancy. This has been accomplished successfully by many investigators.[5,6,20,35,48,100] However, even though falling estriol values may form a basis for a decision to terminate the pregnancy either by cesarean section or induction of labor, it is indeed difficult to evaluate the estriol level in diabetic patients. This is due mainly to the day-to-day variation in estriol values which is sometimes so large that it is difficult to establish the mean value. The fluctuating estriol values are probably caused by the variation in urine volume, and this is evidently associated with the severity of the diabetes. Nevertheless, estriol values are of great help when sufficient serial assays are available to establish a secure mean. Values falling significantly below this level seem to indicate that it is dangerous for the fetus to remain in utero. As reported earlier, we have found that two falling values on two consecutive days at a time of pregnancy when the fetus is considered mature enough to be delivered is an indication to terminate the pregnancy.[5,6] Since the interpretation of falling values is relatively difficult, it is important in diabetic patients that all available clinical data are considered in relation to the estriol values before any decision to terminate is made.

Estriol assays have also been used to monitor patients with pre-eclamptic toxemia. Long-standing toxemia which is characterized by a low estriol level all through the pregnancy requires frequent estriol determinations to evaluate the condition of the fetus. In toxemia, the fetus can apparently survive in the uterus with a very low estriol level, and it seems that as long as the level is horizontal, or shows a small increase, the fetus is not in any immediate danger. Thus, it has been found that the fetus may be doing well in the uterus even at a level as low as 2–3 mg of estriol at the 28th to 36th week. An example of this is shown in Figure 3-4, where the estriol curve from a pregnancy with long-standing toxemia is presented. In the 36th week a surviving infant (weighing 1450 gm) was delivered by induction of labor.

It seems that as long as the estriol level does not fall, the fetus may be better off in the uterus than outside. A horizontal curve in a toxemic pregnancy does not provide any information about the optimum time for delivery, and a low level per se does not indicate immediate danger for the fetus. While the fetus may not grow anymore, it will at least gain in maturity. Falling values, on the other hand, indicate that induction of labor is necessary as soon as the fetus is mature enough.

Many of the factors responsible for the maintenance of the estriol level during pregnancy are unknown at the present time. However, it seems that determining estriol excretion in the urine is a positive approach to

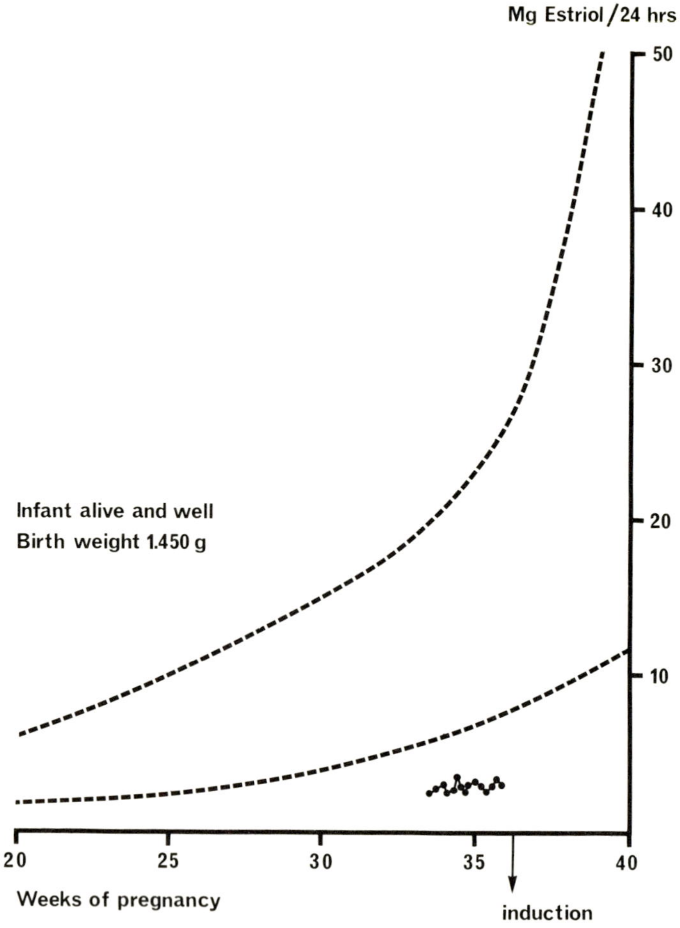

Fig. 3-4. Estriol excretion in a long-standing toxemia of pregnancy. The upper and lower dashed lines are 95% confidence limits of the estriol excretion during normal pregnancy.

the study of the fetal well-being. Future studies may prove that the estriol level in the blood and other estrogen metabolites reflect the condition of the fetus more closely. Until the methodological problems associated with these other assays have been solved, however, the urinary estriol assay will maintain its place in clinical obstetrics.

A wider use of the estriol assays is well justified. We are in full agreement with the idea of Beischer *et al.* who suggested instituting urinary estriol measurements as routine screening tests for all patients at approximately the 30th and 36th week of gestation.[4] They also suggested performing more frequent determinations on patients who show a low level of estriol.

REFERENCES

1. Aitken, E. H., Preedy, J. R., Eton, B., and Short, R. V. Oestrogen and progesterone levels in foetal and maternal plasma at parturition. *Lancet 2*:1096, 1958.
2. Baggett, B., Engel, L. L., Balderas, L., Lanman, G., Savard, K., and Dorfman, R. Conversion of C^{14}-testosterone to C^{14}-estrogenic steroids by endocrine tissues. *Endocrinology 64*:600, 1959.
3. Baulieu, E. E., and Dray, F. Conversion of H^3-dehydroisoandrosterone (3β-hydroxy-Δ^5-androsten-17-one) sulfate to H^3-estrogens in normal pregnant women. *J. Clin. Endocr. 23*:1298, 1963.
4. Beischer, N. A., Bhargava, V. L., Brown, J. B., and Smith, M. A. The Incidence and significance of low oestriol excretion in an obstetric population. *J. Obstet. Gynaec. Brit. Comm. 75*:1024, 1968.
5. Beling, C. G. Gel filtration of conjugated urinary oestrogens and its application in clinical assays. *Acta Endocr.* (Kobenhavn) *Suppl. 79,* 1963.
6. Beling, C. G. Estriol excretion in pregnancy and its application to clinical problems. In *Advances in Obstetrics and Gynecology,* S. C. Marcus and C. C. Marcus (Eds.), Williams & Wilkins, Baltimore, 1967, p. 88.
7. Benegiano, G., Mancuso, S., Mancuso, F. P., Wiqvist, N., and Diczfalusy, E. Studies on the metabolism of C-19 steroids in the human foeto-placental unit. 3. Dehydrogenation and reduction products formed by previable foetuses perfused with androstenedione and testosterone. *Acta Endocr.* (Kobenhavn) *57*:187, 1968.
8. Bloch, K. The biological conversion of cholesterol to pregnanediol. *J. Biol. Chem. 157*:661, 1945.
9. Bolté, E., Mancuso, S., Dray, F., Baulieu, E. E., and Diczfalusy, E. Conversion of testosterone-17α-^{3}H into 17β-estradiol-17α-^{3}H by human placentas perfused *in situ. Steroids 4*:613, 1964.
10. Bolté, E., Mancuso, S., Eriksson, G., Wiqvist, N., and Diczfalusy, E. Studies on the aromatisation of neutral steroids in pregnant women. 1. Aromatisation of C-19 steroids by placentas perfused *in situ. Acta Endocr.* (Kobenhavn) *45*:535, 1964.
11. Bolté, E., Mancuso, S., Eriksson, G., Wiqvist, N., and Diczfalusy, E. Studies on the aromatisation of neutral steroids in pregnant women. 2. Aromatisation of dehydroepiandrosterone and of its sulphate administered simultaneously into a uterine artery. *Acta Endocr.* (Kobenhavn) *45*:560, 1964.
12. Bolté, E., Mancuso, S., Eriksson, G., Wiqvist, N., and Diczfalusy, E. Studies on the aromatisation of neutral steroids in pregnant women. 3. Over-all aromatisation of dehydroepiandrosterone sulphate circulating in

the foetal and maternal compartments. *Acta Endocr.* (Kobenhavn) *45:*576, 1964.

13. Bolté, E., Wiqvist, N., and Diczfalusy, E. Metabolism of dehydroepiandrosterone and dehydroepiandrosterone sulphate by perfusion of human foetus at midpregnancy. *Acta Endocr.* (Kobenhavn) *52:*583, 1966.
14. Brown, J. B. Urinary excretion of oestrogens during pregnancy, lactation and the reestablishment of menstruation. *Lancet 270:*704, 1956.
15. Brown, J. B., and Coyle, M. Urinary excretion of oestriol during pregnancy. 1—A shortened procedure. *J. Obstet. Gynaec. Brit. Comm. 70:*219, 1963.
16. Cassmer, O. Hormone production of the isolated human placenta. *Acta Endocr.* (Kobenhavn) *Suppl. 45:*66, 1959.
17. Cedard, L., Varangot, J., and Yannotti, S. Biosynthèse de l'oestriol dans les placentas humains perfusés *in vitro:* Formation à partir de certains stéroides neutres phénoliques hydroxylés sur le carbone 16. *C. R. Acad. Sci.* (Paris) *254:*3896, 1962.
18. Cedard, L., Varangot, J., and Yannotti, S. Biosynthèse des oestrogènes dans les placentas humains perfusés *in vitro:* Formation d'oestrone et d'oestradiol à partir de stéroides neutres ou substitués. *C. R. Acad. Sci.* (Paris) *257:*2725, 1963.
19. Colás, A., Heinrichs, W. L., and Tatum, H. J. Pettenkofer chromogens in the maternal and fetal circulations: detection of 3β, 16α-dihydroxyandrost-5-en-17-one in umbilical cord blood. *Steroids 3:*417, 1964.
20. Coyle, M. G., and Brown, J. B. Urinary excretion of oestriol during pregnancy. *J. Obstet. Gynaec. Brit. Comm. 70:*225, 1963.
21. Dell'Acqua, S., Mancuso, E., Eriksson, G., Ruse, J. L., Solomon, S., and Diczfalusy, E. Studies on the aromatisation of neutral steroids in pregnant women. 6. Aromatisation of 16α-hydroxylated C-19 steroids by midterm placentas perfused in situ. *Acta Endocr.* (Kobenhavn) *55:*401, 1967.
22. Dell'Acqua, S., Mancuso, S., Wiqvist, N., Ruse, J. L., Solomon, S., and Diczfalusy, E. Studies on the aromatisation of neutral steroids in pregnant women. 5. Metabolism of androst-5-ene-3β, 16α, 17β-triol in the intact foeto-placental unit at midpregnancy. *Acta Endocr.* (Kobenhavn) *55:*389, 1967.
23. Diczfalusy, E. Endocrinology of the foetus. *Acta Obstet. Gynec. Scand.* (*Suppl. 1*) *41:*45, 1962.
24. Diczfalusy, E. Endocrine functions of the human fetoplacental unit. *Fed. Proc. 23:*791, 1964.
25. Diczfalusy, E., Cassmer, O., Alonso, C., and DeMiguel, M. Estrogen metabolism in the human fetus and newborn. *Recent Progr. Hormone Res. 17:*147, 1961.
26. Diczfalusy, E., Cassmer, O., Alonso, C., DeMiguel, M., and Westin, B. Oestrogen metabolism in the human foetus. *Acta Endocr.,* (Kobenhavn) *38:*31, 1961.
27. Diczfalusy, E., and Magnusson, A. M. Tissue concentration of oestrone, oestradiol-17β and oestriol in the human foetus. *Acta Endocr.* (Kobenhavn) *28:*169, 1958.

28. Eberlein, W. R. Steroids secreted by the fetal adrenal cortex. *J. Clin. Invest. 43:*1255, 1964.

29. Eberlein, W. R., Bongiovanni, A. M., Francis, C. M. A simplified method for the routine measurement of urinary estriol. *J. Clin. Endocr. 18:*1274, 1958.

30. Emerman, S., Dancis, J., Levitz, M., Wiqvist, N., and Diczfalusy, E. Metabolism of estrone-6,7-H^3 sulphate-S^{35} in the human perfused fetus. *J. Clin. Endocr. 25:*639, 1965.

31. Engel, L. L., Baggett, B., and Halla, M. In vitro metabolism of estradiol-17β by human fetal liver: formation of estriol, 16-epiestriol, estrone, and estriol glucusiduronic acid. *Endocrinology 70:*907, 1962.

32. Finkelstein, M. Fluorometric determination of micro amounts of oestrone-oestradiol and oestriol in urine. *Acta Endocr.* (Kobenhavn) *10:*149, 1952.

33. Fishman, J. Brown, J. B., Hellman, L., Zumoff, B., and Gallagher, T. F. Estrogen metabolism in normal and pregnant women. *J. Biol. Chem. 237:*1489, 1962.

34. Frandsen, V. A. In *Urinary Excretion of Estriol During Normal Pregnancy,* Munksgaard, Copenhagen, 1963.

35. Frandsen, V. A. The site of production of oestrogenic hormones in human pregnancy. *Europ. Rev. Endocr. 1:*227, 1965.

36. Frandsen, V. R., and Lundwall, F. The excretion of oestrone-oestradiol and oestriol in normal pregnancy. *Acta Endocr.* (Kobenhavn) *53:*93, 1966.

37. Frandsen, V. A., and Stakemann, G. The site of production of oestrogenic hormones in human pregnancy. *Acta Endocr.* (Kobenhavn) *38:*383, 1962.

38. Fuchs, F. Endocrine factors in the maintenance of pregnancy. *Acta Obstet. Gynec. Scand. (Suppl. 1) 41:*7, 1962.

39. Govaerts-Videtzky, M. Elimination urinaire des oestrogènes au cours de la grossesse normale. *Rev. Franc. Etud Clin. Biol. 10:*815, 1965.

40. Greene, J. W., and Touchstone, J. C. Urinary estriol as an index of placental function. *Amer. J. Obstet. Gynec. 85:*1, 1963.

41. Gual, C., Mozato, T., Hyano, M., Gut, M., and Dorfman, R. I. Biosynthesis of estrogens. *Endocrinology 71:*920, 1962.

42. Gurpide, E., Angers, M., Vande Wiele, R. L., and Lieberman, S. Determination of secretory rates of estrogens in pregnant and nonpregnant women from the specific activities of urinary metabolites. *J. Clin. Endocr. 22:*935, 1962.

43. Gustafsson, P. O., and Beling, C. G. Estradiol-induced changes in Beagle pups: effect of prenatal and postnatal administration. *Endocrinology, 85:*481, 1969.

44. Haynes, R. C., Mikhail, G., Eriksson, G., Wiqvist, N., and Diczfalusy, E. Oestradiol metabolism in the previable human foetus and in the foeto-placental unit. *Acta Endocr.* (Kobenhavn) *45:*297, 1964.

45. Hobkirk, R., and Nilsen, M. Observations on the occurrence of six estrogen fractions in human pregnancy urine. *J. Clin. Endocr. 22:*134, 1962.

46. Hollander, N. Role of 19-hydroxy-Δ^4-androstene-3, 17-dione as an intermediate for aromatization of Δ^4-androstene-3, 17-dione by placental microsomes. *Endocrinology 71:*723, 1962.

47. Jaffe, R., Pion, R., Eriksson, G., Wiqvist, N., and Diczfalusy, E. Studies on the aromatisation of neutral steroids in pregnant women. IV. Lack of oestrogen formation from progesterone. *Acta Endocr.* (Kobenhavn) *48:*413, 1965.

48. Jayle, M. F., Scholler, R., Veyrin-Forrer, F. and Mege, F. Clinical importance of oestrogen and pregnanediol estimations in pathological pregnancies. *Europ. Rev. Endocr. 1:*87, 1964.

49. Kirschner, M. A., Wiqvist, N., and Diczfalusy, E. Studies on oestriol synthesis from dehydroepiandrosterone sulphate in human pregnancy. *Acta Endocr.* (Kobenhavn) *53:*584, 1966.

50. Klopper, A. The assessment of feto-placental function by estriol assay. *Obstet. Gynec. Survey 23:*813, 1968.

51. Klopper, A., and Billewicz, W. Urinary excretion of oestriol and pregnanediol during normal pregnancy. *J. Obstet. Gynaec. Brit. Comm.* 70: 1024, 1963.

52. Klopper, A., and Wilson, G. A method for the assay of oestriol in pregnancy urine. *J. Obstet. Gynaec. Brit. Comm. 69:*533, 1962.

53. Lamb, E., Mancuso, S., Dell'Acqua, S., Wiqvist, N., and Diczfalusy, E. Studies on the metabolism of C-19 steroids in the human foeto-placental unit. *Acta Endocr.* (Kobenhavn) *55:*263, 1967.

54. Levitz, M. Conjugation and transfer of fetal-placental steroid hormones. *J. Clin. Endocr. 26:*773, 1966.

55. Levitz, M., Condon, G. P., and Dancis, J. Sulphurylation of estrogens by the human fetus. *Endocrinology 68:*825, 1961.

56. Levitz, M., Emerman, S., and Dancis, J. Sterol synthesis in perfused human placenta. *Excerpta med. (Amst) 51:*266, 1962.

57. Little, B., and Shaw, A. The conversion of progesterone to 17-alpha-hydroxy-progesterone by human placenta *in vitro. Acta Endocr.* (Kobenhavn) *Suppl. 51:*713, 1960.

58. Little, B., Shaw, A., and Purdy, R. The conversion of progesterone to 16α-hydroxy-pregn-4-ene-3, 20-dione and androst-4-ene-3, 17-dione by human placenta *in vitro. Acta Endocr.* (Kobenhavn) *43:*510, 1963.

59. Longchampt, J. E., Gual, C., Ehrenstein, M., and Dorfman, R. I. 19-hydroxy-Δ^4-androstene-3, 17-dione an intermediate in estrogen biosynthesis. *Endocrinology 66:*416, 1960.

60. Lundwall, F., and Stakemann, G. The urinary excretion of oestriol in postmaturity. *Acta Obstet. Gynec. Scand. 45:*301, 1966.

61. MacDonald, P. C., and Siiteri, P. K. Origin of estrogen in women pregnant with an anencephalic fetus. *J. Clin. Invest. 44:*465, 1965.

62. Magendantz, H. G., and Ryan, K. J. Isolation of a new estriol precursor. *Fed. Proc. 23:*275, 1964.

63. Magendantz, H. G., and Ryan, K. J. Isolation of an estriol precursor, 16α-hydroxydehydroepiandrosterone, from human umbilical sera. *J. Clin. Endocr. 24:*1155, 1964.

64. Mahesh, V. B. A paper chromatographic method for estrogen determination. *Steroids 3:*647, 1964.

65. Mancuso, S., Benagiano, G., Dell'Acqua, S., Shapiro, M., Wiqvist, N., and Diczfalusy, E. Studies on the metabolism of C-19 steroids in the human foetal-placental unit. 4. Aromatisation and hydroxylation products formed by previable foetuses perfused with androstenedione and testosterone. *Acta Endocr.* (Kobenhavn) *57:*208, 1968.

66. Mancuso, S., Dell'Acqua, S., Eriksson, G., Wiqvist, N., and Diczfalusy, E. Aromatisation of androstenedione and testosterone by the human fetus. *Steroids 5:*183, 1965.

67. McLeod, S. C., Brown, J. B., Beisher, N. A., and Smith, M. A. The value of urinary oestriol measurements during pregnancy. *Aust. New Zeal. J. Obstet. Gynaec.* (Melbourne) *7:*25, 1967.

68. Merkatz, I., and Beling, C. G. Urinary excretion of oestrogens and pregnanediol in the pregnant baboon. *J. Reprod. Fert. Suppl. 6:*129, 1969.

69. Meyer, A. S. Conversion of 19-hydroxy-Δ^4-androstene-3, 17-dione to estrone by endocrine tissue. *Biochem. Biophys. Acta 17:*441, 1955.

70. Migeon, C. J., Keller, A. R., and Holmstrom, E. G. Dehydroepiandrosterone, Androsterone and 17-hydroxycorticosteroid levels in maternal and cord plasma in cases of vaginal delivery. *Bull. Hopkins Hosp. 97:*415, 1955.

71. Mikhail, G., Wiqvist, N., and Diczfalusy, E. Oestriol metabolism in the previable human foetus. *Acta Endocr.* (Kobenhavn) *42:*519, 1963.

72. Morato, T., Lemus, A. E., and Gual, C. Efficiency of dehydroepiandrosterone sulphate as an estrogen precursor. *Steroids (Suppl.) 1:*59, 1965.

73. Nachtigall, L., Bassett, M., Hogsander, U., Slagle, S., and Levitz, M. A rapid method for the assay of plasma estriol in pregnancy. *J. Endocr. 26:*941, 1966.

74. Neher, R., and Stark, G. Nachweis von Corticosteroiden in menschlicher Placenta und Isolierung von 16α-Hydroxytestosteron. *Experimentia 17:*510, 1961.

75. Oakey, R. E., Bradshaw, L. R. A., Eccles, S. S., Stitch, S. R., and Hays, R. F. The rapid estimation of oestrogens in pregnancy to monitor foetal risk. *Clin. Chim. Acta 15:*35, 1967.

76. Pion, R., Conrad, S., and Wolf, B. Pregnenolone sulphate—An efficient precursor for the placental production of progesterone. *J. Clin. Endocr. 26:*225, 1966.

77. Preedy, J. R., and Aitken, E. H. The determination of estrone, estradiol-17β, and estriol in urine and plasma with column partition chromatography. *J. Biol. Chem. 236:*1300, 1961.

78. Pulkkinen, M. O. Arylsulphatase and the hydrolysis of some steroid sulphates in developing organism and placenta. *Acta Physiol. Scand. (Suppl.) 52:*180, 1961.

79. Reynolds, J. W., Mancuso, S., Wiqvist, N., and Diczfalusy, E. Studies on the aromatisation of neutral steroids in pregnant women. 7. Aromatisation of 3β, 17β-dihydroxy-androst-5-en-16-one by placentas perfused in situ at midpregnancy. *Acta Endocr.* (Kobenhavn) *58:*377, 1968.

80. Roy, E. J., and Brown, J. B. A method for the estimation of oestriol,

oestrone and oestradiol-17β in the blood of pregnant women and of the foetus. *J. Endocr. 21:*9, 1960.

81. Roy, E. J., and MacKay, R. The concentration of oestrogens in blood during pregnancy. *J. Obstet. Gynaec. Brit. Comm. 70:*1034, 1963.
82. Roy, E. V., and Harkness, R. A. The concentration of oestrogens in maternal peripheral blood during and after labor. *J. Obstet. Gynaec. Brit. Comm. 70:*1034, 1963.
83. Ryan, K. J. Conversion of Δ^5-androstene-3β, 16α, 17β-triol to estriol by human placenta. *Endocrinology 63:*392, 1958.
84. Ryan, K. J. Conversion of androstene-dione to estrone by placental microsomes. *Biochim. Biophys. Acta 27:*658, 1958.
85. Ryan, K. J. Metabolism of C-16-oxygenated steroids by human placenta: the formation of estriol. *J. Biol. Chem. 234:*2006, 1959.
86. Ryan, K. J. Metabolism of 16-ketoestrone by human placenta. *Endocrinology 66:*491, 1960.
87. Ryan, K. J. Hormones of the placenta. *Amer. J. Obstet. Gynec. 84:*1695, 1962.
88. Schindler, A. E., and Herrmann, W. L. Estriol in pregnancy urine and amniotic fluid. *Amer. J. Obstet. Gynec. 95:*301, 1966.
89. Schwers, J. In *Les Oestrogenes au Cours de la Seconde Moitié de la Grossesse* (thesis) Arscia S. A. (Ed.) , Brussels, 1965.
90. Schwers, J., Eriksson, G., and Diczfalusy, E. Metabolism of oestrone and oestradiol in the human foeto-placental unit at midpregnancy. *Acta Endocr.* (Kobenhavn) *49:*65, 1965.
91. Schwers, J., Eriksson, G., Wiqvist, N., and Diczfalusy, E. 15α-Hydroxylation: A new pathway of estrogen metabolism in the human fetus and newborn. *Biochim. Biophys. Acta 100:*313, 1965.
92. Schwers, J., Govaerts-Videtzky, M., Wiqvist, N., and Diczfalusy, E. Metabolism of oestrone sulphate by the previable human foetus. *Acta Endocr.* (Kobenhavn) *50:*597, 1965.
93. Siiteri, P. K., and MacDonald, P. C. The utilization of circulating dehydroisoandrosterone sulfate for estrogen synthesis during human pregnancy. *Steroids 2:*713, 1963.
94. Siiteri, P. K., and MacDonald, P. C. Placental estriol biosynthesis during human pregnancy. *J. Clin. Endocr. 26:*751, 1966.
95. Simmer, H. H., Easterling, W. E., Pion, R., and Digman, W. J. Neutral C_{19}-steroids and steroid sulfates in human pregnancy. *Steroids 4:*125, 1964.
96. Smith, O. W., and Arai, K. Blood estrogens in late pregnancy: An evaluation of methods with improved recovery. *J. Clin. Endocr. 23:*1141, 1963.
97. Smith, O. W., and Hagerman, D. D. Quantitative estimation of estrogen conjugates in late pregnancy plasma. *J. Clin. Endocr. 25:*732, 1965.
98. Solomon, S., Lenz, A. L., Vande Wiele, R. L., and Lieberman, S. Pregnenolone, an intermediate in the biosynthesis of progesterone and the adrenocortical hormones. *Proc. Amer. Chem. Soc.,* New York, 1954, p. 290.
99. Taylor, E. S., Bruns, P. D., Duncan, I. W., Drose, V. E. Urinary estriol determinations in normal pregnancy. *Amer. J. Obstet. Gynec. 81:*625, 1961.

100. Touchstone, J. C., Greene, J. W., Jr., McElroy, R. C., and Murawec, T. Blood estriol conjugation during human pregnancy. *Biochemistry* (Wash.) *2*:653, 1963.

101. Vande Wiele, R. L., and Jailer, J. W. Placental steroids. *Ann. N. Y. Acad. Sci. 75*:889, 1959.

102. Varangot, J., and Seeman, A. L'influence de l'accouchement sur le taux des oestrogènes sanguins. *C. R. Soc. Biol.* (Paris) *152*:43, 1958.

103. Villee, D. B., Engel, L. L., Loring, J. M., and Villee, C. A. Steroid hydroxylation in human fetal adrenals: Formation of 16α-hydroxyprogesterone, 17-hydroxyprogesterone and deoxycorticosterone. *Endocrinology 69*:354, 1961.

104. Villee, D. B., and Villee, C. A. Synthesis of corticosteroids in the fetal-placental unit. *Exerpta Med. Int. Cong. Sr. 83*:709, 1964.

105. Warren, J. C., and Cheatum, S. G. Demonstration of a steroid 17-20-desmolase in the human placenta. *Canad. J. Biochem. 42*:143, 1964.

106. Warren, J. C., and Timberlake, C. E. Steroid sulfatase in the human placenta. *J. Clin. Endocr. 22*:1148, 1962.

107. Warren, J. C., and Timberlake, C. E. Biosynthesis of estrogens in pregnancy: Precursor role of plasma dehydroisoandrosterone. *Obstet. Gynec. 23*:689, 1964.

108. Wengle, B. Studies on ester sulphates. 21. On sulphate conjugation in foetal human tissue extracts. *Acta Soc. Med. Upsal. 69*:105, 1964.

109. Wilcox, R. B., and Engel, L. L. Kinetic studies on the role of 19 hydroxy-androst-4-ene, 17-dione in estrogen biosynthesis. *Steroids* (*Suppl.*) *1*:49, 1965.

110. Wilson, R., Eriksson, G., and Diczfalusy, E. Oestriol metabolism in pregnant women. *Acta Endocr.* (Kobenhavn) *46*:525, 1964.

111. Wotiz, W. H., and Martin, H. F. Studies in steroid metabolism. XI. Gas chromatographic determination of estrogens in human pregnancy urine. *Anal. Biochem. 3*:97, 1962.

112. Yousem, H. L. Simple gas chromatographic method for estimation of urinary estriol in pregnant women. *Amer. J. Obstet. Gynec. 88*:375, 1964.

Chapter Four

Progesterone and Related Neutral Steroids

Samuel Solomon and Fritz Fuchs

Progesterone and a number of chemically related neutral steroids have been identified in human pregnancy, both in the maternal body fluids and in the feto-placental unit. Besides progesterone, two of the related compounds, the 20α- and 20β-dihydroprogesterones, are biologically active; together, these steroids are often referred to as progestins or progestagens. The terminology refers to their role in the establishment of gestation. However, clarification of the physiological function of these compounds has lagged considerably behind their identification, and the study of their biosynthesis and metabolism.

This chapter deals with recent findings concerning the formation and metabolism of neutral steroids in pregnancy. It is not intended to be an extensive review of the literature. Rather, it emphasizes the formation and metabolism of classical steroids such as progesterone, pregnenolone, and the more recently isolated steroids such as 15α-hydroxyprogesterone, 15α-hydroxyandrostenedione, 14α-hydroxyprogesterone, and 14α-hydroxytestosterone.

CHEMISTRY

Corner and Allen isolated progesterone from the corpus luteum in 1929.[70] Some years later, other investigators (Diczfalusy,[19] Pearlman and

Supported by grants from the U.S.P.H.S. (AM-04329) and the Medical Research Council of Canada (MT-1658).

Cerceo,[82] and Salhanick *et al.*[90]) demonstrated that the human placenta contains and secretes progesterone. Progesterone is an unsaturated C_{21}-diketone with a two-carbon side chain in the 17β position. The keto group of the side chain can be reduced with the rest of the steroid molecule remaining intact, resulting in 20α- or 20β-dihydroprogesterone. Both isomers have been isolated from the human placenta. The chemical structure of progesterone and its reduction products, as well as newly isolated steroids, is shown in Figure 4-1.

PRODUCTION SITES

The corpus luteum appears to be the major source of progesterone during the initial phase of pregnancy. Subsequently, the placental trophoblast produces progesterone. Mikhail and Allen measured ovarian and peripheral venous blood concentration of progesterone throughout pregnancy.[69] The arteriovenous difference indicated that the corpus luteum is the major source of progesterone during the first twelve weeks of pregnancy. Zander *et al.* have demonstrated that progesterone is present in the corpus luteum throughout pregnancy.[125] This finding has been confirmed by histological and biological studies of the corpus luteum at different stages of pregnancy.[30,55,77] However, as pregnancy progresses, ovarian production of progesterone is no longer necessary for maintenance of the pregnancy. Excision of the corpus luteum or oophorectomy is not normally followed by abortion.[34]

Yoshimi *et al.* measured levels of progesterone, 17-hydroxyprogesterone, and HCG serially in plasma during early pregnancy in patients who conceived after induction of ovulation with gonadotrophin.[120] Both steroids reached a peak concentration three to four weeks after ovulation. Plasma progesterone concentration reached a nadir at six to eight weeks after ovulation and then increased again, while 17-hydroxyprogesterone did not (Fig. 4-2). Since the placenta has limited capacity for 17-hydroxylation,[78,79] these findings suggest that the first peak reflects the function of the corpus luteum, while the second peak not containing 17-hydroxylated progesterone reflects placental secretion. The function of the corpus luteum of pregnancy, therefore, appears to be maximum during the first four weeks after ovulation with subsequent decline. If the second rising phase of the progesterone curve is extrapolated back to zero on Figure 4-2, it would indicate that the trophoblast begins to secrete progesterone between three and six weeks after ovulation. The role of HCG in maintaining the corpus luteum during pregnancy is not clear, since peripheral plasma levels of HCG continue to rise throughout the period when steroid levels decline.

There is some evidence for the production of progesterone by the adult

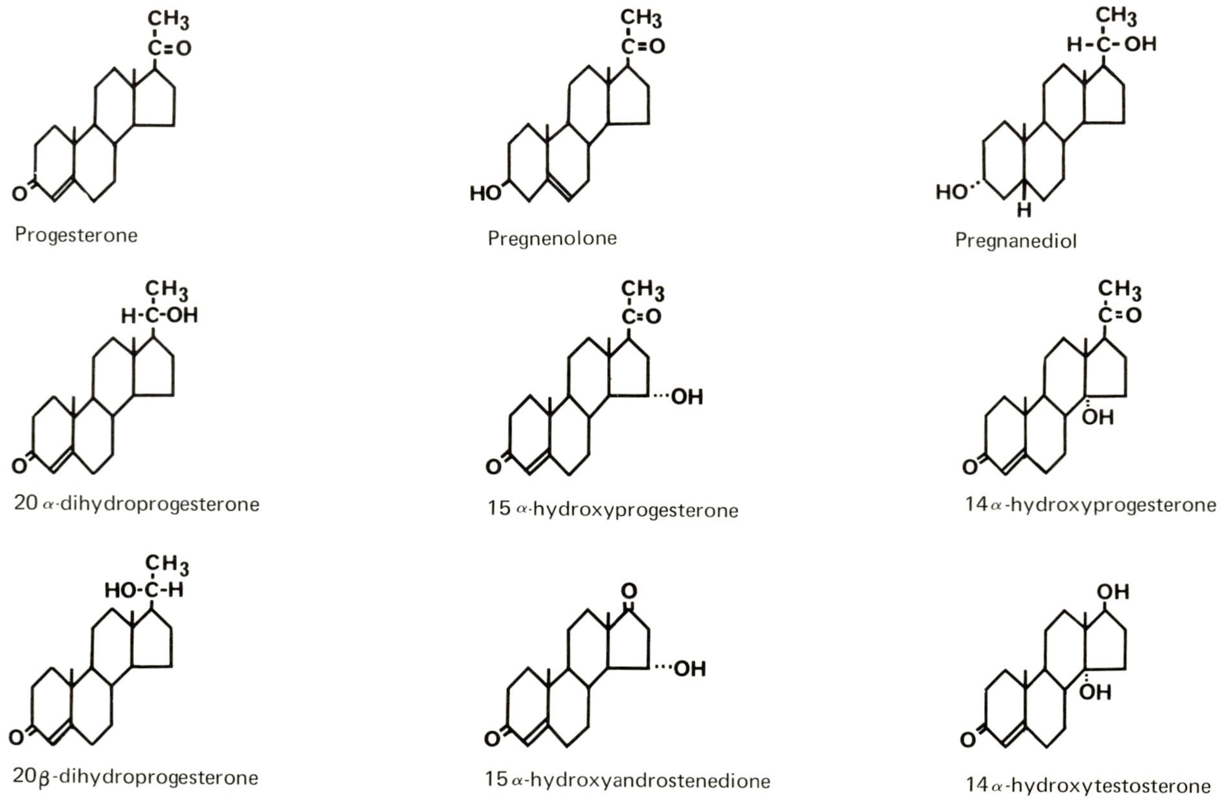

Fig. 4-1. Chemical structure of progesterone and related steroids.

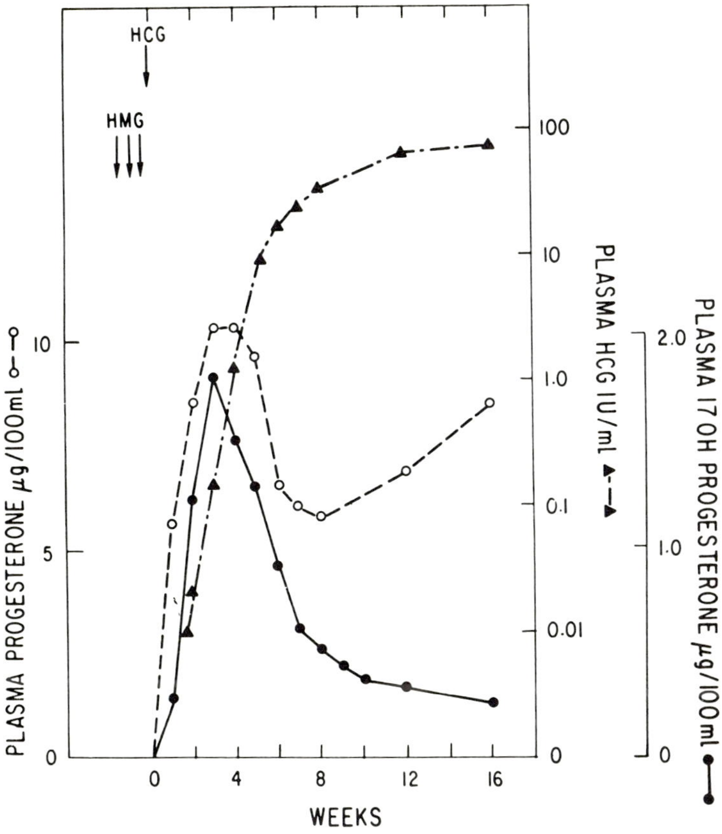

Fig. 4-2. Mean plasma levels of progesterone, 17-hydroxyprogesterone, and HCG following induction of ovulation with HMG-HCG and subsequent conception. (From Yoshimi, Strott, Marshall, and Lipsett. *J. Clin. Endocr. 29*:255, 1969.)

adrenal, but there is no reason to assume that the human adrenal cortex produces amounts of any significance in comparison with the placenta.[59] In summary, the evidence for the production of progesterone by the placenta is as follows:[21, 88]

1. Progesterone, as well as 20α- and 20β-dihydroprogesterone, has been isolated from placental extracts. A high level of progesterone is present in the maternal blood as long as the placenta is attached to the uterine wall, and the concentration increases with increasing placental weight.
2. The concentration of progesterone is higher in the umbilical and uterine venous blood than in peripheral maternal blood.

3. Pregnanediol, a metabolite of progesterone, is excreted in increasing amounts during pregnancy. The level is not significantly changed by hypophysectomy, oophorectomy, or adrenalectomy during pregnancy.
4. Spontaneous or induced intrauterine fetal death results in moderate reduction of pregnanediol excretion, as long as the placenta remains intact.
5. The placenta has the capacity of converting various precursors to progesterone as demonstrated by in situ and in vitro perfusion studies.[89]

Histochemical studies indicate that progesterone is produced in the syncytial cells of the trophoblast.[17] It has not been possible to demonstrate progesterone formation in placental tissue culture[14] or in implanted[109] placental tissue.

BIOSYNTHESIS AND PRODUCTION RATES

The metabolism of placental progesterone has been reviewed recently.[104] The placenta at term transforms acetate to cholesterol in very small quantities under in vitro conditions.[128] It is questionable whether this conversion would account for the large amounts of cholesterol needed for formation of neutral steroids.

The placenta has the capacity to transform cholesterol to pregnenolone and progesterone,[74,103] and maternal cholesterol is efficiently converted to urinary pregnanediol during late pregnancy.[9] Thus, cholesterol appears to be the main precursor of placental progesterone and pregnenolone.

Large amounts of progesterone are elaborated by the human placenta during pregnancy, but an exact assessment of the amount secreted into the fetal and maternal compartments is not yet available. Several attempts have been made to estimate the production rate of progesterone in the maternal compartment. Pearlman, using labeled progesterone, was the first to measure production rates.[81] He estimated that in late pregnancy approximately 250 mg of progesterone are produced per day. Solomon *et al.* found secretion rates of 92 mg daily in early pregnancy, 263 mg at midpregnancy, and 322 mg during the last trimester.[106] These values are higher than the 76 mg daily at midpregnancy and 264 mg daily in the last trimester reported by Bengtsson and Ejarque.[5,23] In one twin pregnancy the secretion rate at term was found by the latter authors to be as high as 521 mg daily.[5] All these measurements may not be valid at the present time because of problems presented by the multiple origin of progesterone and anatomical compartmentalization.

More recently, Little *et al.* have studied the blood level, production rate, and metabolic clearance rate of progesterone in pregnant and oophorectomized women and also in men.[59] The findings presented in Table 4-1 indicate that in late pregnancy the urinary production rate (p^1 observed) obtained by injecting labeled progesterone and then measuring the specific activity of urinary pregnanediol is very similar to the production rate obtained by using the metabolic clearance rate (MCR) and the blood concentration (i). This suggests that placental progesterone in late pregnancy is quantitatively the most important precursor of urinary pregnanediol and not other precursors, as suggested by Arcos *et al.*[4] This is not true in males nor in ovariectomized females, as is evident from the divergent values for production rates obtained from the urinary specific activity (p^1 observed) and those calculated from the MCR. The urinary production rates found in late pregnancy confirm that large amounts of progesterone are elaborated by the placenta.

TABLE 4-1
METABOLIC CLEARANCE RATE AND PRODUCTION RATE OF PROGESTERONE

	Number of subjects	Metabolic clearance rate (MCR) (liter/day)	Plasma progesterone concentration (i) (μg/100 ml)	Production rate (mg/day)	
				p^1 calculated*	p^1 observed
Male	10	2081 ± 137	0.028 ± 0.004	0.59 ± 0.05	3.39 ± 0.51
Ovariectomized female	11	2173 ± 175	0.038 ± 0.004	0.80 ± 0.07	1.06 ± 0.88
Pregnant female	16	2292 ± 210	12.48 ± 1.30	285.6 ± 56.2	290.7 ± 26.2

* p^1 calculated = metabolic clearance rate (MCR) × plasma concentration (i)
(From Little *et al. Excerpta Med. Internat. Congr. Sr. 11:*150, 1966.)

The values for progesterone production in pregnancy are in agreement with the calculations of Zander and von Münstermann.[126] By taking into consideration the arterial and venous uterine blood concentrations of progesterone and the available estimate of uterine blood flow, they calculated that 190–280 mg of progesterone per 24 hours are secreted into the maternal circulation at the end of pregnancy. The amount going to the fetus was estimated to be 75 mg per 24 hours.[124]

METABOLISM IN THE FETOPLACENTAL UNIT

Harbert *et al.* found that at term the concentration of progesterone in the umbilical vein was 72 μg/100 ml of plasma, and in the umbilical artery the concentration was 44 μg/100 ml. The fetus can therefore metabolize about 30 μg of progesterone for every 100 ml of plasma reaching it from the placenta. More recent experiments have demonstrated that progesterone serves as a precursor for a number of other steroids in the fetus. In these experiments 6 μc of progesterone-4-^{14}C in ethanol-isotonic saline solution (1:1) was infused into the umbilical vein at the time of laparotomy in midpregnancy, and the fetal circulation was left intact for 15 minutes. The placenta, umbilical cord, and fetal tissues from two male fetuses (gestation age 21 weeks) were taken for the isolation of metabolites. Each tissue was processed as described earlier,[7] and evidence for radiochemical purity of each metabolite was obtained. In Table 4-2 the reduced metabolites isolated from each tissue are shown. The small amounts of progesterone recovered from the adrenals, liver, testes, and residue suggest that these tissues are very active sites of metabolism. Hydroxylated metabolites isolated from each tissue are shown in Table 4-3, and conjugated metabolites are shown in Table 4-4. The most abundant conjugates isolated in these experiments were deoxycorticosterone sulfate from the adrenal and pregnanediol glucuronide from the liver.

Following injection of labeled progesterone into the intact feto-placental unit some metabolites were found in the cord and placenta. These

TABLE 4-2

PER CENT OF TOTAL RADIOACTIVITY IN EACH FETAL TISSUE DUE TO PROGESTERONE AND REDUCED METABOLITES ISOLATED AFTER INJECTION OF PROGESTERONE-4-^{14}C INTO THE UMBILICAL VEIN AT 21 WEEKS GESTATION

	Metabolites isolated				
Tissue	Progesterone	Pregnanolone	3β-Hydroxy-5α-pregnan-20-one	20α-Dihydro-progesterone	Pregnanediol
Adrenal	15.0*	—†	—	2.8	—
Liver	1.5	0.8	0.5	0.9	38.9
Heart	43.4	4.7	2.7	1.7	17.1
Lungs	35.4	0.4	3.8	1.3	1.0
Kidneys	30.8	0.6	7.3	4.3	1.5
Intestines	43.0	7.3	—	1.7	6.0
Testes	15.3	8.5	—	4.7	—
Thymus	38.9	24.4	—	2.9	—
Thyroid	81.4	10.5	—	—	—
Residue	23.7	1.2	8.2	0.7	1.7
Cord	50.5	—	0.6	0.9	1.1
Placenta	30.0	3.0	2.8	1.6	1.1

* These percentages were computed when radiochemical homogeneity had been achieved in each of the metabolites shown.

† A dash indicates that the metabolite was looked for but not found.

TABLE 4-3

HYDROXYLATED METABOLITES ISOLATED FROM TISSUES OF THE FETUS AFTER THE INJECTION OF PROGESTERONE-4-^{14}C INTO THE UMBILICAL VEIN

Metabolite	Per cent of total radioactivity in each tissue						
	Adrenal	Testes	Lung	Kid-ney	Intes-tine	Residue	Cord
6β-Hydroxyprogesterone	3.5*	—†	0.4	0.7	2.4	0.3	3.7
16α-Hydroxyprogesterone	6.6	—	—	—	—	0.8	—
17α-Hydroxyprogesterone	6.1	17.0	—	—	—	0.5	—
Deoxycorticosterone	—	—	—	—	—	—	—
Corticosterone	—	—	—	—	—	—	—
Hydrocortisone	0.9	—	—	—	—	—	—

* These percentages were computed using the final specific activity when radiochemical homogeneity had been achieved in each of the metabolites shown.

† A dash indicates that the metabolite was looked for but not found. The hydroxylated metabolites were not isolated from liver, heart, thyroid, thymus, and placenta.

TABLE 4-4

CONJUGATED METABOLITES ISOLATED FROM TISSUES AFTER THE INJECTION OF PROGESTERONE-4-^{14}C INTO THE UMBILICAL VEIN

Metabolite	Per cent of total radioactivity in each tissue		
	Adrenal	Liver	Residue
Pregnanolone	—*	0.6†	0.2
3β-Hydroxy-5α-pregnan-20-one-sulfate	—	—	0.4
Pregnanediol sulfate	—	0.7	0.2
Pregnanediol glucuronidate	—	1.6	0.8
Deoxycorticosterone sulfate	1.9	—	—
Corticosterone sulfate	0.9	—	—
11-Dehydrocorticosterone sulfate	0.5	—	—
Hydrocortisone sulfate	0.4	—	—

† These percentages were computed using the final specific activtity when radiochemical homogeneity had been achieved in each of the metabolites shown.

* A dash indicates that the metabolit was looked for but not found.

metabolites have previously been isolated from the tissues after perfusion of the fetus.[7] In these previous studies, pregnanediol was isolated only from the liver of the perfused fetus; in this study it was isolated in large amounts not only from the liver, but also from the heart, residue, umbilical cord, and placenta. Thus, it appears that in the intact feto-placental unit pregnanediol is formed in the liver, enters the circulation, and is transported to other tissues. Support for this view comes from the isolation of pregnanediol from the umbilical cord and the placenta.

Palmer *et al.*, however, failed to isolate pregnanediol after perfusion of midterm placenta in situ with labeled progesterone.[79]

Unconjugated metabolites isolated from the fetal tissues in the present study were the same as those isolated from the tissues of the perfused fetus. Tissue stereospecificity in the reduction of progesterone to pregnanolone and 3β-hydroxy-5α-pregnan-20-one was not observed in these studies, but was seen in the perfused fetus.[7]

The only hydroxylated metabolite isolated from the fetal testes was 17α-hydroxyprogesterone (Table 4-3). Following incubation of progesterone with a mince[1] or homogenate[8] of human fetal testes, not only was 17α-hydroxyprogesterone isolated but also testosterone, androstenedione, 16α-hydroxyprogesterone, 20α-dihydroprogesterone, and 17α,20α-dihydroxypregn-4-en-20-one. It is of interest that in the present study hydroxylated metabolites, such as 6β-hydroxyprogesterone, 16α-hydroxyprogesterone, and 17α-hydroxyprogesterone were isolated from the residual fetal tissues. Whether these steroids are synthesized in tissues other than the adrenals and testes, or transported to these tissues via the fetal circulation, remains to be determined. Only hydrocortisone was isolated from the adrenals; deoxycorticosterone and corticosterone were not detected. 20α-Dihydroprogesterone was isolated from all the fetal tissues with the exception of the thyroid.

Palmer *et al.* perfused human placentas at midterm with labeled progesterone and 20α-dihydroprogesterone; a sizable conversion of 20α-dihydroprogesterone to progesterone, but only a minute conversion of progesterone to 20α-dihydroprogesterone, was found.[79] Progesterone elaborated in the placenta is transported to the fetus, where it is reduced by a number of fetal tissues to 20α-dihydroprogesterone. The 20-reduced metabolite is oxidized to progesterone when it reaches the placenta. This metabolic pathway may be used by the feto-placental unit to conserve progesterone.

17α-Hydroxyprogesterone

Labeled 17α-hydroxyprogesterone-4-^{14}C (6μc) was injected into the umbilical vein of two male fetuses of 14 and 22 weeks gestation at the time of laparotomy for therapeutic abortion and tubal ligation (Ling, Solomon, Macnaughton, and Coutts, unpublished data). The umbilical circulation was interrupted three minutes after injection; the fetal tissues and the placenta were analyzed. Metabolites isolated from these studies are shown in Table 4-5. Cortisol, 11-deoxycortisol, 11β-hydroxyandrostenedione, 5β-androstanedione, and 5α-androstanedione were looked for but were not isolated. However, androstenedione and testosterone were isolated from fetal adrenals and testes of the older of the two fetuses. The possibility

TABLE 4-5

UNCONJUGATED METABOLITES ISOLATED FROM TISSUES OF THE HUMAN FETUS AFTER THE INJECTION OF 17α-HYDROXYPROGESTERONE-4-^{14}C INTO THE UMBILICAL VEIN (EXPRESSED AS THE PERCENTAGE OF TOTAL RADIOACTIVITY IN THE INDIVIDUAL TISSUE)

Metabolite	Adrenals	Testes	Liver
17α-Hydroxyprogesterone	3.65*	4.04	0.13
17α,20α-Dihydroxypregn-4-en-3-one	2.92	3.01	—
3α,17α-Dihydroxy-5β-pregnan-20-one	—†	—	25.74
5β-Pregnane-3α,17α,20α-triol	—	—	22.82
5β-Pregnane-3α,17α,20β-triol	—	—	4.53
Cortisol	—	—	—
11-Deoxycortisol	—	—	—
11β-Hydroxyandrostenedione	—	—	—
Androstenedione	1.90	3.62	—
Testosterone	1.23	4.17	—
5β-Androstenedione	—	—	—
5α-Androstanedione	—	—	—

* These percentages were computed using the final specific activity when radiochemical homogenity had been achieved in each of the metabolites shown.

† A dash indicates that the metabolite was looked for but not found.

exists, therefore, that with advancing gestation a small conversion of 17α-hydroxyprogesterone to testosterone and androstenedione takes place in the fetus.

Pregnenolone and Pregnenolone Sulfate

Pregnenolone and progesterone are formed from cholesterol by the human placenta.[74,103] Under normal circumstances both steroids would reach the fetus. It is of interest, therefore, to discuss the metabolic pathways of pregnenolone and pregnenolone sulfate in the feto-placental unit. A total of 19.8×10^6 cpm of pregnenolone-4-^{14}C (in 0.3 ml of ethanol and 2 ml of 5% dextrose) was injected into the umbilical vein at the time of laparotomy for therapeutic abortion at 13 weeks of gestation. The cord was clamped 20 seconds after the injection; the fetus as well as the placenta were then removed and analyzed. Table 4-6 shows the total radioactivity in each fetal tissue as well as the per cent of radioactivity in the aqueous phase after ether-water partition. It is of interest to note that within 20 seconds of intact umbilical circulation, radioactive material entered the maternal circulation as is evident by its presence in the maternal urine. A sizable portion of the radioactivity in the adrenals, liver, lung, and intestine was found to be water soluble, whereas most of the radioactivity in the kidney, placenta, and the residue was found to be ether soluble.

The metabolites of pregnenolone isolated from the fetal tissues and

TABLE 4-6

RADIOACTIVITY FROM TISSUES OF FETUSES AFTER INJECTION OF LABELED STEROIDS INTO THE UMBILICAL VEIN

	Pregnenolone-4-^{14}C (13 weeks gestation)		Pregnenolone-4-^{14}C sulfate (18 weeks gestation)	
Source	Total radioactivity (cpm $\times$ 10^5)	Per cent in aqueous phase	Total radioactivity (cpm $\times$ 10^5)	Per cent in aqueous phase
Adrenal	2.14	63.7	0.15	96.5
Liver	3.34	39.0	27.30	98.1
Lung	0.62	34.1	0.22	97.9
Kidney	1.31	17.3	0.29	99.0
Intestine	2.22	32.9	0.29	98.5
Residue	22.07	11.6	12.17	70.8
Placenta	1.34	10.0	8.07	12.9
Maternal urine (4 days)	5.30	—	0.83	—

TABLE 4-7

METABOLITES ISOLATED FROM TISSUE OF A FETUS AFTER INJECTION OF PREGNENOLONE-4-^{14}C INTO THE UMBILICAL VEIN AT 13 WEEKS GESTATION

	Per cent of total radioactivity in each tissue						
Metabolite	Adrenal	Liver	Lung	Kid-ney	Intes-tine	Resi-due	Placenta
Pregnenolone	14.6*	34.8	47.3	67.6	43.1	63.8	31.7
20α-Dihydropregnenolone	—†	7.6	—	—	—	1.0	—
16α-Hydroxypregnenolone	—	2.6	—	—	—	—	—
Dehydroisoandrosterone	2.8	—	—	—	—	—	—
Progesterone	—	—	—	—	—	—	31.6
20α-Dihydroprogesterone	—	—	—	—	—	—	2.0
Pregnenolone sulfate	17.0	9.5	17.5	10.5	23.9	8.4	—
20α-Dihydropregnenolone sulfate	—	9.2	—	—	—	—	
17α-Hydroxypregnenolone sulfate	2.3	—	—	—	—	—	
Dehydroisoandrosterone	12.5	—	—	—	—	0.6	

* These percentages were computed using the final specific activity when radiochemical homogeneity had been achieved in each of the metabolites shown.

† A dash indicates that the metabolite was looked for but not found.

placenta are shown in Table 4-7. Metabolites with a Δ^4-3-ketone were isolated only from the placenta. No 3β-hydroxysteroid dehydrogenase appears to be present in fetal tissue at midpregnancy, whereas this enzyme system is present in the placenta. These observations are in agreement with the results from perfusion studies of previable human fetuses with estrone, estradiol, and estriol[20,38,70,93] and also with the findings of Wengle,[111] who demonstrated an extensive sulfokinase activity in incubation studies in vitro with human fetal tissues.

The isolation of unconjugated 16α-hydroxypregnenolone from the liver only, suggests that C_{21}, 3β-hydroxy-Δ^5-steroids are 16α-hydroxylated by this tissue. This observation is in keeping with the isolation by Bolté, Wiqvist and Diczfalusy, of double-labeled androst-5-ene-3β, 16α, 17β-triol from aqueous extract of fetal liver after perfusion of the previable human fetus with ^{14}C-labeled dehydroisoandrosterone and ^{3}H-labeled dehydroisoandrosterone sulfate.[10] Slaunwhite *et al.* have also isolated androst-5-ene-3β, 16α, 17β-triol in fetal liver incubation studies with dehydroisoandrosterone.[101] Thus 16α-hydroxylation of C_{21} steroids with Δ^4-3-ketone occurs in fetal adrenal and residual tissues; 16α-hydroxylation of C_{19} and C_{21} steroids with a 3β-hydroxy-Δ^5 grouping occurs in the fetal liver.

Because of the sizable amounts of sulfate conjugates isolated from the fetal tissues following injection of pregnenolone into the umbilical vein, it was of interest to study the metabolism of pregnenolone sulfate. Accordingly, 15.1×10^6 cpm of pregnenolone-7α-^3H sulfate (in 0.5 ml of ethanol and 10 ml of isotonic saline) was injected over a period of 2 minutes into the umbilical vein at 18 weeks of pregnancy at the time of laparotomy for therapeutic abortion. The cord was clamped 5 minutes after the injection; a female fetus was then delivered. The fetal tissues and placenta were analyzed. In Table 4-6 the total radioactivity in each tissue as well as the per cent of total radioactivity present in the aqueous phase after ether-water partition are shown. Following administration of labeled pregnenolone sulfate into the umbilical cord, less radioactive material appeared in the maternal urine than after injection of the labeled pregnenolone. These results indicate that unconjugated pregnenolone entering the placenta is more readily transported to the maternal circulation than pregnenolone sulfate. Goebelsmann *et al.* found that estriol is transported from the fetal to the maternal circulation more rapidly than estriol-3-sulfate or estriol-16-glucosiduronate.[31]

The metabolites of pregnenolone sulfate isolated from the fetal tissues are shown in Table 4-8. Pregnenolone sulfate was isolated from all tissues analyzed, whereas pregnenolone was isolated only from the liver. This finding suggests that steroid sulfatase activity is absent in fetal tissues, as previously demonstrated by Pulkkinen[84] as well as by French and Warren.[24] Pregnenolone sulfate, pregnenolone, progesterone, and 20α-dihydroprogesterone were isolated from the placenta. This suggests that most of the pregnenolone sulfate reaching the placenta from the fetus is hydrolyzed to pregnenolone and then converted to progesterone and 20α-dihydroprogesterone. Pregnenolone and progesterone were isolated from

TABLE 4-8

METABOLITES ISOLATED FROM TISSUES OF A HUMAN FETUS AFTER INJECTION OF PREGNENOLONE-7α-^{3}H SULFATE INTO THE UMBILICAL VEIN AT 18 WEEKS GESTATION

Tissue	Per cent of total radioactivity in each tissue			
	Pregnenolone sulfate	Pregnenolone	Progesterone	20α-Dihydroprogesterone
Adrenal	46.6*	—†	—	—
Liver	48.6	0.4	—	—
Lung	46.1	—	—	—
Kidney	35.3	—	—	—
Intestine	59.4	—	—	—
Residue	16.2	—	—	—
Placenta	1.2	7.4	19.5	4.6

* These percentages were computed using the final specific activity when radiochemical homogeneity had been achieved in each of the metabolites shown.

† A dash indicates that the metabolite was looked for but not found.

the midterm placenta following perfusion of this tissue with labeled pregnenolone sulfate when it was still attached to the uterus.[80] Some of the very polar $C_{21}O_5$ and $C_{21}O_4$ hydroxylated pregnenolone sulfates isolated from blood from term placenta by Eberlein[22] were not found in fetal tissues or placenta in the studies reported here. This difference may be explained by altered metabolism of pregnenolone and its sulfate in the term fetus as compared to the fetus at midpregnancy.

15α-Hydroxyprogesterone and 15-Hydroxylated Estrogens

In the last five years a number of publications have appeared dealing with the isolation and origin of 15-hydroxysteroids (Table 4-9 and Fig. 4-3). Knuppen, Haupt, and Breuer found that 15α-hydroxyestrone is present in human pregnancy urine.[49] 15β-Hydroxyestrone as well as 15β-

TABLE 4-9

15-HYDROXYSTEROIDS ISOLATED FROM URINE OF PREGNANT WOMEN AND NEWBORNS

Steroid	Author
15α-Hydroxyestrone	Knuppen, Haupt, and Breuer[49]
15β-Hydroxyestrone	Knuppen, Haupt, and Breuer[51]
15β-Hydroxyestradiol	Knuppen, Haupt, and Breuer[51]
15α-Hydroxyestradiol	Lisboa, Goebelsmann, and Diczfalusy[57] Knuppen and Breuer[48]
15α-Hydroxyestriol	Hagen, Barr, and Diczfalusy[35] Zucconi *et al.*[129]
15α-Hydroxyprogesterone	Giannopoulos and Solomon[28]

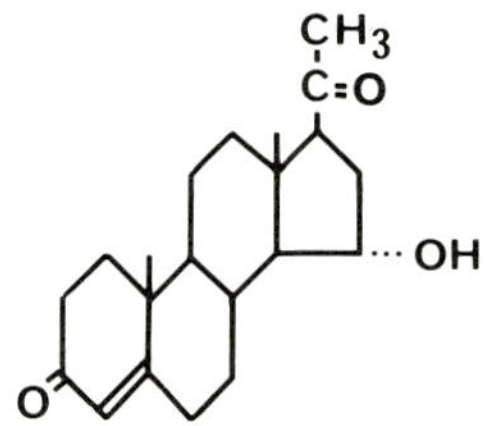

15α-hydroxy-progesterone

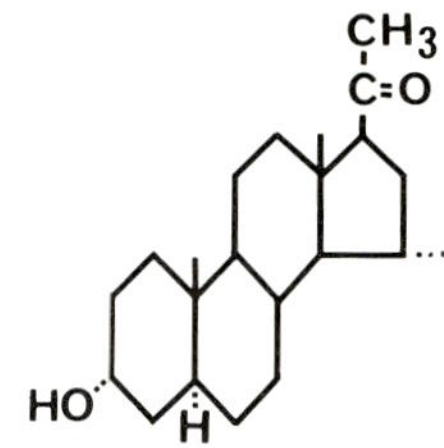

3α, 15α-dihydroxy-5α-pregnan-20-one

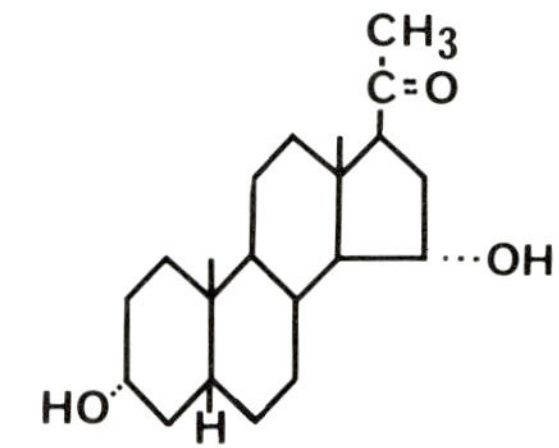

3α,15α-dihydroxy-5β-pregnan-20-one

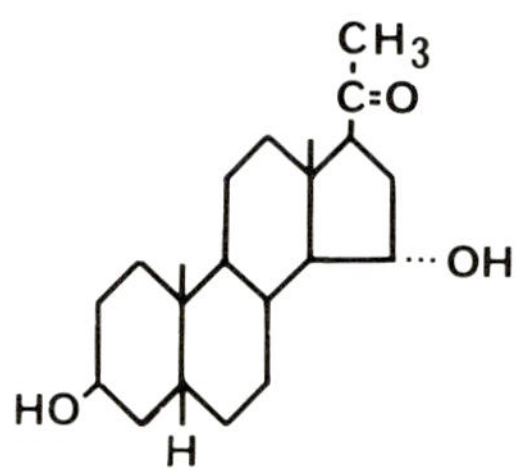

3β,15α-dihydroxy-5β-pregnan-20-one

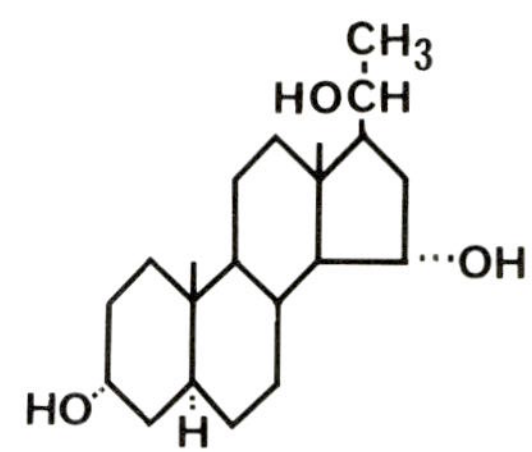

5α-pregnane-3α,15α,20β-triol

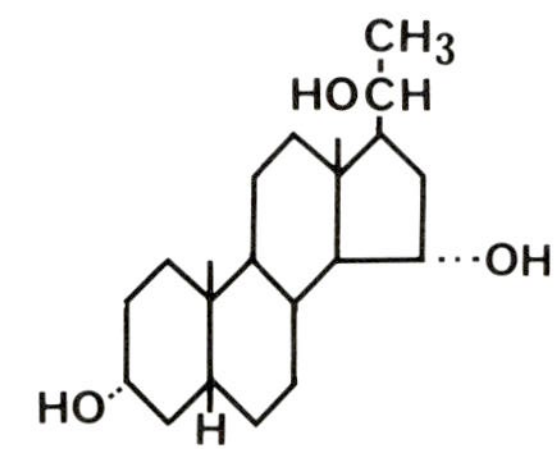

5β-pregnane-3α,15α,20β-triol

Fig. 4-3. The chemical structure of a number of 15-hydroxysteroids.

hydroxyestradiol have also been isolated from this source by Knuppen, Haupt, and Breuer.[51] Lisboa, Goebelsmann, and Diczfalusy[57] as well as Knuppen and Breuer[48] have isolated 15α-hydroxyestradiol from human pregnancy urine. The tetrol, 15α-hydroxyestriol (estetrol) has been isolated from human newborn urine by Hagen, Barr, and Diczfalusy[35] and from pregnancy urine by Zucconi *et al.*[129] In addition to these metabolites, 15α-hydroxyprogesterone has been isolated from human late pregnancy urine by Giannopoulos and Solomon.[28]

The 15α-hydroxyestrogens are formed in vivo and in vitro by a variety of tissues as is shown in Table 4-10. Some caution must be applied when interpreting the results shown in Tables 4-9 and 4-10. The in vitro demonstration of 15α-hydroxylation of precursors by tissues such as human adrenals and liver does not necessarily mean that 15α-hydroxysteroids are formed in vivo in the nonpregnant female. Indeed, it would seem that in vivo 15α-hydroxysteriods are uniquely or almost entirely formed in the fetus.

Following the isolation of 15α-hydroxyprogesterone, a study was undertaken to determine the origin of this steroid during late pregnancy. In the first of these investigations, ^{3}H-progesterone was infused into the peritoneal cavity of the fetus at the time of intraperitoneal blood transfusion for Rh incompatibility; 4-^{14}C-progesterone was injected intravenously in the mother. The 15α-hydroxyprogesterone isolated from the maternal urine in two such studies contained ^{3}H but not ^{14}C. This indicated that

TABLE 4-10

FORMATION OF 15α-HYDROXYESTROGENS

Precursor	Tissue	Product	Author
Estrone	Bovine adrenals	15α-hydroxyestrone	Knuppen and Breuer[47]
Estrone	Human adrenals	15α-hydroxyestradiol	Knuppen, Haupt, and Breuer[50]
Estrone	Human liver	15α-hydroxyestradiol	Breuer, Knuppen, and Haupt[11]
Estrone Estradiol Estrone sulfate	Liver (perfused) Human fetus	15α-hydroxyestradiol	Schwers *et al.*[92]
Testosterone Androstenedione	Liver (perfused) Human fetus	15α-hydroxyestradiol	Mancuso *et al.*[67]
Estradiol	Bovine adrenals (perfused)	15α-hydroxyestradiol	Levy *et al.*[56]
Estradiol	Human fetal tissues	15α-hydroxyestriol	Gurpide *et al.*[33]
Estriol	Human fetal tissues	15α-hydroxyestriol	Schwers *et al.*[94]
Estrone sulfate	Human bile	15α-hydroxyestrone	Jirku, Hogsander, and Levitz[43]
Estrone	Bovine adrenals	14α-hydroxyestrone	Knuppen, Haupt, and Breuer[52]

15α-hydroxyprogesterone was elaborated in the fetoplacental unit but not in the maternal compartment. In a second study, ^{3}H-progesterone was infused into the peritoneal cavity of the fetus; ^{14}C-15α-hydroxyprogesterone was injected intravenously in the mother. From the ^{3}H/^{14}C ratio of the 15α-hydroxyprogesterone isolated from the urine, an 0.08 per cent conversion of progesterone to urinary 15α-hydroxyprogesterone during late pregnancy was calculated. Thus, assuming that 75–125 mg of progesterone is transported from the placenta to the fetus during late pregnancy, then 60–100 μg of 15α-hydroxyprogesterone is elaborated by the fetus at this stage of gestation.

METABOLIC PATHWAYS IN THE MATERNAL COMPARTMENT

The metabolic pathway for progesterone in pregnant women is the same as in nonpregnant women. The most important metabolite formed is pregnanediol (5β-pregnane-3α, 20α-diol) which is derived from progesterone and 20α-dihydroprogesterone. The conversion rate of progesterone to pregnanediol is of the order of 10–15 per cent and seems to be the same in pregnant and nonpregnant women. Pregnanediol is excreted in the urine as well as in the bile, and it is possible that the ratio between the routes of excretion varies. It is excreted in the urine as the 3-glucuronidate. The urine of pregnant women also contains conjugates of C_{21} steroids such as pregnanolone, 5α-pregnane-3,20-dione, 3α-hydroxy-5α-pregnan-20-one, 3β-hydroxy-5α-pregnan-20-one, 5α-pregnane-3α,20α-diol, and 3α,6α-dihydroxy-5α-pregnan-20-one and its 3β-isomer.

The concentration of 15α-hydroxyprogesterone was measured in urine by a double-isotope procedure. Tritium-labeled 15α-hydroxyprogesterone of known specific activity was added to urine. The isolated steroid was acetylated with ^{14}C-acetic anhydride and the acetate purified to a constant ^{3}H/^{14}C ratio. 15α-Hydroxyprogesterone is excreted in the urine in largest amounts during the third trimester of pregnancy (28–34 μg/day); lesser amounts are present during the second trimester (5–6 μg/day), whereas negligible amounts are found during the first trimester of pregnancy. None is detected in the urine during the normal menstrual cycle. Negligible amounts of 15α-hydroxyprogesterone were found in two pools of urine from newborns. These findings suggest that 15α-hydroxyprogesterone is probably elaborated in the second and third trimesters of pregnancy, and is uniquely formed by the fetus. Future studies on the origin of 15α-hydroxyprogesterone had to be conducted during the third trimester of pregnancy.

Once it was determined that 15α-hydroxyprogesterone is uniquely formed in the fetus, an examination of the metabolism of this steroid in the maternal compartment was made. The first task was to isolate sufficiently large amounts of the metabolites of 15α-hydroxyprogesterone for chemical characterization. Nonlabeled 15α-hydroxyprogesterone was therefore administered by mouth to normal males in one study, labeled steroid was administered intravenously at the same time. Six steroids were isolated from the urine and identified; these are shown in Figure 4-3.

A tracer dose of the ^{14}C-labeled steroid was then administered to a pregnant female in the third trimester, and to a normal female in the luteal phase of the menstrual cycle. The specific activities of the metabolites isolated from the urine of the two subjects are shown in Table 4-11. The specific activities of the five steroids isolated from the urine of the nonpregnant subject were essentially the same as the specific activity of the injected steroid. In the pregnant subject the specific activities of the urinary steroids were 20–40 times lower than the specific activity of the injected steroid. These results suggest that there was no endogenous production of 15α-hydroxyprogesterone in the nonpregnant female, but production of 15α-hydroxyprogesterone in the nonpregnant female, but that in the pregnant female these metabolites are normal urinary constituents, probably derived from endogenously produced 15α-hydroxyprogesterone. These findings confirm earlier reports that no 15α-hydroxyprogesterone could be detected in the urine from nonpregnant females. Only 3β,15α-dihydroxy-5β-pregnan-20-one was isolated from the "sulfate" fraction of the urine following solvolysis of the urinary conjugates; the remaining steroids shown in Table 4-12 were isolated from the glucosiduronate fraction. Thus, it is likely that 15α-hydroxyprogesterone is excreted in the urine after being conjugated to glucuronic acid at C-15.

Table 4-13 shows the minimum per cent of conversion of the injected steroid to the urinary metabolites isolated in a radiochemically pure form. It appears that 15α-hydroxyprogesterone was a major urinary product in the normal male who was given a tracer dose of the steroid intravenously and ingested 800 mg of carrier steroid. In addition, large amounts of the

TABLE 4-11
URINARY METABOLITES OF ADMINISTERED (4-^{14}C) 15α-HYDROXYPROGESTERONE*

Metabolite	Specific activity (dpm/μg)	
	Pregnant female	Nonpregnant female
15α-Hydroxyprogesterone	1.56×10^4	3.31×10^5
3α, 15α-Dihydroxy-5α-pregnan-20-one	7.90×10^3	3.45×10^5
3α, 15α-Dihydroxy-5β-pregnan-20-one	9.70×10^3	3.52×10^5
3β-15α-Dihydroxy-5β-pregnan-20-one	8.66×10^3	3.06×10^5
5α-Pregnane-3α, 15α, 20-β-triol	8.68×10^3	3.35×10^5

* Specific activity of injected (4-^{14}C) 15α-hydroxyprogesterone = 3.66×10^5 dpm/μg.

TABLE 4-12
NEW HYDROXYSTEROIDS IN LATE PREGNANCY URINE

Steroid	Excretion rate (μg/day)	Production rate (μg/day)
15α-Hydroxyandrostenedione	4.4–5.2	10.2, 13.1
15α-Hydroxytestosterone	0.48, 0.64	—
15α-Hydroxyprogesterone	28–34	80
15α-Hydroxyestradiol	110	—
15α-Hydroxyestriol	520	—
14α-Hydroxytestosterone	0.11, 0.21	—
14α-Hydroxyprogesterone	0.52	—

two dihydroxy-ketones were excreted; only small amounts of the triol were isolated. The urinary products isolated from the normal female given a tracer dose of the steroid were similar to those observed for the male who ingested 15α-hydroxyprogesterone. In the pregnant female the most abundant urinary product was 15α-hydroxyprogesterone followed by the dihydroxy-ketones; a small amount of the triol was isolated. It can therefore be concluded that the 15α-hydroxy group partially inhibits the reduction of the A/B ring of the steroid nucleus, as well as the 20-ketone, and that when the 20-ketone is reduced the alcohol has a β orientation. It has been possible to isolate five 15α-hydroxysteroids and two 14α-hydroxysteroids from late pregnancy. These new urinary metabolites are shown in Table 4-12 along with their excretion rates and estimations of the production rates of 15α-hydroxyandrostenedione and 15α-hydroxyprogesterone. The urinary steroids excreted in the largest amount were 15α-hydroxyestriol,[122, 129] 15α-hydroxyestradiol,[48, 122] and 15α-hydroxyprogesterone;[28] 15α-hydroxyandrostenedione and 15α-hydroxytestosterone were excreted in small amounts.[29] In addition, very small amounts of 14α-hydroxytestosterone[64] and 14α-hydroxyprogesterone[6] are found in late pregnancy urine.

It seems probable that the 15α- and 14α-hydroxysteroids are all formed

TABLE 4-13
CONVERSION OF 15α-HYDROXYPROGESTERONE TO URINARY METABOLITES

Metabolite	Per cent conversion		
	Normal male	Normal female	Pregnant female
15α-Hydroxyprogesterone (unconverted)	12.9	5.8	18.7
3α, 15α-Dihydroxy-5α-pregnan-20-one	8.7	7.1	2.9
3α, 15α-Dihydroxy-5β-pregnan-20-one	7.9	7.4	7.5
3β, 15α-Dihydroxy-5β-pregnan-20-one	—	0.4	1.0
5α-Pregnane-3α, 15α, 20β-triol	1.4	2.3	1.8

in the fetus and not in the maternal compartment. Recently, it has been found that 15α-hydroxyandrostenedione can be aromatised by the placenta to form 15α-hydroxyestrone and 15α-hydroxyestradiol,[108] and that 15α-hydroxyandrostenedione is a very effective precursor of urinary 15α-hydroxyestriol.[122] The physiological role of 14α- and 15α-hydroxysteroids in the fetus is not known at present. Further investigations will reveal whether they play a role in the control and maintenance of the developing human fetus.

ASSAYS OF PROGESTERONE IN BLOOD AND OTHER BODY FLUIDS

Before 1950, attempts to measure progesterone in blood were based upon bioassays of crude extracts. Bioassays developed by McGinty, Anderson, and McCullough,[68] and by Hooker and Forbes[41] depended on the effect of extracts injected into the uterus of immature rabbits or rats. The sensitivity was superior to some of the later chemical assays, but the precision and specificity was quite low. These methods have lost their practical significance for progesterone assay, although they continue to be of value for assessment of progestational properties of synthetic progestagens.

The rapid progress in steroid analysis has included the development of several sensitive and accurate methods of detection and quantitative determination of progesterone in blood and other body fluids. These assays are based on chemical extraction and determination by various physicochemical techniques. Table 4-14, adapted from van der Molen and Aakvaag,[72] summarizes methods used by different investigators. The most recent method, based upon the competitive protein-binding technique of Murphy,[75] has many advantages and may well become the method of choice.

PREGNANEDIOL EXCRETION DURING PREGNANCY

Pregnanediol, the chief metabolite of progesterone in urine, may be determined by various methods.[45] The fluorometric method described by Klopper, Michie, and Brown[46] is commonly used, although gas chromatographic techniques[42] have become available recently. Klopper and Macnaughton have shown that the fluorimetric method can also be used for determining pregnanediol in bile, feces, and amniotic fluid.[45a] Adlercreutz and Luukkainen used gas chromatography for studies of pregnanediol in bile.[2]

For many years our knowledge of progesterone metabolism during

TABLE 4-14

PHYSICO-CHEMICAL METHODS FOR QUANTITATIVE DETERMINATION OF PROGESTERONE IN BLOOD AND OTHER BIOLOGICAL FLUIDS WITH INDICATION OF SENSITIVITY*

Principle of detection	Sensitivity (μg)	Author
U.V. absorption of progesterone	0.3–0.5	Zander and Simmer;[127] Short[96]
Abosorption of dinitrophenylhydrazone derivative	0.1–0.2	Hinsberg, Pelzer, and Seuken[40]
Absorption of isonicotinic acid hydrazide derivative	0.5–1.0	Sommerville and Deshpande[107]
Absorption of sulphuric acid-ethanol chromogen	0.3–0.5	Oertel, Weiss, and Eik-Nes[78]
Absorption of thiosemicarbazide derivative	0.1–0.2	Pearlman and Cerceo;[83] Simmer and Simmer[100]
KOH-sulphuric acid fluorescence	0.05–0.10	Touchstone and Murawec;[110] Short and Levett[98]
Sulphuric acid fluorescence after conversion to 20β-dihydroprogesterone	0.003–0.005	Heap[39]
Double-isotope derivative (^3H and ^{14}C) measuring 20-^3H-20β-dihydroprogesterone	$\leq$0.10	Woolever and Goldfien[116]
Double isotope derivative (^3H and ^{35}S) measuring progesterone-^{35}S-thiosemicarbazide-2′, 4′-diacetate	0.002	Riondel *et al.*[85]
Double isotope derivative (^3H and ^{14}C) measuring 20β-dihydroprogesterone-^3H-acetate	0.01–0.02	Wiest;[114] Wiest, Kerenyi, and Csapo;[115] Gandy[27]
Argon ionization detection after gas-liquid chromatography	0.01–0.10	Collins and Sommerville;[15] Carlson, Meyer, and Blair[12]
Flame ionization detection after gas-liquid chromatography	0.005–0.10	Yannone, McComas, and Goldfien;[117] Luisi *et al.*;[61] Lurie and Villee[65]
Electron capture detection of the chloroacetate derivative of 20β-dihydroprogesterone	0.001	van der Molen and Groen[73]
Competitive protein-binding radioassay	0.0002	Neill *et al.*[76]

* Adapted from van der Molen and Aakvaag, *Hormones in Blood*, Academic Press, London, 1967.

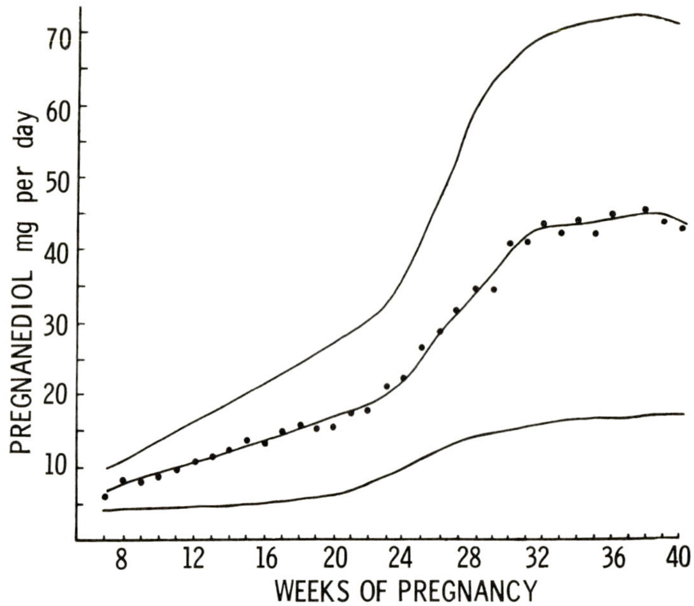

Fig. 4-4. Pregnanediol excretion in normal pregnancy. The dots represent observed means, the central line fitted means. The upper and lower lines show the 95% probability limits. (From Shearman. *J. Obstet. Gynec. Brit. Comm. 66*:1, 1959.)

pregnancy was based almost entirely upon assay of pregnanediol in urine in particular and, to a minor extent, its determination in feces. It was thought that pregnanediol excretion reflected the endocrine function of the placenta. Using the method of Klopper, Michie, and Brown,[46] Shearman[95] studied the urinary excretion of pregnanediol in a large number of normal pregnancies. These results are plotted on Figure 4-4, representing mean values and 95 per cent confidence limits.

Because the quantity of pregnanediol excreted in the urine varies over a broad range, and since its excretion does not reflect the physiological disposition of the fetus, pregnanediol assays have not been quite as useful as anticipated in the monitoring of high-risk pregnancies. This will be discussed further in Chapter Fourteen.

PROGESTERONE IN BLOOD DURING PREGNANCY

The enhanced production rate of progesterone with advancing gestation is associated with an increasing concentration in maternal and presumably also in fetal blood. Zander was the first to obtain reliable estimations of plasma progesterone during pregnancy with chemical assays.[124] Subsequently, rising levels have been clearly demonstrated by a number of investigators, although the shape of the curve showing the average values varies considerably from author to author. Short and Eton found levels of progesterone to be approximately 5 μg/100 ml of plasma in the first and second trimesters and around 15 μg/100 ml in the last trimester.[97] Yannone, McCurdy, and Goldfien,[118] using gas chromatography, found a linear rise throughout pregnancy, from around 2 μg/100 ml at 8 weeks to about 14 μg/100 ml at 40 weeks. Levels reported by Gandy of 1 μg/100 ml during the first trimester with a gradual rise to 12 μg/100 ml at the onset of labor are somewhat lower than those found by others.[27] Her values for progesterone are shown in Figure 4-5, and those for 20α-dihydroprogesterone are shown in Figure 4-6.

Table 4-15 shows values for blood progesterone reported by different investigators. The table includes values from each trimester as well as values from the umbilical vein and artery. It is obvious that the umbilical vein has a higher concentration of progesterone than the artery, and that the umbilical artery has a higher concentration of progesterone than peripheral maternal blood. However, this is due to a large extent to the rapid disappearance of progesterone from the maternal circulation. Fuchs, Fuchs, and Short have reported that the uterine venous blood in midpregnancy contained 9–10 times as much progesterone as the peripheral venous blood (see Fig. 13-2 in Chapter Thirteen).[25] The concentration in uterine venous blood remained high after intra-amniotic injection of 20 per cent saline solution in midpregnancy until long after the onset of strong myometrial contractions.[99]

The concentration of progesterone in the maternal plasma is usually rising toward term, and several investigators have found that labor can start in spite of rising levels of progesterone[3,18,53,71,97,100] and progresses without any relationship to the peripheral progesterone concentrations. Llauro, Runnebaum, and Zander[60] recently made a detailed study of progesterone concentrations at term. They found no fall before the onset of labor, but approximately a 10 per cent fall until a cervical dilatation of 5 cm, and another 10 per cent fall until full dilatation (see Fig. 13-3, Chapter Thirteen). This does not indicate that a fall in the maternal blood level of progesterone is a prerequisite for the initiation and maintenance of labor.

Wiest[114] has determined the progesterone concentrations in placenta, membranes, amniotic fluid, myometrium, and maternal peripheral plasma at delivery with the double-isotope derivative assay.[113,115] The values obtained are shown in Table 4-16. Wiest, [114] as well as Lurie, Reid, and Villee,[63] has studied the diurnal variations of the maternal blood con-

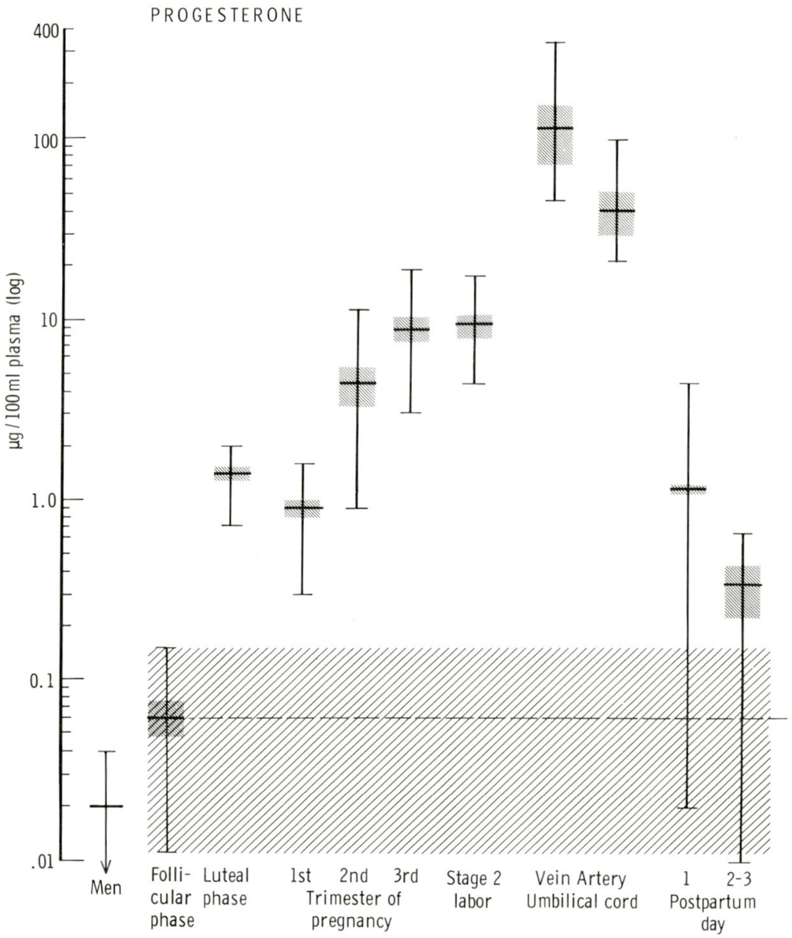

Fig. 4-5. Peripheral plasma concentration of progesterone in 6 women studied during the course of pregnancy, compared to the levels in normal men and nonpregnant women, plotted on a log scale. The means and the standard deviations are represented by the horizontal bars and hatched areas, respectively. The plasma concentration in 8 other mothers in labor are compared with the cord levels at birth. (Courtesy of Dr. Hortense M. Gandy.)

centrations. No consistent pattern was apparent, but the variations over a 24-hour period were considerable. These variations underscore the need for caution in the interpretation of changes in progesterone levels during labor or saline-induced abortion.

Lurie and Weiss[66] looked for progesterone in the cerebrospinal fluid during pregnancy, using the same method as for plasma.[62] In two cases

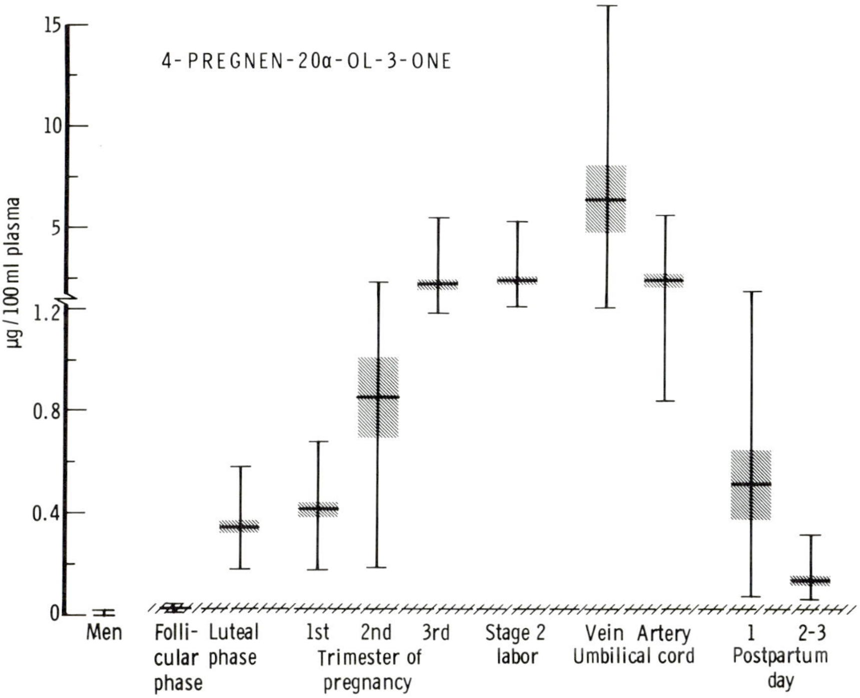

Fig. 4-6. Peripheral plasma concentration of 20α-dihydroprogesterone in 6 women studied during the course of pregnancy, compared to the levels in men and nonpregnant women, plotted on a broken arithmetic scale. The means and the standard deviations are represented by the horizontal bars and hatched areas, respectively. The plasma concentration in 8 other mothers in labor are compared with the cord levels at birth. (Courtesy of Dr. Hortense M. Gandy.)

the concentration was 0.30 and 0.55 µg/100 ml, respectively, in two other cases progesterone was undetectable.

Deshpande, Turner, and Sommerville[18] and Lauritzen and Lehmann[54] have studied the pregnanediol concentrations in maternal blood toward the end of pregnancy, during labor, and after delivery, as well as in the cord blood. Both groups found quite high values in the maternal plasma, higher than the concentrations of progesterone. Deshpande, Turner, and Sommerville found an increase of the ratio of pregnanediol to progesterone before or during labor.[18] The pregnanediol levels in the cord blood were of the same order of magnitude as in the maternal blood. The pregnanediol values found by Lauritzen and Lehmann were generally lower than those of the other group;[54] progesterone was not measured simultaneously in their series.

TABLE 4-15

CONCENTRATION OF PROGESTERONE IN μg/100 ML in PERIPHERAL PLASMA OF PREGNANT WOMEN AND IN UMBILICAL VENOUS AND ARTERIAL PLASMA AT BIRTH

	Trimester of pregnancy						Umbilical			
Author	N*	First	N	Second	N	Third	N	Vein	N	Artery
Zander;[123] Runnebaum and Zander[87]						4 − 27	7	37.2 ± 6.0	5	14.8 ± 1.8
Short;[96] Short and Eton[97]		2 − 6		2 − 10		6 − 28	7	46 ± 11		
Sommerville and Deshpande[107]						7 − 13		24 − 83		
Greig *et al.*[32]			10	3 − 9	180	2 − 27	8	40 − 187	8	22 − 80
Harbert *et al.*[36]						0 − 40	49	72.4 ± 29.5	32	43.6 ± 32.9
Lurie and Villee[64]						7.5 − 17.1		60 − 80		
van der Molen[71]	7	<5 − 7	29	<5 − 21	30	4 − 26	7	49		
Kumar, Ward, and Barnes[53]					31	3 − 25				
Wiest[113]			7	3 − 18	6	14 − 21				
Gandy[27]	11	0.9 ± 0.12	12	4.47 ± 1.09	14	8.71 ± 1.42	7	109.1 ± 38.6	7	41.96 ± 10.6

* N = number of subjects studied.

TABLE 4-16

PROGESTERONE CONCENTRATIONS DURING LATE HUMAN PREGNANCY IN MATERNAL PLASMA, PLACENTA, MYOMETRIUM, MEMBRANES, AND AMNIOTIC FLUID*

		Progesterone concentration (μg/100 ml or 100 gm wet tissue)				
Patient	Weeks gestation	Peripheral Plasma	Placenta	Myometrium†	Fetal membranes†	Amniotic Fluid
G.P.	35	16.0	181	40	52	16.7
R.S.‡	37	28.5	305	57	115	12.3
P.	37	13.9	277	22	27	—
M.D.	38	17.7	213	19	76	8.3
P.S.	39	9.1	119	—	53	—
S.L.	40	—	327	19	50	—

*Samples obtained through or at Cesarean sectioning. Quantities of tissue analyzed: placenta, 0.5 gm; fetal membranes and myometrium, 1.0 gm; amniotic fluid and plasma, 3 ml. Values are averages of duplicate determinations. (From Wiest, *Steroids 10*:279, 1967.)

† Material selected without regard to proximity to the placenta.

‡ Twin pregnancy.

Progesterone, like several other steroids, circulates bound to various proteins, including albumin, transcortin, and orosomucoid.[105,112] Only 1–2 per cent is found in the free form. Transcortin has the highest affinity for cortisol, but the affinity for progesterone is not insignificant, and the increasing concentration of progesterone in pregnancy may lead to some competition with cortisol for the binding sites on transcortin.[86] In the cord blood where the binding systems are of lower capacity, considerable displacement of cortisol by progesterone may occur as evidenced by the very high unbound cortisol concentrations in cord blood.[86]

The binding of progesterone to plasma proteins does not seem to impede the transfer of progesterone across the placenta. Haskins and Soiva injected progesterone-4-^{14}C intravenously into human mothers at term.[37] Determination of radioactivity in the maternal and fetal plasma indicated a free passage; the activity was identified as progesterone and pregnanediol.

CONCLUDING REMARKS

This chapter has emphasized some of the more recent advances in our understanding of the formation and metabolism of progesterone in human pregnancy. In addition, some of the classical and newer methods of analysis of progesterone and pregnanediol have been listed. It is immediately evident that we have made considerable progress in our understanding of how progesterone is formed in the placenta, metabolized by the fetal tissues, and returned to the placenta for further conversions. This body of knowledge indicates that the fetus plays an active role in building complex molecules such as hydrocortisone from progesterone which reaches it from the placenta. In addition, fetal tissues conjugate the neutral steroids, largely with sulfuric acid and to a minor extent with glucuronic acid. It is also evident that pregnenolone formed in the placenta plays a vital role as precursor of the neutral steroids utilized by the placenta in the formation of estrogens. This duality of function led to the use of the term "feto-placental unit" in describing steroid metabolism in human pregnancy. The functional significance of the complementary activity of the fetus and placenta is not yet fully understood, however.

The newly detected 15- and 14-hydroxysteroids are obviously endogenous products formed during late pregnancy. These interesting new steroids also deserve investigation as to their physiological role in human pregnancy.

The salient questions concerning the role of progesterone in the maintenance of the growth and development of the fetus, in the defense mechanism of the myometrium, as a mediator of biochemical events in mother and fetus during gestation, and in the preparation of the breasts for lactation, have not been touched upon directly. Some of these questions will be discussed in Chapter Thirteen. While recent advances in our knowledge of the endocrinology of pregnancy have complicated the picture by adding new compounds to an already complex situation, they have also provided a better basis for the elucidation of some of the physiological problems.

REFERENCES

1. Acevedo, H. F., Axelrod, L. R., Ishikawa, E., and Takaki, F. Studies in fetal metabolism. II. Metabolism of progesterone-4-C^{14} and pregnenolone-7α-H^3 in human fetal testes. *J. Clin. Endocr. 23:*885, 1963.
2. Adlercreutz, H., and Luukkainen, T. Gas chromatographic identification of pregnanediol and some of its isomers in bile of pregnant women. *Ann. Med. Exp. Biol. Fenn. 42:*161, 1964.
3. Aitken, E. H., Preedy, J. R. K., Eton, B., and Short, R. V. Oestrogen and progesterone levels in foetal and maternal plasma at parturition. *Lancet 2:*1096, 1958.
4. Arcos, M., Gurpide, E., Vande Wiele, R. L., and Lieberman, S. Precursors of urinary pregnanediol and their influence on the determination of the secretory rate of progesterone. *J. Clin. Endocr. 24:*237, 1964.
5. Bengtsson, L. P., and Ejarque, P. M. Production rate of progesterone in the last month of human pregnancy. *Acta Obstet. Gynec. Scand. 43:*49, 1964.

6. BHAVNANI, B. R., YOUNGLAI, E. V., and SOLOMON, S. Synthesis of 14α-hydroxy-progesterone and its isolation from human late pregnancy urine. *Biochemistry 8:*2105, 1969.
7. BIRD, C. E., WIQVIST, N., DICZFALUSY, E., and SOLOMON, S. Metabolism of progesterone by the perfused previable human fetus. *J. Clin. Endocr. 26:*1144, 1966.
8. BLOCH, E. Metabolism of 4-^{14}C-progesterone by human fetal testis and ovaries. *Endocrinology 74:*833, 1964.
9. BLOCH, K. The biological conversion of cholesterol to pregnanediol. *J. Biol. Chem. 157:*661, 1945.
10. BOLTÉ, E., WIQVIST, N., and DICZFALUSY, E. Metabolism of dehydroepiandrosterone and dehydroepiandrosterone sulphate by the human fetus at mid-pregnancy. *Acta Endocr.* (Kobenhavn) *52:*583, 1966.
11. BREUER, H., KNUPPEN, R., and HAUPT, M. Metabolism of estrone and estradiol-17β in human liver *in vitro. Nature* (London) *212:*76, 1966.
12. CARLSON, J. H., MEYER, R. K., and BLAIR, A. J. The analysis of progestational compounds by gas liquid chromatography. *Clin. Res. 12:*351, 1964.
13. CHAMBERLAIN, J., KNIGHTS, B. A., and THOMAS, G. H. A system of analysis by gas chromatography of 17α- and 17β-pregnane-3,20-diols and their identification as metabolites of progesterone in man, the monkey, rabbit and guinea-pig. *J. Endocr. 28:*235, 1964.
14. DECLERCK, P. Contribution à la cytophysiologie du placenta à terme; Les possibités d'une survie et d'une croissance in vitro du syncytiotrophoblaste. Notes préliminaires. *Bull. Soc. Roy. Belg. Gynec. Obstet. 26:*493, 1956.
15. COLLINS, W. P., and SOMMERVILLE, I. F. Quantitative determination of progesterone in human plasma by thin-layer and gas-liquid radiochromatography. *Nature* (London) *203:*836, 1964.
16. CORNER, G. W., and ALLEN, W. M. Physiology of corpus luteum; production of special uterine reaction (progestational proliferation) by extracts of corpus luteum. *Amer. J. Physiol. 88:*326, 1929.
17. DEANE, H. W., and SELIGMAN, A. M. Evaluation of procedures for cytological localization of ketosteroids. *Vitamins Hormones* (N.Y.) *11:*173, 1953.
18. DESHPANDE, G. N., TURNER, A. K., and SOMMERVILLE, I. F. Plasma progesterone and pregnanediol in human pregnancy, during labour and postpartum. *J. Obstet. Gynaec. Brit. Comm. 67:*954, 1960.
19. DICZFALUSY, E. Progesterone in human placental tissue. *Acta Endocr.* (Kobenhavn) *10:*373, 1952.
20. DICZFALUSY, E., CASSMER, O., ALONSO, C., and DE MIGUEL, M. Estrogen metabolism in the human fetus and newborn. *Recent Prog. Hormone Res. 17:*147, 1961.
21. DICZFALUSY, E., and TROEN, P. Endocrine functions of the human placenta. *Vitamins Hormones* (N.Y.) *19:*229, 1961.
22. EBERLEIN, W. R. Steroids and sterols in umbilical cord blood. *J. Clin. Endocr. 25:*1101, 1965.
23. EJARQUE, P. M., and BENGTSSON, L. P. Production rate of progesterone in human midpregnancy. *Acta Endocr.* (Kobenhavn) *41:*521, 1962.

24. French, A. P., and Warren, J. C. Steroid-3β-sulfatase in fetal and placental tissues. *Steroids 6:*865, 1965.

25. Fuchs, F., Fuchs, A.-R., and Short, R. V. Progesterone in the uterine venous blood of women during the first half of gestation. *J. Endocr. 27:*333, 1963.

26. Futterweit, W., McNiven, N. L., and Dorfman, R. I. Gas-chromatographic identification of progesterone in human pregnancy plasma. *Biochim. Biophys. Acta 71:*474, 1962.

27. Gandy, H. M. Concentration of testosterone, androstenedione, dehydroepiandrostenedione, dehydroepiandrostenedione sulfate, pregnenolone, pregnenolone sulfate and progesterone and its isomers in maternal venous and umbilical venous and arterial plasma. *Excerpta Med. Int. Congr. Sr. 157:*172, 1968.

28. Giannopoulos, G., and Solomon, S. Isolation of 15α-hydroxyprogesterone from human pregnancy urine. *Biochemistry 6:*1226, 1967.

29. Giannopoulos, G., and Solomon, S. The isolation of 15α-hydroxytestosterone and 15α-hydroxyandrostenedione from human pregnancy urine. In preparation.

30. Gillman, J., and Stein, H. B. The human corpus luteum of pregnancy. *Surg. Gynec. Obstet. 72:*129, 1941.

31. Goebelsmann, U., Wiqvist, N., Diczfalusy, E., Levitz, M., Condon, G. P., and Dancis, J. Fate of intra-amniotically administered oestriol-15-^{3}H-3-sulphate and oestriol-16-^{14}C-16-glucosiduronate in pregnant women at midterm. *Acta Endocr.* (Kobenhavn) *52:*550, 1966.

32. Greig, M., Coyle, M. G., Cooper, W., and Walker, J. Plasma progesterone in mother and foetus in the second half of human pregnancy. *J. Obstet. Gynaec. Brit. Comm. 69:*772, 1962.

33. Gurpide, E., Schwers, J., Welch, M. T., Vande Wiele, R. L., and Lieberman, S. Fetal and maternal metabolism of estradiol during pregnancy. *J. Clin. Endocr. 26:*1355, 1966.

34. Hall, R. E. Removal of the corpus luteum in early pregnancy. *Bull. Sloane Hosp. Women 1:*49, 1955.

35. Hagen, A. A., Barr, M., and Diczfalusy, E. Metabolism of 17β-oestradiol-4-^{14}C in early infancy. *Acta Endocr.* (Kobenhavn) *49:*207, 1965.

36. Harbert, G. M., Jr., McGaughey, H. S., Jr., Scoggin, W. A., and Thornton, W. M. Concentration of progesterone in newborn and maternal circulations at delivery. *Obstet. Gynec. 23:*413, 1964.

37. Haskins, A. L., and Soiva, K. U. The placental transfer of progesterone-4-C^{14} in human term pregnancy. *Amer. J. Obstet. Gynec. 79:*674, 1960.

38. Haynes, R. C., Jr., Mikhail, C., Eriksson, G., Wiqvist, N., and Diczfalusy, E. Oestradiol metabolism in the previable human foetus and in the foetoplacental unit. *Acta Endocr.* (Kobenhavn) *45:*297, 1964.

39. Heap, R. B. A fluorescence assay of progesterone. *J. Endocr. 30:*293, 1964.

40. Hinsberg, K., Pelzer, H., and Seuken, A. Bestimmung sehr kleiner Mengen Progesteron im menschlichem Plasma. *Biochem. Z. 328:*117, 1956.

41. Hooker, C. W., and Forbes, T. R. Bio-assay for minute amounts of progesterone. *Endocrinology 41:*158, 1947.

42. HORNING, E. C., LUUKKAINEN, T., HAAHTI, E. O. A., CREECH, B. G., and VANDEN HEUVEL, W., JR. Studies of human steroidal hormones by gas chromatographic techniques. *Recent Prog. Hormone Res. 19:*57, 1963.
43. JIRKU, H., HOGSANDER, U., and LEVITZ, M. 15α-Hydroxy-estrone sulfate in the non-pregnant female. *Biochim. Biophys. Acta 137:*588, 1967.
44. JUNGMANN, R. A., and SCHWEPPE, J. S. Biosynthesis and metabolism of neutral steroids by human midterm placenta and fetal liver. *J. Clin. Endocr. 27:*1151, 1967.
45. KLOPPER, A. I. "Pregnanediol (5β-pregnane-3α, 20α-diol) and Pregnanetriol (5β-pregnane-3α, 17α, 20α-triol)." In *Methods in Hormone Research,* Vol. 1, R. I. Dorfman (Ed.), Academic Press, New York, 1968, p. 229.
45a. KLOPPER, A. I., and MACNAUGHTON, M. C. The identification of pregnanediol in liquor amnii, bile and faeces. *J. Endocr. 18:*319, 1959.
46. KLOPPER, A., MICHIE, E. M., and BROWN, J. B. Method for determination of urinary pregnanediol. *J. Endocr. 12:*209, 1955.
47. KNUPPEN, R., and BREUER, H. 15α-Hydroxylierung von Ostron in der Nebenniere. *Hoppe Seyler Zs. Physiol. Chem. 337:*159, 1964.
48. KNUPPEN, R., and BREUER, H. Isolierung von 15α-hydroxyoestradiol-(17β) aus dem Urin schwangerer Frauen. *Hoppe Seyler Zs. Physiol. Chem. 348:*581, 1967.
49. KNUPPEN, R., HAUPT, O., and BREUER, H. Isolation and identification of 15α-hydroxyestrone from the urine of pregnant women. *Biochem. J. 96:*33c, 1965.
50. KNUPPEN, R., HAUPT, M., and BREUER, H. Formation of 15α-hydroxyoestradiol-17β and 18-hydroxyoestrone by human adrenal tissue. *J. Endocr. 33:*529, 1965.
51. KNUPPEN, R., HAUPT, O., and BREUER, H. Isolation and identification of 15α-hydroxyesterone and 15β-hydroxyestradiol from the urine of pregnant women. *Steroids 8:*403, 1966.
52. KNUPPEN, R., HAUPT, O., and BREUER, H. 14α-hydroxyoestrone, a new oestrogen metabolite. *Biochem. J. 105:*971, 1967.
53. KUMAR, A., WARD, E. F., and BARNES, A. C. Serial plasma progesterone levels and onset of labor. *Amer. J. Obstet. Gynec. 90:*1360, 1964.
54. LAURITZEN, C., and LEHMANN, W. D. Pregnandiolbestimmungen in Plasma vor, während und nach der Entbindung. *Z. Geburtsh. Gynaek. 162:*159, 1964.
55. LEMAIRE, W. J., RICE, B. F., and SAVARD, K. Steroid hormone formation in the human ovary: V. Synthesis of progesterone *in vitro* in corpora lutea during the reproductive cycle. *J. Clin. Endocr. 28:*1249, 1968.
56. LEVY, H., HOOD, B., CHA, C. H., and CARLO, J. J. The monohydroxylation of 17β-estradiol at the 15α-, 16α, and 16β-positions by bovine adrenal perfusion. *Steroids 5:*677, 1965.
57. LISBOA, B. P., GOEBELSMANN, U., and DICZFALUSY, E. Isolation of 15α-hydroxyoestradiol from human pregnancy urine. *Acta Endocr.* (Kobenhavn) *54:*467, 1967.
58. LITTLE, B., DIMARTINS, J., and NYHOLM, B. The conversion of progesterone

to Δ^4-pregnene-20α-ol-3-one by human placenta *in vitro. Acta Endocr.* (Kobenhavn) *30:*530, 1959.

59. LITTLE, B., TAIT, J. F., TAIT, S. A. S., and ERLENMEYER, F. Progesterone clearance in non-pregnant and pregnant subjects. *Excerpta Med. Int. Congr. Sr. 111:*150, 1966.

60. LLAURO, J. L., RUNNEBAUM, B., and ZANDER, J. Progesterone in human peripheral blood before, during, and after labor. *Amer. J. Obstet. Gynec. 101:*867, 1968.

61. LUISI, M., GAMBASI, G., MARESCOTTI, V., SAVI, C., and POLVANI, F. A gas-chromatographic method for the quantitative determination of progesterone in human plasma. *J. Chromatogr. 18:*278, 1965.

62. LURIE, A. O., REID, D. E., and VILLEE, C. A. Progesterone in blood. A quantitative method employing gas liquid chromatography. *J. Clin. Endocr. 26:*742, 1966.

63. LURIE, A. O., REID, D. E., and VILLEE, C. A. The role of the fetus and placenta in maintenance of plasma progesterone. *Amer. J. Obstet. Gynec. 96:*670, 1966.

64. LURIE, A. O., and VILLEE, C. A. Selium: a common contaminant of samples prepared for gas-liquid chromatography. *J. Chromatogr. 21:*113, 1966.

65. LURIE, A. O., and VILLEE, C. A. Device for the injection of dry samples prepared for gas-liquid chromatography. *J. Gas Chromatogr. 4:*160, 1966.

66. LURIE, A. O., and WEISS, J. B. Progesterone in cerebrospinal fluid during human pregnancy. *Nature* (London) *215:*1178, 1967.

67. MANCUSO, S., BENAGIANO, G., DELL'ACQUA, S., SHAPIRO, M., WIQVIST, N., and DICZFALUSY, E. Studies on the metabolism of C_{19} steroids in the human foeto-placental unit. IV. Aromatization and hydroxylation products formed by previable foetuses perfused with androstenedione and testosterone. *Acta Endocr.* (Kobenhavn) *57:*208, 1968.

68. MCGINTY, D. A., ANDERSON, L. P., and MCCULLOUGH, N. B. Effect of local application of progesterone on rabbit uterus. *Endocrinology 24:*829, 1939.

69. MIKHAIL, G., and ALLEN, W. M. Ovarian function in human pregnancy. *Amer. J. Obstet. Gynec. 99:*308, 1967.

70. MIKHAIL, G., WIQVIST, N., and DICZFALUSY, E. Oestriol metabolism in the previable human foetus. *Acta Endocr.* (Kobenhavn) *42:*519, 1963.

71. VAN DER MOLEN, H. J. Determination of plasma progesterone during pregnancy. *Clin. Chim. Acta 8:*943, 1963.

72. VAN DER MOLEN, H. J., and AAKVAAG, A. "Progesterone." In *Hormones in Blood,* C. H. Gray and A. L. Bacharach (Eds.), Academic Press, New York, 1967, p. 221.

73. VAN DER MOLEN, H. J., and GROEN, D. Determination of progesterone in human peripheral blood using gas-liquid chromatography with electron capture detection. *J. Clin. Endocr. 25:*1625, 1965.

74. MORRISON, G., MEIGS, R. A., and RYAN, K. J. Biosynthesis of progesterone by the human placenta. *Steroids* (*Suppl. 2*) *6:*117, 1965.

75. MURPHY, B. E. P. Some studies of the protein-binding of steroids and their application to the routine micro and ultramicro measurement of various

steroids in body fluids by competitive protein-binding radioassay. *J. Clin. Endocr. 27:*973, 1963.

76. Neill, J. D., Johansson, E. D. B., Datta, J. K., and Knobil, E. Relationship between the plasma levels of luteinizing hormone and progesterone during the normal menstrual cycle. *J. Clin. Endocr. 27:*1167, 1967.
77. Nelson, W. W., and Greene, R. R. Some observations on the histology of the human ovary during pregnancy. *Amer. J. Obstet. Gynec. 76:*66, 1958.
78. Oertel, G. W., Weiss, S. P., and Eik-Nes, K. B. Determination of progesterone in human blood plasma. *J. Clin. Endocr. 19:*213, 1959.
79. Palmer, R., Blair, J. A., Eriksson, G., and Diczfalusy, E. Studies on the metabolism of C_{21} steroids in the human foetoplacental unit. 3. Metabolism of progesterone and 20α- and 20β-dihydroprogesterone by midterm placentas perfused *in situ. Acta Endocr.* (Kobenhavn) *53:*407, 1966.
80. Palmer, R., Eriksson, G., Wiqvist, N., and Diczfalusy, E. Studies on the metabolism of C_{21} steroids in the human fetoplacental unit. 2. Metabolism of pregnenolone sulphate by midterm placentas perfused *in situ. Acta Endocr.* (Kobenhavn) *52:*598, 1966.
81. Pearlman, W. H. (16-^{3}H) Progesterone metabolism in advanced pregnancy and in oophorectomized-hysterectomized women. *Biochem. J. 67:*1, 1957.
82. Pearlman, W. H., and Cerceo, E. J. Isolation of progesterone from human placenta. *J. Biol. Chem. 198:*79, 1952.
83. Pearlman, W. H., and Cerceo, E. Estimation of saturated and α, β-unsaturated ketonic compounds in placental extracts. *J. Biol. Chem. 203:*127, 1953.
84. Pulkkinen, M. O. Arylsulphatase and the hydrolysis of some steroid sulphates in developing organism and placenta. *Acta Physiol. Scand. (Suppl. 180) 52:*71, 1961.
85. Riondel, A., Tait, J. F., Tait, S. A. S., and Gut, M., and Little, B. Estimation of progesterone in human peripheral blood using ^{35}S-thiosemicarbazide. *J. Clin. Endocr. 25:*229, 1965.
86. Rosenthal, H. E., Slaunwhite, W. R., and Sandberg, A. A. Transcortin: a corticosteroid-binding protein of plasma. X. Cortisol and progesterone interplay and unbound levels of these steroids in pregnancy. *J. Clin. Endocr. 29:*352, 1969.
87. Runnebaum, B., and Zander, J. Progesterone, Δ^4-pregnen-20α-ol-3-on, Δ-4-pregnen-20β-ol-3-on und 17α-Hydroxyprogesteron im Plasma der Nabelvene und der Nabelarterien. *Klin. Wschr. 40:*453, 1962.
88. Ryan, K. J. Hormones of the placenta. *Amer. J. Obstet. Gynec. 84:*1695, 1962.
89. Ryan, K. J., Meigs, R., and Petro, Z. The formation of progesterone by human placenta. *Amer. J. Obstet. Gynec. 96:*676, 1966.
90. Salhanick, H. A., Noall, M. W., Zarrow, M. X., and Samuels, L. T. Isolation of progesterone from human placentae. *Science 115:*708, 1952.
91. Schindler, A. E., and Siiteri, P. K. Isolation and quantitation of steroids from normal human amniotic fluid. *J. Clin. Endocr. 28:*1189, 1968.
92. Schwers, J., Eriksson, G., Wiqvist, N., and Diczfalusy, E. 15α-Hydroxyla-

tion: a new pathway of oestrogen metabolism in the human foetus and newborn. *Biochim. Biophys. Acta 100:*313, 1965.

93. Schwers, J., Govaerts-Videtsky, M., Wiqvist, N., and Diczfalusy, E. Metabolism of oestrone sulphate by the previable human foetus. *Acta Endocr.* (Kobenhavn) *50:*597, 1965.
94. Schwers, J., Gurpide, E., Vande Wiele, R. L., and Lieberman, S. Urinary metabolites of estradiol and estriol administered intra-amniotically. *J. Clin. Endocr. 27:*1403, 1967.
95. Shearman, R. P. Some aspects of the urinary excretion of pregnanediol in pregnancy. *J. Obstet. Gynaec. Brit. Comm. 64:*1, 1959.
96. Short, R. V. Progesterone in blood. I. The chemical determination of progesterone in peripheral blood. *J. Endocr. 16:*415, 1958.
97. Short, R. V., and Eton, B. Progesterone in blood. III. Progesterone in the peripheral blood of pregnant women. *J. Endocr. 18:*418, 1959.
98. Short, R. V., and Levett, I. The fluorimetric determination of progesterone in human plasma during pregnancy and the menstrual cycle. *J. Endocr. 25:*239, 1962.
99. Short, R. V., Wagner, G., Fuchs, A.-R., and Fuchs, F. Progesterone concentrations in uterine venous blood after intra-amniotic injection of hypertonic saline in midpregnancy. *Amer. J. Obstet. Gynec. 19:*132, 1965.
100. Simmer, H. H., and Simmer, I. Progesterone in the peripheral venous blood of pregnant women with late gestoses. *Klin. Wschr. 37:*971, 1959.
101. Slaunwhite, N. R., Jr., Karsay, M. A., Hollmer, A., Sandberg, A. A., and Niswander, K. Fetal liver as an endocrine tissue. *Steroids* (*Suppl. 2*) *6:*211, 1965.
102. Solomon, S. The formation and metabolism of neutral steroids in the human fetus and placenta. *Excerpta Med. Int. Congr. Sr. 132:*653, 1966.
103. Solomon, S. "Synthesis of Steroids by the Placenta." In *The Placenta and Fetal Membranes,* C. A. Villee (Ed.), Williams & Wilkins, Baltimore, 1960, p. 201.
104. Solomon, S. The formation and metabolism of neutral steroids in the human placenta and fetus. *J. Clin. Endocr. 26:*762, 1966.
105. Solomon, S., and Friesen, H. G. Endocrine relations between mother and fetus. *Ann. Rev. Med. 19:*399, 1968.
106. Solomon, S., Watanabe, M., Dominguez, O. V., Gray, M. J., Meeker, C. I., and Sims, E. A. H. "Progesterone and Aldosterone Secretion Rates in Pregnancy." In *Biological and Clinical Aspects of Placental Steroidogenesis,* F. Polvani and A. Bompiani (Eds.), Williams & Wilkins, Baltimore, 1964, p. 32.
107. Sommerville, I. F., and Deshpande, G. N. The quantitative determination of progesterone and pregnanediol in human plasma. *J. Clin. Endocr. 18:*1223, 1958.
108. Stern, M., Givner, M. L., and Solomon, S. Aromatization of 15α-hydroxyandrostenedione by human placental tissue. *Endocrinology 83:*348, 1968.
109. Stewart, H. L., Jr. Hormone secretion by human placenta grown in the eyes of rabbits. *Amer. J. Obstet. Gynec. 61:*990, 1951.

110. Touchstone, J. C., and Murawec, T. Enhancement of the fluorescence of progesterone (and other steroids) in sulfuric acid. *Anal. Chem. 32:*822, 1960.

111. Wengle, B. Distribution of some steroid sulphokinases in foetal human tissues. *Acta Endocr.* (Kobenhavn) *52:*607, 1966.

112. Westphal, W., Firschein, H. E., and Pearce, E. M. Transport of cortisol-4-C^{14} and progesterone-4-C^{14} by serum protein as demonstrated by paper electrophoresis and paper chromatography. *Amer. J. Physiol. 185:*54, 1956.

113. Wiest, W. G. Estimations of progesterone in biological tissues and fluids from pregnant women by double isotope derivative assay. *Steroids 10:*279, 1967.

114. Wiest, W. G. A double isotope derivative assay for progesterone and 20α-hydroxy pregn-4-en-3-one. *Steroids 10:*257, 1967.

115. Wiest, W. G., Kerenyi, T., and Csapo, A. I. A double isotope derivative dilution assay for progesterone in biological fluids and tissues. *Excerpta Med. Int. Congr. Sr. 111:*114, 1966.

116. Woolever, C. A., and Goldfien, A. A double-isotope derivative method for plasma progesterone assay. *Int. J. Appl. Radiat. 14:*163, 1963.

117. Yannone, M. E., McComas, D. B., and Goldfien, A. The assay of plasma progesterone. *J. Gas Chromatogr. 2:*30, 1964.

118. Yannone, M. E., McGurdy, J. R., and Goldfien, A. Plasma progesterone levels in normal pregnancy, labor and the puerperium. *Amer. J. Obstet. Gynec. 101:*1058, 1968.

119. Yoshimi, T., and Lipsett, M. B. The measurement of plasma progesterone. *Steroids 11:*527, 1968.

120. Yoshimi, T., Strott, C. A., Marshall, J. R., and Lipsett, M. B. Corpus luteum function in early pregnancy. *J. Clin. Endocr. 29:*225, 1969.

121. YoungLai, E. V., Bhavnani, B., and Solomon, S. Isolation of 14α-hydroxy-testosterone from human late pregnancy urine. *J. Clin. Endocr. 29:*101, 1969.

122. YoungLai, E. V., and Solomon, S. The formation of estra-1, 3, 5 (10)-triene-3, 15α, 16α, 17β-tetrol (estetrol) and estra-1,3,5 (10)-triene-3, 15α, 17β-triol from neutral precursors. *J. Clin. Endocr. 28:*1611, 1968.

123. Zander, J. Progesteron in menschlichem Blut und Geweben; Progesteron im peripheren venosen Blut der Frau. *Klin. Wschr. 33:*697, 1955.

124. Zander, J. "Gestagens in Human Pregnancy." In *Recent Progress in the Endocrinology of Reproduction*, C. W. Lloyd (Ed.), Academic Press, New York, 1959, p. 255.

125. Zander, J., Forbes, T. R., von Münstermann, A. M., and Neher, R. Δ^4-3-ketopregnene-20α-ol and Δ^4-3-ketopregnene-20β-ol, two naturally occurring metabolites of progesterone. Isolation, identification, biologic activity and concentration in human tissues. *J. Clin. Endocr. 18:*337, 1958.

126. Zander, J., and von Münstermann, A. M. Weitere Untersuchungen über Progesterone in menschlichem Blut und Geweben. *Klin. Wschr. 32:*894, 1954.

127. Zander, J., and Simmer, H. Die chemische Bestimmung von Progesterone in organischen Substraten. *Klin. Wschr. 32*:528, 1954.

128. Zelewski, L., and Villee, C. A. The biosynthesis of squalene, lanosterol and cholesterol by minced human placenta. *Biochemistry 5*:1805, 1966.

129. Zucconi, G., Lisboa, B. P., Simonitsch, E., Roth, L., Hagen, A. A., and Diczfalusy, E. Isolation of 15α-hydroxyestriol from pregnancy urine and from the urine of newborn infants. *Acta Endocr.* (Kobenhavn) *56*:413, 1967.

Chapter Five

Androgens

Hortense M. Gandy

This chapter is concerned with the concentration of testosterone, androstenedione, dehydroepiandrosterone (DHA), and dehydroepiandrosterone sulfate (DHAS), 16α-OH-dehydroepiandrosterone (16α-OH-DHA), and 16α-OH-dehydroepiandrosterone sulfate (16α-OH-DHAS) in the maternal and feto-placental circulations. Discussion of biosynthesis of these C_{19} steroids, usually referred to as androgens, is limited to evidence that they are secreted by the human adrenals, gonads, and placenta as there is increasing evidence that steroidogenesis in pregnancy differs in various animal species. These C_{19} steroids have biological properties of their own, but are also precursors of estrogens. The concentration and metabolism of C_{19} steroids present in peripheral plasma has been reviewed by Mitchell[186] and Eberlein, Winter, and Rosenfield.[74]

The term "androgen" is applied to a substance, usually a C_{19} steroid, with certain physiological functions and biological activities. In the male, these are: development and maintenance of the prostate and seminal vesicles, production of sexual hair growth pattern, voice changes, beard growth, and increase in the size of the phallus.[241] Androgens promote protein metabolism, somatic growth, and accelerate ossification[11,101,119,145] as well as influence sexual behavior in both sexes.[108] Nitrogen, phosphorous, and potassium retention and lowering of the respiratory quotient occur following administration of such C_{19} steroids as testosterone.[69] Production, transport, and metabolism of C_{19} steroids have an important role in the function and maintenance of the feto-placental

* Supported in part by U.S.P.H.S. Research Grant AM07328 and GRSG-FR0536.

unit. These steroids most likely have a role in the sex development of the fetus.

Androgenicity of a steroid appears to be dependent on the presence of a hydroxyl group at C-17 in the equatorial configuration or a ketone at C-17 available to such a hydroxyl group.[244] Potency of C_{19} steroids are assessed by different parameters in man and animals. Animal assays in use measure the effect of steroids on such target organs as: (1) the capon or chick's comb, (2) bone maturation in mice, or (3) the rat seminal vesicle, ventral prostate, or levator ani. These techniques have been reviewed by Dorfman.[67, 68] The results of bioassay studies indicate that testosterone is probably the most potent naturally occurring C_{19} steroid known. The relative potency of other natural C_{19} steroids in relation to testosterone is shown in Table 5-1. Comparison of animal assay data is of limited value due to differences in the species of animals used, season, vehicle and route of administration, and end point. Studies of potency in man are concerned with the parameters of nitrogen retention or effect on creatine, creatinine, and calcium excretion.

TABLE 5-1

RELATIVE ANDROGENIC POTENCY OF NATURAL C_{19} STEROIDS

Steroid	Seminal vesicles	Capon's comb	Bone maturation
Testosterone	100	100	100
5α-Androstane-17β-ol-3-one	200	75	
Androstanediol	33	75	
Androstenedione	20	12	
DHA	3	16	42
Androsterone	10	10	
Etiocholanolone	0	0	
Epitestosterone	0	0	
DHAS			100

There are few relative data that suggest that the relative potencies of steroids cited in Table 5-1 are similar in man. Androstenedione, DHA, and DHAS do not appear to be significant androgens in man in terms of anabolic activity although they are known precursors of testosterone and estrogens. McSwiney *et al.* administered androstenedione, DHA, and 11-β-OH-Δ^4-androstenedione, successively, in doses of 100 mg/day to subjects for various test periods.[179] No significant anabolic effect could be demonstrated for any of these C_{19} steroids except in two experiments with androstenedione that was contaminated with testosterone. Neither Segaloff *et al.*[245] nor Lipsett, Coffman, and Nixon[159] were able to demonstrate nitrogen retention following the administration of DHA or DHAS.

Recently Baird *et al.* have suggested that such compounds as androstenedione, DHA, and DHAS be classified as prehormones since these compounds have little known biological potency but are converted to more biologically active compounds such as testosterone and the estrogens.[7]

BIOSYNTHESIS OF C_{19} STEROIDS BY THE ADULT ADRENAL CORTEX AND THE GONADS

Dorfman and Ungar[70] as well as Samuels and Uchikawa[227] have recently reviewed the synthesis of C_{19} steroids. Information on the synthesis of C_{19} steroids by the gonads and the adrenals is based upon data obtained from: (1) isolation of these steroids from gonadal and adrenal cortical tissue, (2) incubation of gland tissue with steroid precursors, (3) tissue culture, (4) organ perfusion, and (5) intravenous infusion of an isotopically labeled steroid precursor. Such in vitro studies do not demonstrate actual biosynthetic systems in the intact organism but do suggest that the pathways of synthesis of C_{19} steroids by the gonads and the adrenal cortex are qualitatively similar but quantitatively different.

The Adrenal Gland

C_{19} steroids are probably derived from acetate which is converted to cholesterol (Figure 5-1). Adrenal cortical tissue has the capacity to form unconjugated C_{19} steroids from acetate[23,24,25,267] as well as from mevalonate or cholesterol.[217] The primary conversion of cholesterol appears to be to pregnenolone; reduced nicotinamide adenine dinucleotide phosphate (NADPH) is required for this transformation step. Conversion of cholesterol to pregnenolone is a mitochondrial function. Pathways involved in synthesis of C_{19} steroids from cholesterol are: (1) pregnenolone $\longrightarrow$ progesterone $\longrightarrow$ 17α-OH-progesterone $\longrightarrow$ androstenedione $\longrightarrow$ testosterone, and (2) pregnenolone $\longrightarrow$ 17α-OH-pregnenolone $\longrightarrow$ DHA that can be converted to androstenedione or reduced to Δ^5-androstene-3β, 17β-diol. The latter pathways appears to be the main route of DHA synthesis. The conversion of pregnenolone to progesterone takes place in the presence of Δ^5-isomerase and 3β-hydroxy steroid dehydrogenase. The 17-hydroxylation of progesterone and pregnenolone is a microsomal function. All hydroxylation reactions require molecular oxygen and NADPH. The 17-desmolase is necessary for conversion of 17α-OH-pregnenolone to DHA. Conversion of DHA to testosterone involves: (1) oxidation of the 3β-hydroxyl group to a 3-ketone with the 3β-hydroxy steroid dehydrogenase; dinucleotide phosphate is required, and (2) migration of the double bond from the 5-6 position to the 4-5 position requiring the Δ^5-

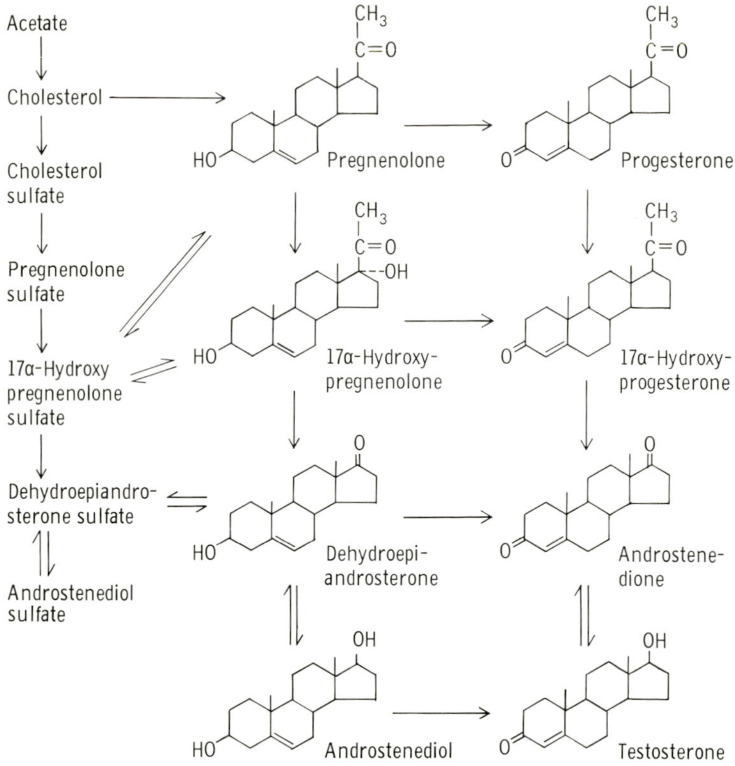

Fig. 5-1. Most probable routes of biosynthesis of C_{19} steroids by the adrenal gland.

isomerase without a known cofactor. Reduction of the 17-ketone of androstenedione to the 17β-hydroxyl of testosterone occurs in the presence of 17β-hydroxy steroid dehydrogenase.

Normal adrenal cortical tissue also has the capacity to form C_{19} steroids from the following precursors as well as from cholesterol: pregnenolone,[71] 17α-OH-pregnenolone,[259, 272] progesterone,[127, 272] 17α-OH-progesterone,[135] or from other C_{19} steroids.[2, 44, 48, 190] Adrenal cortical tumor tissue can also convert these precursors,[35, 48, 52, 58, 103, 274] as well as pregnenolone sulfate,[36, 103] to C_{19} steroids. Since adrenal cortical tissue contains the enzymes involved in the formation of the active nucleotide sulfate as well as an active sulfokinase which transfers sulfate from adenosine-3′-phosphate-5′-phosphosulfate, this tissue has the capacity to form DHAS. This conjugate can be formed from cholesterol and its sulfate,[35, 217] 20α-OH-cholesterol,[246] pregnenolone,[103] 17α-OH-pregnenolone and its sulfate,[36, 154] androstenediol sulfate,[14] or DHA.[240] Sulfurylation of DHA also occurs in the liver, intestinal wall, and other tissues of the body.[31, 240, 282]

The Gonads

Ovary

The ovary is a heterogeneous organ with various cell types with selective capacities for elaboration of different groups of steroids. It has the capacity to convert isotopically labeled acetate into C_{19} steroids.[207,209,224] Huang and Pearlman studied steroidogenesis by isolated corpora lutea with radioactive acetate as the substrate.[121] Progesterone was the major steroid formed; there was no evidence for formation of C_{19} steroids or estrogens. However, Savard, Marsh, and Rice recovered androstenedione and estrogens in addition to progesterone, 4-pregnen-20α-ol-3-one, and 17α-OH-progesterone from corpora lutea incubated with radioactive acetate.[234] More recently Ryan, Petro, and Kaiser have studied steroidogenesis in isolated granulosa and theca cells from human ovarian follicles from subjects pretreated with human menopausal gonadotrophin (HMG) and human chorionic gonadotrophin (HCG).[222,223] Follicle size and steroid production were enhanced. Granulosa cells formed DHA, androstenedione, pregnenolone, cholesterol, progesterone, 17α-OH-progesterone, and estrone. The theca cells formed androstenedione, pregnenolone, progesterone, 17α-OH-progesterone, estrone, and estradiol. There are few studies of steroidogenesis with ovarian cortical tissue devoid of corpora lutea. Rice, Hammerstein, and Savard have demonstrated that stroma from ovaries from women at different stages of the menstrual cycle and in early pregnancy have the capacity to produce androstenedione, testosterone, DHA, 17α-OH-pregnenolone, pregnenolone, estrone, and estradiol with acetate-1-C^{14} as substrate.[207,209] C_{19} steroids were the major compounds produced. Hilar cells from polycystic ovaries have the capacity to form DHA from radioactive acetate.[192]

Studies of ovarian tissue preparations with various substrates and the steroids formed by each preparation are summarized in Table 5-2. The presence of C_{19} steroids in follicular cyst fluids is also indicative of the capacity of the ovary to secrete C_{19} steroids. Formation of DHAS by normal ovarian tissue has not been demonstrated.

Testis

Pathways of synthesis of C_{19} steroids by the testis are similar to those described for the ovary and the adrenal. De novo synthesis of testosterone, DHA, and androstenedione from acetate-1-^{14}C by testis slice preparations has been demonstrated in vitro.[206,232] These findings have been confirmed in vivo by Knapstein *et al.* who obtained labeled DHA and testosterone from spermatic venous plasma following injection of acetate-1-^{14}C and cholesterol-^{3}H into the spermatic artery.[143] The normal testis is also

TABLE 5-2

FORMATION OF C_{19} STEROIDS BY THE HUMAN OVARY

Precursor	Tissue preparation	Pathology	Product formed	Author
Acetate	Mince, follicular cyst lining	None	DHA, androstenedione, 17α-OH-progesterone, 17α-OH-pregnenolone, estrone, estradiol, pregnenolone	Ryan and Smith[224]
	Mince, cortex and medula	None, polycystic	DHA	Noall, Alexander, and Allen[192]
	Slice	Polycystic	Testosterone	Leon, Castro, and Dorfman[155]
	Slice, stroma	None	Testosterone	Rice, Hammerstein, and Savard[207]
	Slice, stroma	None, pregnant, polycystic, postmenopause	DHA, testosterone; androstenedione, 17α-OH-pregnenolone, estrone, estradiol, pregnenolone	Rice and Savard[209]
	Granulosa cell	None (HMG pretreatment)	DHA, androstenedione, pregnenolone, cholesterol, estrone, 17α-OH-progesterone, progesterone	Ryan, Petro, and Kaiser[223]
	Theca cell		Cholesterol, progesterone, 17α-OH-progesterone, pregnenolone, androstenedione, estrone, estradiol	
	Combined theca and granulosa		Cholesterol, progesterone, 17α-OH-progesterone, pregnenolone, androstenedione, estrone, estradiol	
Pregnenolone	Granulosa cell	None (HMG pretreatment)	No C_{19} steroids, progesterone, 17α-OH-progesterone	Ryan and Petro[222]
	Theca mince		Androstenedione, progesterone, 17α-OH-progesterone, estradiol	
	Homogenate	None, polycystic	DHA, androstenedione, testosterone	Axelrod and Goldzieher[5]
	Mince	None, days 1–27 of menstrual cycle	DHA, testosterone, androstenedione, progesterone 17α-OH-progesterone, 17α-OH-pregnenolone	Kumari and Goldzieher[149]
	Slice	Granulosa cell tumor	DHA	MacAulay and Welsky[168]

Progesterone	Homogenate	Arrhenoblastoma	Androstenedione, 17α-OH-progesterone	Wiest, Zander, and Holmstrom[284]
	Mince	None, polycystic	Androstenedione, 17α-OH-progesterone, 17α, 20α-dihydroxy-4-pregnene-3-one, 4-pregnen-20α-ol-3-one, 4-pregnen-20β-ol-3-one	Warren and Salhanick[278]
	Homogenate	None	Androstenedione, testosterone	Kase, Forchielli, and Dorfman[134]
	Slice	Arrhenoblastoma	Androstenedione, testosterone, 17α-OH-progesterone 4-pregnen-20α-ol-3-one, 4-pregnen-20β-ol-3-one	Savard *et al.*[233]
	Homogenate	Lipoid cell tumor	Testosterone, androstenedione, 17α-OH-progesterone	Sandberg *et al.*[228]
	Granulosa and theca cells	None	Estrone, 17α-OH-progesterone, estrone, androstenedione, 17α-OH-progesterone, estradiol	Ryan, Petro, and Kaiser[225]
	Mince	None	Androstenedione, testosterone, 17α-OH-progesterone	Kumari and Goldzieher[149]
	Homogenate	Arrhenoblastoma, polycystic	Androstenedione	Sandberg, Jenkins, and Trifon[229]
	Slice	Granulosa cell tumor	Androstenedione	MacAulay and Welsky[168]
17α-OH-progesterone	Homogenate	None	Testosterone, androstenedione	Kase, Forchielli, and Dorfman[134]
	Homogenate	Lipoid cell tumor	Testosterone	Sandberg *et al.*[228]
Androstenedione	Homogenate	Lipoid cell tumor	Testosterone	Sandberg *et al.*[228]
	Mince	None	Testosterone, 6β-OH-Δ^4-androstene,3,17-dione	Huang[120]
	Homogenate	None, polycystic	Testosterone, estrogens	Axelrod and Goldzieher[5]
Testosterone	Homogenate	None, polycystic	Androstenedione, estrogens	Axelrod and Goldzieher[5]
DHA	Slice	None (pregnant)	DHA, testosterone, androstenedione, androstenediol, estrone, estradiol	Flickinger, Wu, and Touchstone[81]
DHAS	Homogenate	Arrhenoblastoma, polycystic	Testosterone, androstenedione	Sandberg, Jenkins, and Trifon[229]

capable of forming C_{19} steroids from pregnenolone[4] or progesterone.[144] Testicular tissue from subjects with testicular feminization, carcinoma of the prostate, or tumor of the testis has the capacity to utilize acetate,[206, 232] cholesterol,[128, 231] pregnenolone,[53, 104, 175, 189, 201] 17α-OH-pregnenolone,[189] progesterone,[53, 65, 86, 144, 175, 189, 231, 255, 262] or 17 -OH-progesterone.[4, 24, 65, 254, 255] Androstenedione, as substrate in testicular incubation studies, gives rise to androstenedione and testosterone sulfate. Normal testis, unlike normal ovarian tissue, has the capacity to produce DHAS as well as androstenedione from DHA[64] Knapstein *et al.* obtained labeled androstenedione, testosterone, and androstenediol from spermatic venous effluent following spermatic arterial infusion of 4-^{14}C-DHA and ^{35}S-DHAS.[142] Dixon, Vincent, and Kase have isolated testosterone sulfate from tissue incubates with DHAS as substrate.[64]

BIOTRANSFORMATION OF C_{19} STEROIDS

Transformation of C_{19} steroids has been recently reviewed by Baulieu[13] and Rosenfeld, Fukushima, and Gallagher.[218] Some of the routes of biotransformation are shown in Figure 5-2. These pathways for biotransformation are largely derived from studies based upon urinary steroid metabolites; thus the picture is far from complete.

The system DHA $\rightleftharpoons$ DHAS is operative in the liver, kidney,

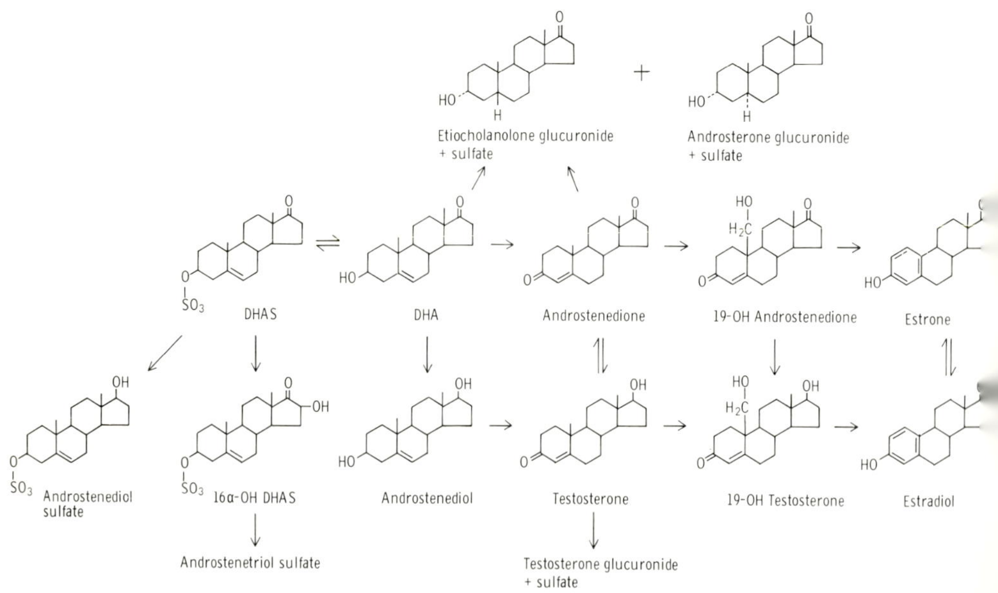

Fig. 5-2. Most probable routes of biotransformation of C_{19} steroids.

skin, skeletal muscles, and in whole blood.[18,106,277] DHA and its ester are largely converted peripherally to 3α-hydroxy steriods of the 5α and 5β series. A small amount of DHA and DHAS is excreted in the urine unchanged. DHA may also be converted to androstenedione and testosterone.[94, 117, 172, 257] This conversion probably occurs in the liver.[147] The contribution of DHA to testosterone is negligible in the adult male but accounts for approximately 15 per cent of circulating testosterone in the adult female.[117, 118, 160, 214] The conversion of DHA to androstenedione occurs by oxidation of the hydroxyl group by a 3β-hydrogenase[32] resulting in a 3-keto-Δ^4 steroid which is transformed to androstenedione. Metabolism of androstenedione proceeds as described later. Approximately 0.03–0.05 per cent of secreted DHA is converted to testosterone glucuroniside.[13, 39]

Transformation of DHA and DHAS in the feto-placental unit results in formation of estradiol as well as 16α-OH-DHA and its ester. Both are precursors of estriol via the intermediates, androst-5-ene, 3β, 16α, 17β-triol, and 16α-OH-testosterone.[15,27,29,249,250,252,279] These conversions account for a large portion of the total amount of estrogens which are produced by the placenta. Siiteri and MacDonald have demonstrated that little, if any, intravenously administered 4-^{14}C-DHAS is converted to estrogens in nonpregnant women whereas conversion of DHAS to estrogens in normal pregnancy rises from 1–2 per cent at seven weeks to 28–45 per cent near term.[249,250] Approximately 15 per cent of injected, labeled DHAS was converted to estriol. Conversion of DHAS to estradiol in women pregnant with anencephalic fetuses was similar to that demonstrated in women with normal pregnancies. Siiteri and MacDonald have also demonstrated that subjects pregnant with hydatidform moles convert 46–50 per cent of injected 4-^{14}C-DHAS to estradiol; conversion was proportional to the amount of molar tissue present.[249,250]

Testosterone and androstenedione are interconvertible in the body.[18,93,116,117] About one-half of the circulating testosterone in the adult female is formed from androstenedione. The contribution of androstenedione to testosterone is negligible in the adult male but approximately one-third of the daily production of androstenedione arises from peripheral conversion of testosterone.[117] Conversion of androstenedione and testosterone to estrone and estradiol, respectively, has been demonstrated in vivo.[170] Approximately 1.8 per cent of circulating androstenedione and 0.5 per cent of testosterone in the normal male are converted to estrone and estradiol, respectively, whereas 0.8 and 0.2 per cent of androstenedione and testosterone, respectively, are converted to estrone and estradiol in the nonpregnant female.[170]

Biotransformation of androstenedione and testosterone results in 5β- and 5α-saturated,-3,17 diketones; this step is accomplished by reduction of the double bond in ring A. A small fraction of these diketones is excreted in the urine, but the major portion is further reduced to the 3-hydroxy-ketosteroids, etiocholanolone, and androsterone. Although these compounds are the major urinary metabolites of testosterone and androstenedione, they are not inert end products. Etiocholanolone, when administered intravenously, is pyrogenic in man. Androsterone has the capacity to lower elevated levels of serum cholesterol.[111, 133] Etiocholanolone and androsterone are both conjugated with glucuronic and sulfuric acid.[12] Both steroids are excreted as glucuronide and as sulfate.[12] These compounds can be further degraded to $3\alpha,17\beta$-diols and subsequently hydroxylated at the C-18 methyl group.

A small amount of circulating testosterone and androstenedione is converted to testosterone glucuroniside.[38, 39, 216] About 20 per cent of this metabolite is excreted unchanged; the remaining conjugate is metabolized to etiocholanediol and androstanolone glucuroniside. There is evidence that some testosterone is conjugated with sulfuric acid in vitro,[64] although the daily production is very small.[40] Whether testosterone sulfate is a degradative metabolite of testosterone or whether it is secreted by the gonad or adrenal is not clear, although it has been isolated from urine.[59] Androstenedione or testosterone may also undergo hydroxylation at C-1, C-6, or C-16 in the liver and be excreted in this form.[242]

BIOSYNTHESIS AND BIOTRANSFORMATION OF C_{19} STEROIDS IN THE FETO-PLACENTAL UNIT

Frandsen and Stakemann were the first to suggest that the fetal adrenal probably produced a substance that could serve as precursor for estrogen biosynthesis in the placenta.[86] Subsequently, C_{19} steroid formation, particularly as precursors of estrogens, has been studied in the feto-placental unit. Methods of study have included: (1) perfusion of the fetus or placenta with isotopically labeled precursor, (2) introduction of labeled tracers into the intact feto-placental circulation, uterine artery, or maternal anticubital vein, and (3) incubation studies with various fetal tissues or placenta with labeled precursors.

The adrenal primordia becomes distinct during the fourth week of development; encapsulation occurs about the seventh week. Chromaffin cells invade the cortex about the eighth week. The fetal adrenal at term is 10–20 times larger than that of the adult. Most of the hypertrophied area, the fetal zone, is composed of a histologically distinct central reticular zone which involutes shortly after birth.[152, 153] The fetal zone is absent or atrophic in anencephalic monsters. Early studies of steroidogenesis by the fetal adrenal failed to demonstrate C_{19} steroid formation,[41] although Bloch, Benirschke, and Rosenberg tentatively identified testosterone, DHA, and 11β-OH-Δ^4-androstenedione in adrenal tissue from 9–21 week old fetuses of both sexes.[22] Concentration of C_{19} steroids per gram of tissue decreased with advancing fetal age. Subsequently, it has been demonstrated that the adrenal gland of the 9–21 week old fetus has the capacity to: (1) synthesize the cyclopentenophenanthrene nucleus, (2) hydroxylate in the 17-, 21-, and 11- positions, (3) replace the C-20, 21 side chain with a 17-ketone, and (4) sulfurylate steroids. These transformations have also been demonstrated with adrenal tissue from the adult. However, the capacity for conversion of acetate to pregnenolone and 17α-OH-pregnenolone is minimal, as is utilization of cholesterol sulfate for steroidogenesis.[258] The fetal adrenal does not possess the necessary enzymes for conversion of DHAS to testosterone or androstenedione.[173] Studies demonstrating C_{19} steroidogenesis by the fetal adrenal are summarized in Table 5-3.

Steroid formation by the fetal adrenal must be considered in relation to the placenta and other fetal organs. Baillie, Ferguson, and Hart have shown that the genital ridge of a 14-mm embryo, approximately 6 weeks of age, has the capacity to produce C_{19} steroids depending upon the availability of DHA or the coexistence of pathways of cholesterol biosynthesis.[6] Testicular tissue from fetuses 9–24 weeks of age is capable of forming androstenedione and testosterone from acetate;[208] DHA is also formed with pregnenolone as precursor.[1] Additional studies are needed to know whether the fetal testis continues to make C_{19} steroids as the fetus progresses in age after the fourth month, since the number of interstitial cells is maximum at that time and then progressively decreases.[101,191] The significance of C_{19} steroid formation by the fetal testis is not known, nor is it known how this formation is controled. C_{19} steroid formation by the fetal ovary, lung, intestine, and kidney has not been demonstrated, although these organs have the capacity to form C_{21} steroids from progesterone.[19,285] The fetal liver has the capacity to aromatize testosterone and also DHA to a lesser extent,[253] as well as the capacity to metabolize C_{19} steroids to their 3α:5β and 3α:5α reduced forms.[54] The fetal liver is also the principal site of 16α-hydroxylation of DHAS and estrone sulfate circulating in the feto-placental unit.[30,243] Foreskin from newborns has the capacity to convert DHAS to testosterone, DHA, and androstenedione.[139]

De novo synthesis of steroids from acetate by the placenta at midterm is limited.[156,157] The placenta has large amounts of sulfatase activity but has little sulfurylating ability, whereas the fetal adrenal has a marked capacity to sulfurylate steroids.[90,91,203,279] Placental tissue forms C_{19} steroids from progesterone, as demonstrated by studies cited in Table 5-4. This tissue also has the capacity to aromatize androstenedione,[17,26,27,109,220] 16α-OH-androstenedione and 16α, 17α-dihydroxy-an-

TABLE 5-3

FORMATION OF C_{19} STEROIDS BY THE FETAL ADRENAL

Precursor	Tissue preparation	Fetus' age (weeks)	Crown-rump (cm)	Product formed	Author
Acetate	Slice	12–22	8–21	DHA, pregnenolone, 11β-OH-Δ^4-androstenedione	Bloch and Benirschke[21]
	Slice	20	Not cited	DHAS, pregnenolone sulfate, cholesterol sulfate, 17α-OH-pregnenolone sulfate	Jaffe, Pérez-Palacios, and Lamont[128]
20α-OH-cholesterol	Slice	Not cited	Not cited	DHA, cortisol, 17α-20α-dihydroxy cholesterol, corticosterone	Shimizu, Shimao, and Tanaka[247]
Pregnenolone	Homogenate, slice	Not cited		DHA	Villee, Loring, and Villee[273]
	Homogenate	Not cited	10	DHA, androstenedione, 16α-OH-DHA, 17α-OH-pregnenolone	Villee and Villee[275]
	Mince	Not cited	10	11β-OH-Δ^4-androstenedione, cortisol, corticosterone, 16α-OH-pregnenolone	
	Homogenate	Not cited	21	DHA, DHAS, pregnenolone sulfate	
	Mince	Not cited	10	Androstenedione, 11β-OH-Δ^4-androstenedione	Villee and Driscoll[271]
	Infusion	Not cited	Not cited	DHA, DHAS, pregnenolone sulfate, 17α-OH-pregnenolone sulfate	Solomon[258]
	Slice	22	Not cited	DHAS, pregnenolone sulfate, 17α-OH-progesterone, 11-desoxycortisol, cortisol	Klein and Giroud[141]
	Homogenate	42	36	DHA, androstenedione, cortisol, cortisosterone, 11-desoxycortisol, 16-OH-progesterone, 17α-OH-progesterone, progesterone	Villee and Loring[272]
Pregnenolone sulfate	Homogenate	12 to 19	Not cited	DHAS, 17-OH-pregnenolone sulfate, 16α-OH-DHAS	Pérez-Palacios, Pérez, and Jaffe[199]
Progesterone	Homogenate	Not cited	Not cited	Androstenedione, 17α-OH-progesterone	Solomon[259]
	Homogenate	Not cited	10	Androstenedione, cortisol, deosycorticosterone, corticosterone	Villee[273]
	Mince	Not cited	10	11β-OH-Δ^4-androstenedione, 16α-OH-progesterone	
	Homogenate	Not cited	21	Androstenedione, DHA, 11β-OH-Δ^4-androstenedione, 16α-OH-pregnenolone	
	Culture	<10	Not cited	Androstenedione	
	Homogenate	42	36	Androstenedione, 16-OH-progesterone, cortisol, 17-OH-progesterone, corticosterone, desoxycorticos-	Villee[272]

TABLE 5-4

FORMATION OF C_{19} STEROIDS BY THE PLACENTA

Precursor	Tissue preparation	Fetus' age (weeks)	Products formed	Author
Acetate	Perfused cotylidone	Term	Lanosterol, cholesterol	Levitz, Emerman, and Dancis[157]
	Mince	Term	Squalene	Leusden and Villee[156]
Mavalonate	Perfused cotylidone	Term	Squalene, ianosterol	Levitz, Emerman, and Dancis[157]
Progesterone	Homogenate	Term	Androstenedione, 16α-OH-progesterone	Little, Shaw, and Purdy[161]
	Homogenate perfusion	Term	Androstenedione	Warren and Cheatum[276]
	Homogenate	20–21	Androstenedione, testosterone	Jungmann and Schweppe[131]
Androstenedione	Homogenate		19-OH-Δ^4-androstenedione	Longchampt *et al.*[166]
	Infusion	Not cited	Estrogens	Bolté *et al.*[27]
	Infusion	18–20	Testosterone	Benagiano *et al.*[17]
DHA	Slice		Androstenedione	Bloch and Newman[25]
	Perfusion	Not cited	Testosterone, androstenedione, estrogens	Bolté *et al.*[27–29]
	Perfusion	Midterm	Testosterone, androstenedione, estrogens	Lamb *et al.*[151]
DHAS	Perfusion	Term	Androstenedione, 19-OH-Δ^4-androstenedione, estrogens	Charreau *et al.*[46]
	Perfusion	Midterm	Androstenedione, testosterone, estrogens, DHAS	Lamb *et al.*[151]
	Perfusion	Not cited	DHA, testosterone, androstenedione, estrogens	Bolté *et al.*[27–29]
	Homogenate	Term	DHA	Warren and Timberlake[279]
Testosterone	Perfusion	Midterm	Androstenedione, estradiol, estrone	Bolté *et al.*[26, 27]
	Perfusion	18–20	Androstenedione	Benagiano *et al.*[17]
	Perfusion	Term	Androstenedione, 19-OH-Δ^4-androstenedione	Charreau *et al.*[46]

drost-4-en-3-one,[221] testosterone,[26,27,221] 16α-OH-testosterone,[221] androstenetriol,[220,221] DHA[27,151,188,221] DHAS[26,27,29,151,188,277] and 16α-OH-DHA[50,171] to estrogens; testosterone sulfate is not aromatized.[47] Progressive increase in placental ability to aromatize occurs from about the tenth week of pregnancy. The placenta lacks 11β-, 16α-, 17α-, and 21-hydroxylase as well as 17-20 desmolase activity, but has a high degree of 3β-ol-dehydrogenase with $\Delta^{4,5}$-isomerase activity, as demonstrated with DHA and androst-5-ene-3β, 17β-diol as substrates.[16,197] The midterm placenta is capable of hydroxylating estrone in the 16α and 16β positions, but the term placenta has little or no ability to hydroxylate at these positions.[16,27,161,253,279]

C_{19} STEROIDS IN ADRENAL VENOUS EFFLUENT

Recent advances in methodology have made it possible to measure the concentration of various C_{19} steroids in adrenal venous effluent. Levels of C_{19} steroids present in adrenal venous plasma obtained from subjects without adrenal disease are summarized in Table 5-5. DHA and DHAS are probably the most abundant C_{19} steroids secreted by the normal adult adrenal. Androstenedione was the first C_{19} steroid identified as a secretion product of the adrenal cortex.[202] Concentration of DHA in adrenal venous plasma ranges from undetectable to 254 μg/100 ml.[98,112,165,248,281,283] Values obtained by use of a colorimetric assay are somewhat lower than the values of 167–254 μg obtained by use of a double isotope dilution derivative method for assay. It is of interest that

TABLE 5-5

CONCENTRATION OF C_{19} STEROIDS IN ADRENAL VENOUS EFFLUENT IN PATIENTS WITHOUT ADRENAL LESIONS (μg/100 ml)

No. of patients	Lesion	DHA	Androstenedione	11β-OH-Δ^4-Androstenedione	Testosterone	Author
12	Breast CA	40.5*	3–5	6.1–135		Lombardo, McMorris, and Hudson[165]
3	None	8–47	3–5	3–8		Hirschman *et al.*[112]
3	Breast CA†	18–42	18–73	39–115		Short[248]
8	None	0–102	0–37		1.1–1.3	Wieland *et al.*[283]
10	None	4.4–23	4–15	14–23		Weinheimer *et al.*[281]
5	Hirsute				0.04–0.88	Burger, Kent, and Kellie[34]
2	None	167–254	20–40	33.5–69	0.95–0.98	Gandy and Peterson[98]

* Present in only 1 case.

† Premedicated with ACTH.

the adrenal venous concentrations of DHA in patients with bilateral adrenal hyperplasia as well as in those with adrenal adenoma are lower than the concentrations in subjects without adrenal disease.[98] Reports of concentration of DHAS in adrenal venous effluent are few. Levels of DHAS of 4–30 μg/100 ml in the three subjects studied by Baulieu *et al.* overlap the range of values for concentration of DHA; however, two of the three patients had renal cancer.[13] These values for DHAS are somewhat lower than levels reported by others.[98,270,283] The concentration of androstenedione in adrenal venous effluent from patients with no apparent adrenal disease ranges from undetectable to 40 μg/100 ml;[98,112,281] subjects that received adrenocorticotropin (ACTH) prior to surgery had higher levels.[248]

There is some evidence that the adrenal also secretes 11β-OH-Δ^4-androstenedione, androsterone, etiocholanolone, testosterone, and androstenediol. The concentration of 11β-OH-Δ^4-androstenedione ranges from 3–135 μg/100 ml;[98,112,165,281] levels in patients receiving ACTH prior to blood sampling are within the same range.[248] Levels of testosterone range from 0.04–1.3 μg/100 ml;[34,97,98,281] androsterone, etiocholanolone, and androstenediol are present in smaller amounts than testosterone.[98,112] The discrepancies among reports cited in Table 5-5 may be due to differences in sample size, sex, age, and health of the subjects, type of anesthesia, technique of blood sampling, and/or assay procedure used.

The precise site of C_{19} steroid production in the adrenal cortex has not been clearly defined, although there is considerable evidence that secretion of C_{19} steroids is probably under the control of ACTH. A variety of evidence suggests that ACTH causes release as well as de novo synthesis of steroids. Action of ACTH on adrenal steroidogenesis is on some rate-limiting step in the biosynthetic sequence between cholesterol and pregnenolone to progesterone. The rate-limiting factor appears to be the availability of reduced pyridine nucleotide coenzymes.[110] Studies on the effect of ACTH on adrenal venous concentration of C_{19} steroids are limited, as evidence is largely indirect and is based upon change in quantity of metabolites of C_{19} steroids excreted in the urine. Levels of DHA, DHAS, and androstenedione in adrenal venous and peripheral plasma increase following administration of ACTH; the level of testosterone does not.[140,281] Glucocorticoids suppress adrenal secretion of C_{19} steroids. This is indicated by such indirect evidence as decrease in peripheral plasma levels of DHA in man,[97,140] DHAS in women,[150] and in excretion of C_{19} metabolites in urine (reported by numerous investigators) as well as decrease in secretion rates of DHA, DHAS, and androstenedione.[158] Peripheral plasma levels of DHA and DHAS decrease significantly following adrenalectomy,[98,150] whereas levels of testosterone and androstenedione do not always decrease.[98]

C_{19} STEROIDS IN OVARIAN VENOUS EFFLUENT

The concentrations of testosterone, DHA, and androstenedione present in ovarian venous and peripheral plasma obtained simultaneously from women without apparent ovarian disease are shown in Table 5-6. Androstenedione appears to be the major C_{19} steroid secreted by the ovary. Levels in peripheral plasma range from 0.126–0.99 μg/100 ml; ovarian venous levels range from 0.45–5.91 μg/100 ml.[97, 98, 115, 213] The amount of testosterone in peripheral and ovarian effluent is considerably less than that of androstenedione. Levels of testosterone range from 0.01–0.11 μg and from undetectable to 1.04 μg/100 ml in peripheral and ovarian effluent, respectively.[97, 98, 115, 213] The concentration of DHA in peripheral plasma ranges from 0.24–1.46 μg/100 ml; ovarian venous levels are approximately twice as high as peripheral levels.[97, 98, 213] Although the number of subjects studied is small, the venous effluent level of these C_{19} steroids in at least one ovary in a given subject is significantly higher than the respective peripheral plasma level. Differences in age, disease state, and phase of the menstrual cycle as well as the sample size may account for the discrepancies in values for steroid concentrations cited. Rivarola *et al.* looked for but could not demonstrate a significant difference in peripheral and ovarian plasma levels of DHAS.[213]

The mean concentration of DHA and androstendione in peripheral and ovarian venous effluent obtained at the time of hysterotomy in four women during midpregnancy are similar to levels in nonpregnant women. The mean concentration of testosterone is higher in pregnant than in nonpregnant women.[95, 96, 180, 187, 211]

In vitro studies suggest that steroid secretion by the ovary is mediated through follicle stimulating (FSH) and luteinizing hormones (LH). The exact site of action or specific role of gonadotrophins in ovarian steroidogenesis is not known, although FSH and LH appear to be necessary for ovulation to occur. Possible sites of LH stimulation of steroidogenesis have been investigated and recently reviewed.[75, 234] Savard, Marsh, and Rice have demonstrated that cyclic adenosine 3′, 5′-monophosphate (3′, 5′-AMP) stimulates ovarian steroidogenesis in vitro, and have suggested that 3′, 5′-AMP may be involved in the mechanism of LH action on steroidogenesis.[234] Antibiotics such as puromycin and actinomycin D have an inhibitory effect on LH stimulation of steroidogenesis in vitro.[234]

FSH stimulates follicular growth;[225] LH is concerned with ovulation of the follicle. Both FSH and LH appear to be necessary for induction of ovulation but their precise role in ovarian function is not clear.

TABLE 5-6

CONCENTRATION OF C_{19} STEROIDS IN OVARIAN AND PERIPHERAL PLASMA OF PREGNANT AND NONPREGNANT WOMEN (μg/100 ml)

No. of patients	Testosterone		Androstenedione		DHA		Author
	Peripheral	Ovarian	Peripheral	Ovarian	Peripheral	Ovarian	
5*	0.047 (0.033–0.062)†	0.074 (0.05–0.095)	0.126 (0.126–0.144	0.822 (0.45–1.2)			Horton, Romanoff, and Walker[115]
4‡	0.054 (0.049–0.059)	0.134 (0.052–0.206)	0.253 (0.243–0.264)	1.87 (0.47–3.56)	0.98 (0.495–1.46)	1.85 (0.76–2.51)	Rivarola *et al*[213]
9§	0.054 (0.01–0.11)	0.33 (0–1.04)	0.40 (0.18–0.99)	2.04 (0.05–5.97)	0.66 (0.24–1.37)	1.15 (0.72–1.74)	Gandy, Moody, and Peterson[97, 98]
4‖	0.13 (0.10–0.28)	0.51 (0.31–0.59)	0.43 (0.31–0.59	2.43 (0.67–4.73)	0.59 (0.45–0.68)	1.84 (0.67–3.78)	Gandy[96]

* 30–64 years of age with metastatic breast CA; menstrual status not stated.

† Mean concentration with range in parenthesis.

‡ 34–47 years of age; one with breast CA.

§ 28–49 years of age; myomata uteri; cyclical menses.

‖ 13–39 years of age; pregnant; hysterotomy 16th–24th week of gestation.

Pituitary synthesis and release of gonadotrophins is regulated by centers in the hypothalamus.[66,76,108,177] There is some evidence that the ovarian-pituitary axis behaves similarly to the adrenal cortical-pituitary axis as demonstrated by the effect of steroids secreted by the ovary on gonadotrophin levels in urine and plasma.[3,137,194,219,237] FSH and LH are present in relatively constant levels in urine and plasma of women with cyclical menses, except at mid-cycle when a discrete elevation of FSH and LH occur which lasts less than 72 hours.[33,42,78,176,182,193,204,235-237] There is one report that FSH in urine is lowest at midcycle.[92] An early follicular rise in plasma FSH has been described by Faiman and Ryan[77] as well as Taymor, Aono, and Pheteplace.[266] Levels of FSH and LH are elevated in untreated castrated and postmenopausal women.[77,137,181,235] Recently Saxena, Gandy, and Peterson,[236] as well as Faiman *et al.*[79] have demonstrated that FSH and HCG-LH levels are elevated early in pregnancy; elevation persists throughout pregnancy. Midgley has reported that FSH is not present in sera of pregnant women.[181] Maternal plasma levels of gonadotrophins decline rapidly after parturition.[79,236] Peripheral plasma concentrations of C_{19} steroids have not been correlated with plasma nor urinary levels of gonadotrophins in normal women. Levels of testosterone and androstenedione are higher at midcycle and during the luteal phase than during the follicular phase.[96,114,164]

Reported studies on the relationship of gonadotrophins on ovarian steroidogenesis in vivo are largely concerned with formation of estrogens or progesterone. Purified human FSH and LH preparations have not been generally available for experimental studies. It is difficult to assess C_{19} steroid formation by the intact ovary since the adrenal also secretes C_{19} steroids, and there is peripheral interconversion of DHA and androstenedione to testosterone.[117,118,169,172,269] Approximately half the testosterone in women is formed from androstenedione secreted by the ovary and about 15 per cent from DHA secreted by the adrenal. Gemzell[100] and others have induced ovulation in women with HMG and HCG; secretion or production of C_{19} steroids was not reported. Korenman, Kirschner, and Lipsett could not demonstrate a significant increase in the blood production rate of testosterone following the administration of 2000 I.U. of HCG twice daily for five days.[146] However, Lloyd *et al.* have reported that plasma levels of testosterone are significantly increased from 0.062 to 0.216 μg/100 ml following the sequential administration of HCG in doses of 600 I.U. daily for six days.[163] Levels of testosterone did not increase following five days of treatment with HMG in doses of 5 mg a day. Lamb *et al.* have also reported an increase in plasma levels of testosterone following HCG.[150] Korenman, Kirschner, and Lipsett were not able to confirm either of these reports.[146]

C_{19} STEROIDS IN TESTICULAR VENOUS EFFLUENT

Testosterone, the major C_{19} steroid secreted by the testis, is present in testicular venous effluent in the range of 4–89 μg/100 ml.[72,98,113,123] The concentration of testosterone can not be correlated with age. The testis of normal men and those with carcinoma of the prostate, as well as of patients with testicular feminization, secrete DHA and androstenedione. Secretion is inferred from the difference in peripheral and spermatic plasma concentration of these two steroids.[98,122,215] The results of secretion and production rate studies also suggest that the normal testis secretes DHA.[45]

Testicular secretion of C_{19} steroids is regulated by gonadotrophins. FSH acts on germinal epithelium to promote and maintain spermatogenesis; LH acts on Leydig cells to secrete androgens and estrogens. The role of FSH in testicular steroidogenesis is not yet clear.[105,129,177,178] Recently, peripheral plasma levels of FSH and LH in normal men have been measured by radioimmunoassay.[137,181,194,235,237] Mean values obtained for FSH and LH by Saxena *et al.*[235] of 16.9 with a range of 3.9–42 and 14 with a range of 2.5–31.5 mIU Second International Reference Preparation of Human Postmenopausal Gonadotrophin/ml, respectively, are somewhat higher than levels obtained by others.[137,181,194,237] These mean values for FSH and LH in men are similar to those present in plasma obtained from women during the follicular and luteal phase of the cycle. There is considerable evidence that there is diurnal variation in peripheral plasma concentration of LH, FSH, and testosterone as well as androstenedione, DHA, and DHAS in normal men.[96,140,235,236,263] Neither Peterson, Midgley, and Jaffe[200] nor Odell, Ross, and Rayford[194] were able to demonstrate diurnal variation in plasma levels of LH or FSH. Administration of synthetic androgens or estrogens results in a decrease in plasma levels of LH as well as Leydig cell function.[82,140,200] The latter is inferred by an 80 per cent decrease in peripheral plasma concentration of testosterone. HCG elicits an increase in Leydig cell secretion of testosterone as inferred from an increase in the peripheral plasma level of testosterone[51,140,160,196] and blood production rates of testosterone in man.[214] The testis in prepubertal boys also responds to stimulation by HCG as manifested by a rise in the peripheral plasma level of testosterone.[226]

The peripheral plasma concentrations of androstenedione and DHA in males are not affected by HCG,[140,196] although there is some evidence that the testis secretes these steroids in small amounts.[45,98,215] Recently, Bardin, Ross and Lipsett have stimulated the Leydig cell-pituitary axis in normal men with clomiphene citrate. Peripheral plasma levels of LH and testosterone increased concomitantly. This response could not be elicited in men with panhypopituitarism. These findings suggest that the level of circulating testosterone probably controls the secretion of LH. Bilateral orchectomy results in a fall in plasma level of testosterone to levels comparable to those present in plasma from normal women,[51,98] and a rise in urinary and plasma levels of gonadotrophins. Hypophysectomy results in a decrease in plasma levels of testosterone, FSH, and LH.

C_{19} STEROIDS IN THE FETO-PLACENTAL UNIT

There has been considerable interest in the identification and measurement of C_{19} steroids in the cord and maternal circulation ever since Frandsen and Stakemann reported that pregnancy with an anencephalic fetus was associated with an abnormally low maternal urinary excretion of estrogens.[86] They postulated that the fetal adrenal was involved in the elaboration of estrogens during pregnancy. Subsequently, Bolté *et al.* suggested that both fetal and maternal C_{19} steroids could serve as precursors for estrogens.[26,27,29] The role of C_{19} steroids in estrogen synthesis by the feto-placental unit has been discussed in Chapter Three.

C_{19} steroids have been measured in cord and maternal plasma samples obtained simultaneously. DHAS is the most abundant C_{19} steroid in cord and maternal plasma.[50,95,184,251,252] Arterial and venous cord effluent levels range from 53–306 μg and from 27–252 μg/100 ml, respectively, arterial levels always being higher than venous levels. These findings suggest that the fetal adrenal secretes DHAS and/or that the placenta takes up DHAS from fetal circulation. Concentration of DHAS in maternal plasma ranges from 17 to 257 μg/100 ml; the mean value of 100 μg/100 ml reported by Simmer *et al.*[252] is approximately three to five times higher than the means values of 16 and 32 μg/100 ml reported by others.[50,95,184] Simmer *et al.* have suggested that there is no significant difference in fetal and maternal levels of DHAS, if DHAS concentration is calculated in terms of whole blood and the hematocrit of each patient.[251] The concentrations of DHAS and 16α-OH-DHAS in maternal and fetal blood of pregnancies with anencephalics are markedly lower than in blood samples from maternal and fetal blood of pregnancies with normal fetuses.[49,73] Maternal plasma levels of DHAS and 16α-OH-DHAS are also markedly decreased in women receiving prednisone or cortisone, and cord levels appear to vary inversely with the dose of corticoids administered.[351] Neither 16α-OH-DHA nor 16α-OH-DHAS was detectable in maternal plasma from these women; urinary excretion of estriol was decreased. These findings suggest that fetal adrenal production of DHAS, a precursor of estriol, can be suppressed by exogeneous corticosteroids. The major metabolic fate of DHAS in normal pregnant women or in women with an anencephalic fetus or hydatidiform mole is placental extraction and conversion to estrogens. Conversion of DHAS to estrogens in nonpregnant subjects is negligible.[15,28,249,250,280] DHAS is more efficiently converted to estrogen than is DHA.[249]

The mean concentrations of DHA in maternal peripheral plasma of 0.67 and 1.01 μg/100 ml at time of delivery are more than twice as high as the mean cord values of 0.25 and 0.38 μg/100 ml, respectively, in two studies.[95,124] There is no significant difference in arterial and venous cord values. These findings suggest that DHA is either not made or is rapidly utilized in the feto-placental unit. DHA and DHAS may have direct roles in fetal growth and development in utero aside from roles as estrogen precursors. Although these two steroids are considerably lower in plasma of prepubescent children than in adults, they are elevated in prepubescent children with congenital adrenal hyperplasia and some children with precocious puberty.[96,98]

Some of the DHAS in the fetal circulation is 16α-hydroxylated in the fetal liver[30,243] and then hydrolyzed, converted into 16α-OH-androstenedione, and subsequently into estriol by the placenta. Cord arterial levels of 16α-OH-DHAS, like DHAS, are higher than venous levels; these values are eight to ten times higher than maternal levels.[171,184] The arterial cord plasma concentration of 16α-OH-DHA is twice as high as cord venous values; levels in maternal plasma are almost half the venous cord levels as shown in Table 5-7. Concentrations of testosterone and androstenedione in maternal and cord effluent are shown in Table 5-8 and 5-9. Mean values for cord levels of testosterone and androstenedione, like DHA, are significantly less than maternal peripheral plasma levels.[95,124,187] Cord venous levels of testosterone and androstenedione are twice as high as arterial levels in subjects studied by Gandy.[95] However, Mizunio *et al.* have reported that the levels of the two hormones are similar.[187] Cord plasma from male infants contained significantly higher levels of androstenedione than from females, although testosterone levels were not significantly different.[187] The presence of low levels of androstenedione and testosterone in cord blood is consistent with the finding of a relative deficiency of 3β-hydroxysteroid dehydrogenase in fetal adrenal tissue. The significance of low levels of androstenedione and testosterone in cord blood in relation to maternal peripheral circulation is not known, although both of these steroids, as well as DHA, are known precursors of estrogens.[26,173,174]

Schindler and Siiteri have isolated and quantitated steroids in pooled

TABLE 5-7

MATERNAL AND CORD PLASMA LEVELS OF DHA, DHAS, 16α-OH-DHA, AND 16α-OH-DHAS (μg/100 ml)

Steroid	No. of patients	Maternal vein		Umbilical				Author
				Vein		Artery		
		Mean	Range	Mean	Range	Mean	Range	
DHA	9	1.016	(0.314–1.8)	*				Rivarola, Forest, and Migeon[211]
	8	0.67	(0.26–1.44)	0.25	(0.13–0.39)	0.27	(0.16–0.42)	Gandy[95]
DHAS	16	16.1		†				Migeon, Keller, and Holmstrom[184]
	20	100	(35–257)	130	(38–252)	162	(82–306)	Simmer *et al.*[252]
	12	32	(17–44)	68	(37–91	81	(59–98)	Colás[50]
	8	32	(17–56.8)	40	(31.2–45.7)	65	(53–83.3)	Gandy[95]
16α-OH-DHA	1	3		8		15		Magendantz and Ryan[171]
16α-OH-DHAS				83‡		112‡		Magendantz and Ryan[171]
	2	4		94	(68–137)	85	(44–129)	
	16‡	<10		87	(31–148)	110	(35–250)	Easterling *et al.*[73]
	12	7	(2–13)	114	(65–68)	147	(69–204)	Colás, Heinrichs, and Tatum[50]

* Mixed cord values 0.071–0.495 with a mean of 0.153.

† Mixed cord, mean value 0.38.

‡ Pooled plasma.

TABLE 5-8

TESTOSTERONE IN MATERNAL AND CORD PLASMA (μg/100 ml)

No. of patients	Maternal vein			No. of patients	Umbilical						Author
					Vein			Artery			
	Mean	SD	Range		Mean	SD	Range	Mean	SD	Range	
7	0.134	± 0.072	(0.068–0.232)	9	0.046	± 0.024	(0.02–0.098)				Rivarola, Forest, and Migeon[211]
12	0.127	± 0.025	(0.094–0.226)	22	0.048	± 0.028	(0.016–0.078)				Mizunio *et al.*[187]
				5*	0.054	± 0.02	(0.026–0.078)	0.043	± 0.012	(0.034–0.058)	
				5†	0.072	± 0.021	(0.024–0.116)	0.057	± 0.022	(0.030–0.087)	
8	0.215	± 0.115	(0.09–0.36)	8	0.088	± 0.055	(0.03–0.18)	0.037	± 0.054	(0.016–0.14)	Gandy[95]

* 5 male infants not included in the 22 infants above. † 5 female infants not included in the 22 infants above.

TABLE 5-9

ANDROSTENEDIONE IN MATERNAL AND CORD PLASMA (μg/100 ml)

No. of patients	Maternal vein			No. of patients	Umbilical						Author
					Vein			Artery			
	Mean	SD	Range		Mean	SD	Range	Mean	SD	Range	
7	0.387	± 0.176	(0.146–0.689)	9	0.126	± 0.058	(0.068–0.248)				Rivarola, Forest, and Migeon[211]
12	0.357	± 0.125	(0.203–0.589)	22	0.099	± 0.026	(0.063–0.153)				Mizuno *et al.*[187]
				5*	0.125	± 0.020	(0.110–0.153)	0.113	± 0.016	(0.096–0.131)	
				5†	0.086	± 0.008	(0.074–0.094)	0.081	± 0.025	(0.048–0.1)	
8	0.565	± 0.176	(0.26–0.82)	8	0.34	± 0.08	(0.12–0.37)	0.18	± 0.12	(0.07–0.39)	Gandy[95]

* 5 male infants not included in the 22 infants above. † 5 female infants not included in the 22 infants above.

amniotic fluid obtained immediately prior to delivery.[239] They found that 16α-OH-DHA was present in quantities of 798 μg/L, whereas only 8.3 μg of DHA was isolated. Levels of 16-ketoandrostenediol and estriol were 575 and 1572 μg/L, respectively. Levels of these steroids, with the exception of DHAS, were lower in amniotic fluid from patients with pregnancies complicated by diabetes, polyhydramnios, anencephaly, or Rh-incompatibility than in normal pregnancies.[238]

More recently, Gandy has studied the concentration of C_{19} steroids in amniotic fluid and cord plasma obtained at the time of hysterotomy.[95, 96] The mean concentrations of C_{19} steroids present in amniotic fluid were as follows: 0.05 μg/100 ml for DHA with a range of 0.04–0.06; 0.54 μg/100 ml for DHAS with a range of 0.48–0.59; 0.12 μg/100 ml for androstenedione with a range of 0.10–0.14; and 0.06 μg/100 ml for testosterone with a range of 0.02–0.04. Mean cord levels of DHA and DHAS were 10 and 100 times, respectively, higher than the mean levels of these steroids in amniotic fluid; androstenedione and testosterone were 3 and 2 times higher, respectively.

The tropic stimulus that causes fetal adrenal hypertrophy and steroidogenesis has not been clearly defined, although roles have been suggested for ACTH and HCG.[55, 130] There are few studies on the concentration of ACTH in maternal and cord plasma samples obtained simultaneously. The concentrations of HCG, LH, and FSH in the cord and peripheral plasma of the newborn are considerably lower than in the mother.[61, 62, 79, 236] This difference in concentration of gonadotrophins in maternal and cord plasma may be related either to a more rapid metabolism of the hormone by the newborn or to an effective placental barrier to passage of the hormone.[62] Maternal plasma levels of FSH, LH, and HCG decline rapidly after parturition.[79, 183, 236] Whether gonadotrophins in maternal circulation affect steroidogenesis in the fetus has not been clearly defined, although exogenous HCG does enhance transformation of testosterone to estrogens.[44] Normal pregnancy and delivery have ensued after surgical hypophysectomy in the mother as early as the 12th week of gestation.[132, 162] ACTH may well be the stimulus for C_{19} steroid formation by the fetal adrenal, although Bloch has demonstrated that ACTH is not necessary for production of DHAS by organ cultures of a 21-week-old fetal adrenal.[20]

SECRETION AND PRODUCTION RATES

Concepts involved in measurement and calculation of secretion and production of hormones are discussed in Chapter One and reviewed recently.[7,264,268] Early studies of the secretion rate of testosterone overestimated secretion. The results of these studies were calculated from the specific activity of urinary testosterone glucuronide following the intravenous administration of isotopically labeled testosterone. However, testosterone glucuronide in urine is not a unique metabolite of secreted testosterone; it is also derived from peripheral conversion of androstenedione and DHA as suggested by Korenman, Wilson, and Lipsett.[148] More recently, the metabolic clearance rate (MCR), blood production rate (PR), and transfer constant (ρ) values of testosterone have been studied.

The MCR of testosterone is approximately 1000 L/day and 700 L/day in males and females, respectively; blood production rates are 7 and 0.4 mg/day.[8,116,117,124,160,214,261] The secretion rate and PR of testosterone are similar in males. About half the testosterone in females is derived from androstenedione in blood by peripheral conversion.[117]

The MCR of androstenedione of 2300 L/day and 2000 L/day in males and females, respectively, are similar. Production rates of 1.7 and 3.5 mg/day in men and women, respectively, are significantly different.[117,213,214] The secretion rate and PR of androstenedione are identical in females. Horton and Tait have demonstrated that less than 25 per cent of androstenedione in the female is derived from the ovary and that the balance is secreted by the adrenal.[117] Approximately one-third of the daily production of androstenedione in the male arises from peripheral conversion of testosterone. Studies of the results of PR and MCR of C_{19} steroids are summarized in Tables 5-10 and 5-11. The primary site of conversion of blood androstenedione to blood testosterone is probably extrasplanchnic.[117]

Early studies of the secretion rate of DHA and DHAS, like those of testosterone, overestimated secretion.[45,269] Horton and Tait have reported that the MCR of DHA, 1694 L/day, and the blood production rate of DHA, 7 mg/day, are similar for men and women. More recently, Lieberman and Gurpide have reported that the secretion rate of DHA is 1–2 mg/day in women and 3–8 mg/day in men.[158] DHA is a minimum precursor of androstenedione and testosterone in the normal adult female.[118]

The secretion rate of DHAS ranges from 5.9–24 mg/day in men and from 5–8 mg/day in nonpregnant women.[158,170] The MCR of DHAS is 7 L/day in nonpregnant women and 30 L/day in pregnant women; clearance in women with toxemia ranges from 8–17 L/day.[126] Most of the studies on MCR, secretion rates, PR, and transfer constants have been performed in subjects with intact adrenals and gonads. Thus, it is difficult to clearly define adrenal versus gonadal contribution. Further studies on

TABLE 5-10

MEAN PRODUCTION RATES OF TESTOSTERONE IN NORMAL SUBJECTS

	Male				Female			
No. of patients	Urine PR (mg/day)	Blood PR (mg/day)	MCR (L/day)	No. of patients	Urine PR (mg/day)	Blood PR (mg/day)	MCR (L/day)	
10			935	7			830	Hudson *et al.*[124]
5	6.5	6.9	980	2	1.9	0.8	800	Horton and Tait[117]
6		7.8	1110	6		0.34	892	Horton, Shinsako, and Forsham[116]
18		6.23	1216	14		0.32	601	Southern *et al.*[261, 263]
6			1240	5		0.23	590	Bardin[8]
2	5.8	5.82	1030	2	0.85	0.32	529	Rivarola *et al.*[214]

TABLE 5-11

MEAN PRODUCTION RATES OF ANDROSTENEDIONE IN NORMAL SUBJECTS

	Male				Female			
No. of patients	Blood PR (mg/day)	MCR L/day	Plasma (μg/100 ml)	No. of patients	Blood PR (mg/day)	MCR (L/day)	Plasma (μg/100 ml)	
6	1.40	2430	0.06	6	3.40	2230	0.14	Horton and Tait[117]
2	2.1	1778	0.12	2	3.1	1338	0.24	Rivarola *et al.*[214]
				5	3.01	1900	0.15	Bardin and Lipsett[8]

MCR and production rate of C_{19} steroids in pregnant subjects would be of value in understanding estrogen production and C_{19} steroid metabolism.

C_{19} STEROIDS IN PERIPHERAL PLASMA OF ADULTS AND PREGNANT WOMEN

Early studies of androgen production were limited to the bioassay of androgens in body fluid and the chemical measurement of steroids with a 17-ketone group in urine. Testosterone, probably the most potent androgen occurring in man, is not a 17-ketosteroid even though its chief metabolites, etiocholanolone and androsterone, are. Only a fraction of urinary 17-ketosteroids arise from testosterone production; the larger portion is derived from adrenal cortical secretion of androstenedione, DHA, and DHAS. Metabolites of this group of steroids account for approximately 67 and 80 per cent of ketosteroids in urine in men and women, respectively.

The concentration of DHAS was the first C_{19} steroid assessed in peripheral plasma. Mean levels reported by various authors reviewed by Vihko[270] range from 87–227 and 41–137 $\mu g/100$ ml in men and women, respectively; maximum concentration occurs in young adults with a gradual decrease in concentration after age thirty. Morning levels of DHAS are higher than those in the late afternoon.[96,185] The concentration of DHAS in maternal peripheral plasma decreases during pregnancy.[95,184,198] This finding is consistent with the suggestion by Siiteri and MacDonald that DHAS in maternal blood is circulated to the placenta and converted to estradiol.[250] A significant increase in maternal plasma concentration of DHAS does not occur during labor, as illustrated in Figures 5-3 and 5-4.

Plasma levels of androsterone sulfate vary from 19–58 $\mu g/100$ ml and from 6–27 $\mu g/100$ ml in men and women, respectively.[57,58,185,195,270] The concentration of etiocholanolone sulfate is somewhat lower than that of androsterone sulfate.

It is difficult to compare reports of plasma concentration of sulfates in that specificity of methods varies from direct assay of sulfate conjugates by colorimetric methods with no correction for losses to quantitation by use of gas liquid chromatography or a double-isotope, dilution derivative method.

Finkelstein, Forchielli, and Dorfman first measured levels of testosterone in peripheral plasma by conversion of testosterone to estrone with a placental enzyme; estrone was measured fluorometrically.[80] Since then, double-isotope derivative techniques, gas chromatography, and

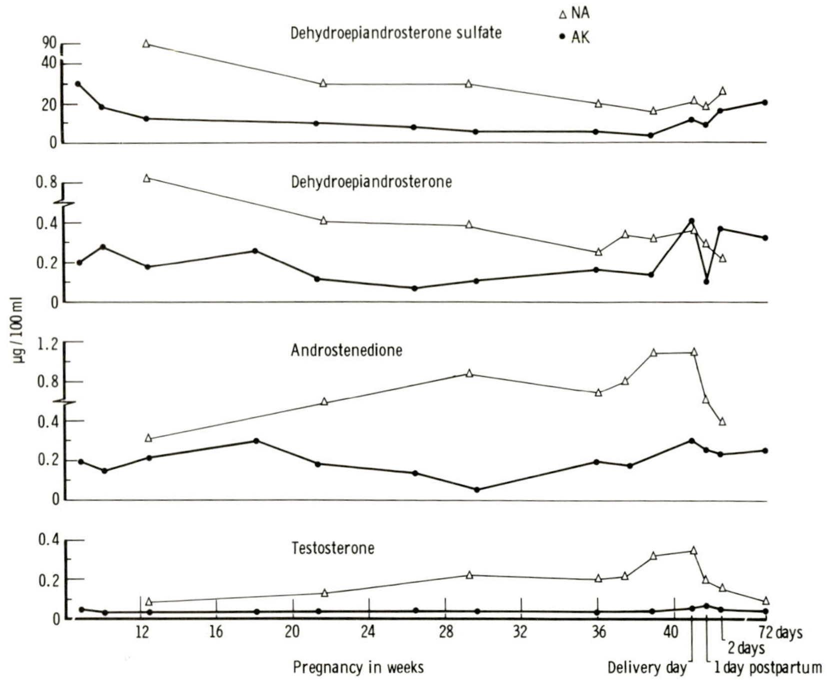

Fig. 5-3. Plasma levels of C_{19} steroids in peripheral plasma of 2 patients during pregnancy, on delivery day at stage 2 of labor, and postpartum.

competitive binding methods have been developed. The mean concentration of testosterone in men is approximately 0.66 μg/100 ml with a range of 0.28–1.44; it remains fairly constant until the eighth decade.[9, 83, 98, 102, 114, 124, 125, 138, 150, 210, 212, 230] Initially, Hudson, Coghlan, and Dulmanis could not demonstrate fluctuation in the plasma concentration of testosterone in men in a given 24-hour period.[122] Subsequently, others have shown that levels of testosterone are higher in the morning than in the afternoon or evening plasma samples.[140, 235, 263] This finding is consistent with the occurrence of diurnal variation in plasma levels of FSH and LH.[235, 236] The peripheral plasma concentration of testosterone in prepubertal males is less than 0.04 μg/100 ml;[87, 98] levels in newborns range from undetectable–0.032 μg/100 ml.[187] The mean level of testosterone in the peripheral plasma of nonpregnant women is 0.038 μg/100 ml. The range and mean values reported by various investigators are summarized in Table 5-12. The highest levels of testosterone occur in nonpregnant women with cyclical menses about the time of ovulation and during the luteal phase.[164] Diurnal variation in levels of testosterone has

TABLE 5-12

PERIPHERAL PLASMA CONCENTRATION OF TESTOSTERONE AND ANDROSTENEDIONE IN NONPREGNANT WOMEN (μg/100 ml)

No. of	Testosterone		No. of	Androstenedione		
patients	Mean	Range	patients	Mean	Range	Author
10	0.12	0.02 –0.26				Forchielli *et al.*[83]
2	0.085	0.059–0.079				Riondel *et al.*[210]
15	0.12	0.05 –0.35				Hudson *et al.*[124, 125]
7	0.059					
57	0.052	0.03 –0.10				Lobotsky *et al.*[164]
10	0.07	0.02 –0.12				Kirschner, Lipsett, and Collins[140]
20	0.11	0.05 –0.29				Lamb *et al.*[150]
			7	0.13*	0.11–0.17	Horton[114]
			10	0.17†	0.1 –0.2	
24	0.017	0.006–0.035	24	0.16	0.02–0.19	Goldfien *et al.*[102]
9	0.047	0.024–0.07	9	0.18	0.1 –0.29	Rivarola and Migeon[212]
20	0.037	0.014–0.058	20	0.16	0.09–0.22	Bardin and Lipsett[9]
20	0.032	0.002–0.07	18	0.13	0.05–0.33	Gandy and Peterson[98]
13	0.068	0.033–0.114	13	0.15	0.06–0.25	Saroff[230]

* Follicular phase of the menstrual cycle.

† Luteal phase of the menstrual cycle.

not been demonstrated in women. There is no overlap in the range of values for normal men and women except in early studies where methodology was not sensitive enough for accurate assay of small amounts of testosterone.

Meeker first reported that levels of testosterone in the peripheral plasma of pregnant women increased as early as the ninth week of pregnancy.[180] Levels in this group of patients ranged from 0.24 μg/100 ml during the first trimester to 1.17 μg/100 ml during the third trimester. These values are significantly higher than levels of 0.068–0.36 μg/100 ml reported by others[56,95,187,211] which overlap the range for men and nonpregnant women. Levels of testosterone are not elevated in all pregnant women as illustrated by subject AK shown in Figure 5-3 as well as in

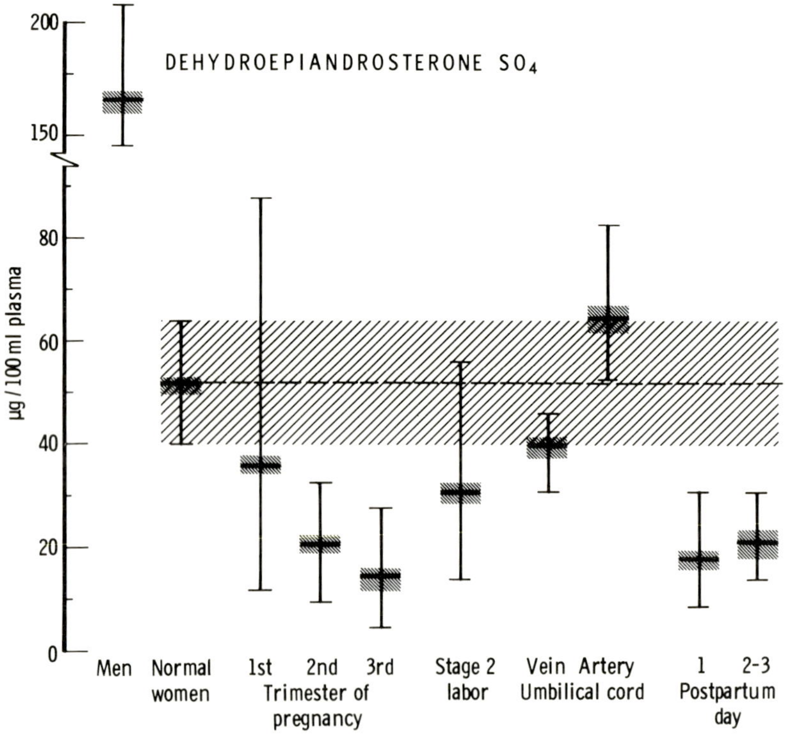

Fig. 5-4. Range of DHAS in maternal peripheral plasma in 6 patients during pregnancy compared to concentration in normal men and nonpregnant women. The mean and the standard error are represented by the horizontal and hatched area, respectively. Concentrations of DHAS in maternal plasma during labor and in the cord in 8 other patients are also illustrated.

pregnant subjects studied by others.[187,211] The mean level of testosterone during the first trimester of pregnancy is twice as high as the mean for nonpregnant women. A second rise in the plasma concentration of testosterone occurs around the 37th week of pregnancy; mean levels at that time range from three to seven times the mean for nonpregnant women. A significant added increase in the concentration of testosterone in maternal peripheral plasma during labor has not been reported. Maternal peripheral plasma levels at the time of delivery are significantly higher than cord arterial or venous values as shown in Table 5-8. Changes in the maternal plasma concentration of testosterone during the course of pregnancy are illustrated in Figure 5-5. The occurrence of masculinization of mothers or fetuses is rare in pregnancy. The sex of the infant can be correlated with neither maternal nor cord levels of testosterone. The

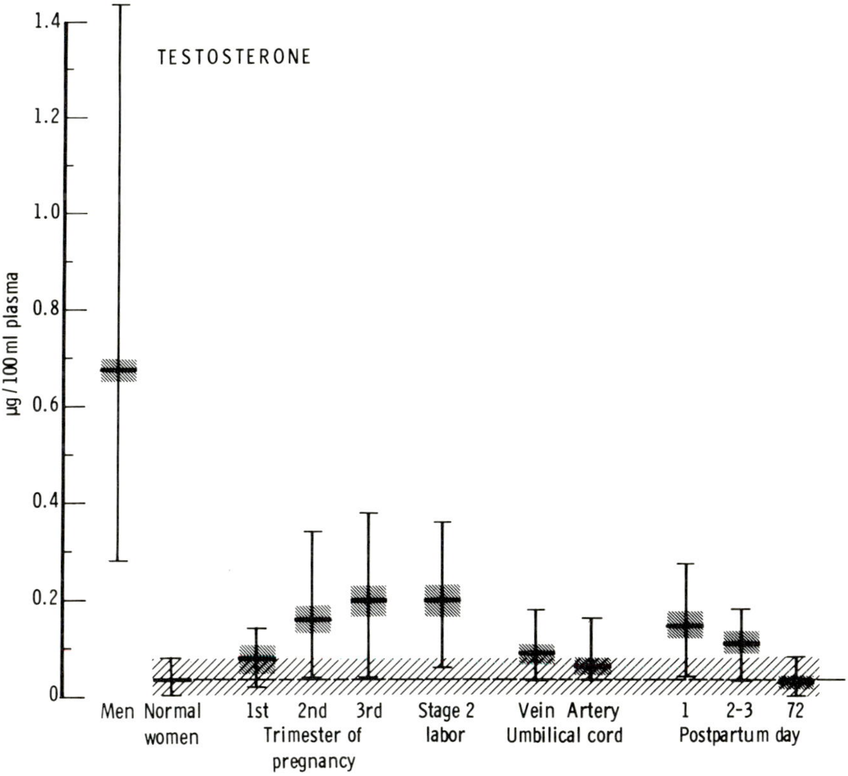

Fig. 5-5. Range of testosterone in peripheral plasma during pregnancy in the same 6 patients shown in Fig. 5-4. The mean and the standard error are represented by the horizontal line and hatched area, respectively.

significance of elevation of maternal plasma levels of testosterone during pregnancy is not known. Elevated levels of testosterone decrease rapidly following parturition.

More than 90 per cent of the testosterone in plasma is bound to a specific protein, a globulin.[136, 198, 211] Testosterone binding protein is increased during pregnancy;[84, 198, 211] it can be increased in men by administering estrogen. This specific binding protein may alter the biological activity of testosterone. Although the total plasma concentration of testosterone in pregnant women is increased, the unbound fraction is not.[124] A rapid fall in the testosterone binding protein, like plasma levels of testosterone, occurs following parturition. Whether or not the difference in plasma concentration of testosterone is simply related to alteration in binding can only be clarified when more information is available on the MCR and PR of testosterone in pregnancy.

Plasma levels of androstenedione in nonpregnant women (0.13–0.18 μg/100 ml) shown in Table 5-9 are slightly higher than those in men (0.06–0.13 μg/100 ml).[9, 98, 102, 114, 212, 230] The levels of androstenedione in women are highest during the luteal phase of the menstrual cycle.[119] Values for androstenedione in men are highest in the morning; levels at 8 P.M. are 35–50 per cent lower than those at 8 A.M.[96] A diurnal variation in the plasma level of androstenedione has not been demonstrated in women.

Rivarola *et al.*[211] have reported that maternal plasma levels of androstenedione are not significantly higher than those in their group of nonpregnant women. Mizunio *et al.*[187] as well as Gandy[95] (Fig. 5-6) have demonstrated that the concentration of androstenedione increases during pregnancy as does testosterone. The initial increase in the maternal plasma level of androstenedione occurs during the first trimester; a second increase occurs around the 37th week of pregnancy. These rises are demonstrated by both patients in Figure 5-3. The ratio of androstenedione to testosterone in plasma in pregnant women of 5.4 is almost twice that in nonpregnant. The significance of this change in ratio is not known. The concentration of androstenedione increases during labor in some subjects by three to four times the levels reported for nonpregnant women, in others the range of values overlaps the range for nonpregnant women. It is difficult to assess the significance of elevation of this steroid in maternal plasma during labor in the absence of knowledge of the role of diurnal variation in steroid concentration in the mother and/or in the fetus, the contribution of the adrenal versus the ovary, or the role of anesthesia on secretion or production of androstenedione and its precursors. Elevated levels of androstenedione in the mother during labor decrease rapidly by the first postpartum day (Fig. 5-6). Elevation of plasma concentration of

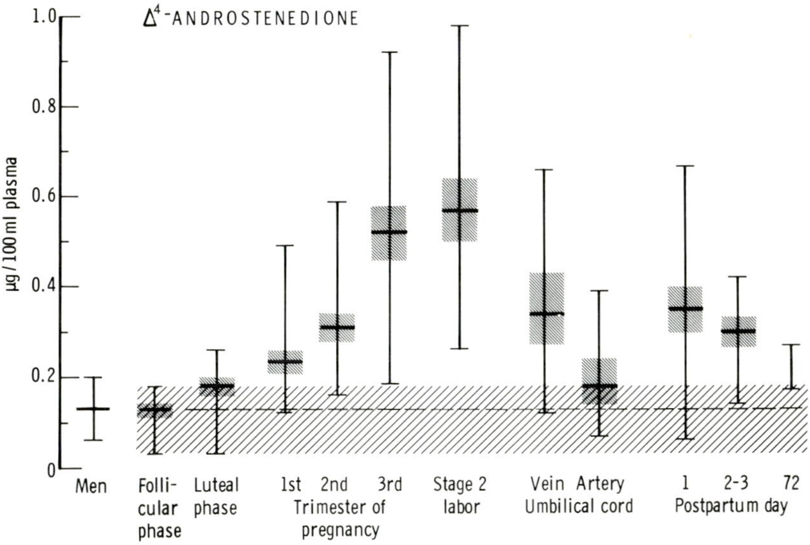

Fig. 5-6. Range of androstenedione in peripheral plasma during pregnancy in the same 6 patients shown in Figs. 5-4 and 5-5. The mean and standard error are represented by the horizontal line and hatched area, respectively.

testosterone and androstenedione during pregnancy with absence of maternal or fetal masculinization is of considerable interest, particularly since cord levels of these steroids are significantly lower than maternal peripheral levels. Bolté *et al.* have suggested that the placenta acts as a two-way barrier, limiting transplacental passage of androgens present in maternal and fetal circulations and converting them into estrogens.[27]

The concentrations of DHA in men and women are similar, although the mean value reported by Kirschner, Lipsett, and Collins[140] of 1.28 μg/100 ml is somewhat higher than the mean values of 0.38–0.51 μg/100 ml reported by others.[98,102,215,230] The concentration of DHA in plasma obtained from men at 8 A.M. is 50–60 per cent higher than levels at 8 P.M.[96,140] Quantities of DHA and its ester in peripheral plasma appear to decrease with aging, particularly in subjects over 50 years of age.[22] The mean concentration of DHA in the plasma of prepubertal children is less than 0.074 μg/100 ml.[98,102,140,215,230]

Levels of DHA in pregnant women are lower, but not significantly so, than the mean for nonpregnant women.[98,219] The decrease in the plasma level of DHA and its ester during pregnancy is illustrated in Figures 5-3 and 5-7. The concentration of DHA in maternal plasma increases during labor and at delivery when compared with levels during pregnancy.[95,211]

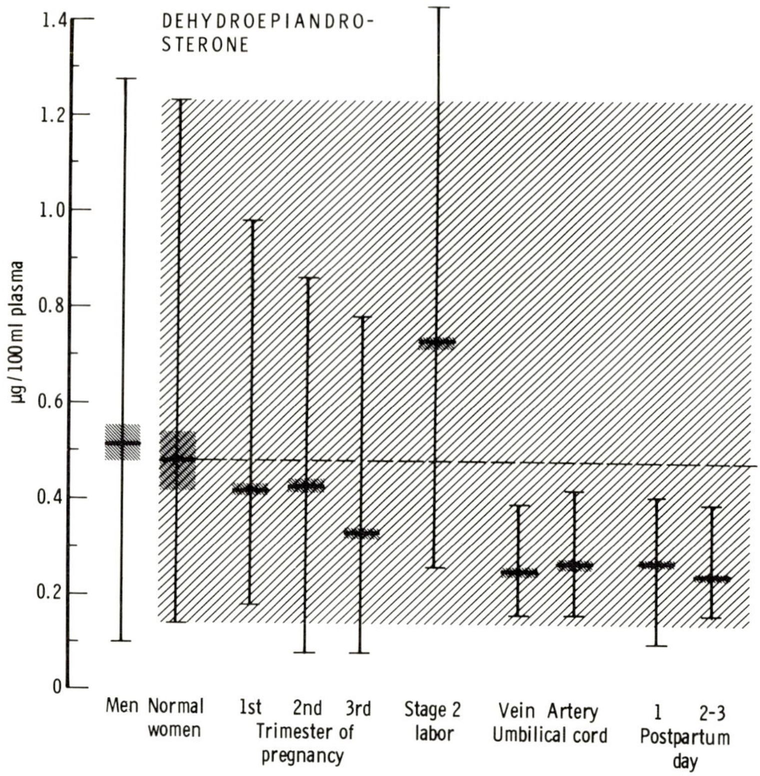

Fig. 5-7. Range of DHA in peripheral plasma during pregnancy in the same 6 patients shown in Figs. 5-4, 5-5, and 5-6. The mean and standard error are represented by the horizontal line and hatched area, respectively.

The significance of the elevation of DHA in maternal periperhal plasma during labor and at the time of delivery is not known. Whether or not maternal peripheral plasma concentration of DHA is influenced by the time of blood sampling or altered adrenal function during labor remains to be clarified. These elevated levels of DHA decrease during the first 24 hours after delivery to levels lower than those present in nonpregnant women. Rivarola, Forest, and Migeon have demonstrated increased binding of DHA during pregnancy.[211] They have suggested that the decrease in total DHA in plasma during pregnancy combined with an increased binding of DHA results in a marked decrease in plasma concentration of unbound DHA. A specific binding protein for DHA has not been characterized. The physiological significance of unbound C_{19} steroids in normal men, nonpregnant women, and pregnant women is not known.

APPENDIX

The following trivial names and abbreviations are used:

melvalonate = 3,5-dihydroxy-3-methyl-pentanoic acid
lanosterol = 4,4′,14α-trimethylcholestra-8(9),24-dien-3β-ol
cholesterol = cholesta-5-en-3β-ol
20α-hydroxycholesterol = cholesta-5-ene-3β,20α-diol
17α,20α-dihydroxy-cholesterol = cholesta-5-ene-3β, 17α-triol
testosterone = 17β-hydroxyandrost-4-en-3-one
androstenedione = androst-4-ene-3,-17-dione
androsterone = 3β-hydroxy-5α-androstan-17-one
etiocholanolone = 3α-hydroxy-5α-androstan-17-one
dehydroepiandrosterone (DHA) = 3β-hydroxyandrost-5-en-17-one
11β-hydroxyandrostenedione (11β-OH-Δ^4-androstenedione) = 11β-hydroxyandrost-4-ene-3,17-dione
16α-hydroxytestosterone = 16α, 17β-dihydroxyandrost-4-ene-3-one
16α-hydroxydehydroepiandrosterone (16α-OH-DHA) = 3β,16α-dihydroxyandrost-5-en-17-one
19-hydroxyandrostenedione (19-OH-androstenedione) = 19-hydroxyandrost-4-ene-3,17-dione
androstanediol = androstane-3α,17β-diol
progesterone = pregn-4-ene-3,20-dione
pregnanolone = 3α-hydroxy-5β-pregnan-20-one
6β-hydroxyprogesterone = 6β-hydroxypregn-4-ene-3,20-dione
16α-hydroxyprogesterone = 16α-hydroxypregn-4-ene-3,20-dione
17α-hydroxyprogesterone (17α-OH-progesterone) = 17α-hydroxy-pregn-4-ene-3,20-dione
pregnenolone = 3β-hydroxypregn-5-en-20-one
16α-hydroxypregnenolone (16α-OH-pregnenolone) = 3β, 16α-dihydroxy-pregn-5-en-20-one
17α-hydroxypregnenolone (17-α-OH-pregnenolone) = 3β, 17α-dihydroxy-pregn-5-en-20-one
estrone = 3-hydroxy-estra-1,3,5(10)-trien-17-one
estradiol = estra-1,3,5(10)-triene-3,17β-diol
estriol = estra-1,3,5(10)-triene-3β, 16α, 17β-triol
dexamethasome (decadron) = 11β, 17α,21-trihydroxy-9α-fluro-16α-methyl-pregna-1,4-diene-3,20-dione
corticosterone = 11β-21-dihydroxypregn-4-ene-3,20-dione
cortisol = 11β,17α,21-trihydroxy-4-pregnene-3,20-dione
dehydroepiandrosterone sulfate (DHAS) = 17-ketoandrost-5-ene-3β-yl-sulfate

16α-dehydroepiandrosterone sulfate (16α-OH-DHAS) = 16α-hydroxy-17-oxoandrost-5-en-3β-yl-sulfate

pregnenolone sulfate = 20-oxo-pregn-5-en-3β-yl-sulfate

17α-hydroxypregnenolone sulfate (17α-OH-pregnenolone sulfate) = 17α-hydroxy-20-oxopregn-5-en-3β-yl-sulfate

16α-hydroxypregnenolone sulfate (16α-OH-pregnenolone sulfate) = 16α-hydroxy-20-oxopregn-5-en-3β-yl-sulfate

REFERENCES

1. Acevedo, H. F., Axelrod, L. R., Ishikawa, E., and Takaki, F. Steroidogenesis in the human fetal testis: the conversion of pregnenolone-7α-H^3 to dehydroepiandrosterone, testosterone and 4-androstene-3, 17-dione. *J. Clin. Endocr. 21:*1611, 1961.
2. Adams, J. B. Formation of steroid sulfates by extracts of human adrenals. *Biochim. Biophys. Acta 71:*243, 1963.
3. Alder, A., Burger, H., Davis, J., Dulmanis, A., Hudson, B., Sarfarty, G., and Straffon, W. Carcinoma of prostate: response of plasma luteinizing hormone and testosterone to estrogen therapy. *Brit. Med. J. 1:*28, 1968.
4. Axelrod, L. R. Metabolic patterns of steroid biosynthesis in young and aged human testis. *Biochim. Biophys. Acta 97:*551, 1965.
5. Axelrod, L. R., and Goldzieher, J. W. The polycystic ovary. VIII. The metabolism of 5-pregnenolone, progesterone, testosterone, 4-androstenedione and oestrone by normal and polycystic ovarian tissues. *Acta Endocr.* (Kobenhavn) *56:*255, 1967.
6. Baillie, A. H., Ferguson, M. M., and Hart, D. M. Histochemical evidence of steroid metabolism in the human genital ridge. *J. Clin. Endocr. 26:*738, 1966.
7. Baird, D., Horton, R., Longcope, C., and Tait, J. F. Steroid prehormones. *Perspect. Biol. Med. 11:*385, 1968.
8. Bardin, C. W., and Lipsett, M. B. Testosterone and androstenedione blood production rates in normal women and women with idiopathic hirsutism or polycystic ovaries. *J. Clin. Invest. 46:*891, 1967.
9. Bardin, C. W., and Lipsett, M. B. Estimation of testosterone and androstenedione in human peripheral plasma. *Steroids 9:*71, 1967.
10. Bardin, C. W., Ross, G. T., and Lipsett, M. B. Site of action of clomophine citrate in men: a study of the pituitary-Leydig cell axis. *J. Clin. Endocr. 27:*1558, 1967.
11. Bartlett, P. D. Rates of protein synthesis, amino acid catabolism and size of nitrogen pool during nitrogen storage induced with testosterone propionate, and testosterone proprionate combined with growth hormone. *Endocrinology 52:*272, 1953.
12. Baulieu, E. E. Three sulfate esters of 17-ketosteroids in the plasma of normal subjects after administration of ACTH. *J. Clin. Endocr. 20:*900, 1960.

13. Baulieu, E. E., Corpéchot, C., Dray, F., Emiliozzi, R., Lebeau, M. C., Mauvais-Jarvis, P., and Robel, P. An adrenal-secreted "androgen": dehydroepiandrosterone sulfate. Its metabolism and a tentative generalization on the metabolism of other conjugates in man. *Recent Prog. Hormone Res. 21:*411, 1965.

14. Baulieu, E. E., Corpéchot, C., and Emiliozzi, R. H^3-androstene-3, 17 diol-S^{35}-3-sulfate to H^3-dehydroisoandrosterone-S^{35} sulfate *in vivo:* an example of the "direct" metabolism of a steroid. *Steroids 2:*429, 1963.

15. Baulieu, E. E., and Dray, F. Conversion of H^3-dehydroepiandrosterone (3β-hydroxy-Δ^5-androsten-17-one) sulfate to H^3-estrogens in normal pregnant women. *J. Clin. Endocr. 23:*1298, 1963.

16. Baulieu, E. E., Wallace, E., and Lieberman, S. The conversion *in vitro* of Δ^5-androstene 3β, 17β-diol-17α-H^3 to testosterone-H^3 by human adrenal and placental testosterone. *J. Biol. Chem. 238:*1316, 1963.

17. Benagiano, G., Kivel, F. W., Zielske, F., Wiqvist, N., and Diczfalusy, E. Studies on the metabolism of C_{19} steroids in the human foeto-placental unit. 2. Metabolism of androstenedione and testosterone in the intact foeto-placental unit. *Acta Endocr.* (Kobenhavn) *56:*203, 1967.

18. Blaquier, J., Forchielli, E., and Dorfman, R. I. *In vitro* metabolism of androgens in whole human blood. *Acta Endocr.* (Kobenhavn) *55:*697, 1967.

19. Bloch, E. Metabolism of 4-^{14}C-progesterone by human fetal testis and ovaries. *Endocrinology 74:*833, 1964.

20. Bloch, E. "Fetal Adrenal Cortex; Function and Steroidogenesis." In *Functions of the Adrenal Cortex,* Vol. 2, K. W. McKerns (Ed.), Appleton-Century-Crofts, New York, 1968, p. 721.

21. Bloch, E., and Benirschke, K. Synthesis *in vitro* of steroids by human fetal adrenal gland slices. *J. Biol. Chem. 234:*1085, 1959.

22. Bloch, E., Benirschke, K., and Rosemberg, E. C_{19} steroids, 17α-hydroxycorticosterone and a sodium retaining factor in human fetal adrenal glands. *Endocrinology 58:*626, 1956.

23. Bloch, E., Dorfman, R. I., and Pincus, G. The conversion of acetate to dehydroepiandrosterone by human adrenal gland slices. *Arch. Biochem. 61:*245, 1956.

24. Bloch, E., Dorfman, R. I., and Pincus, G. The conversion of acetate to C_{19} steroids by human adrenal gland slices. *J. Biol. Chem. 224:*737, 1957.

25. Bloch, E., and Newman, E. Comparative placental steroid synthesis. I. Conversion of 7-H^3-dehydroepiandrosterone to H^3-androstenedione. *Endocrinology 79:*524, 1966.

26. Bolté, E., Mancuso, S., Dray, F., Baulieu, E. E., Diczfalusy, E. Conversion testosterone-17α-^3H into 17β-estradiol-17α-^3H by human placenta perfused *in situ. Steroids 4:*613, 1964.

27. Bolté, E., Mancuso, S., Eriksson, G., Wiqvist, N., and Diczfalusy, E. Studies on the aromatisation of neutral steroids in pregnant women. I. Aromatisation of C_{19} steroids by placentas perfused *in situ. Acta Endocr.* (Kobenhavn) *45:*535, 1964.

28. Bolté, E., Mancuso, S., Eriksson, G., Wiqvist, N., and Diczfalusy, E. Studies on the aromatisation of neutral steroids in pregnant women. II. Aromatisation of dehydroepiandrosterone and of its sulfate administered simultaneously into a uterine artery. *Acta Endocr.* (Kobenhavn) *45:*560, 1964.

29. Bolté, E., Mancuso, S., Eriksson, G., Wiqvist, N., and Diczfalusy, E. Studies on the aromatisation of neutral steroids in pregnant women. III. Overall aromatisation of dehydroepiandrosterone sulfate circulating in the fetal and maternal compartments. *Acta Endocr.* (Kobenhavn) *45:*576, 1964.

30. Bolté, E. Wiqvist, N., and Diczfalusy, E. Metabolism of dehydroepiandrosterone sulphate by the human foetus at midpregnancy. *Acta Endocr.* (Kobenhavn) *52:*583, 1966.

31. Boström, H., Franksson, C., and Wengle, B. On phenol and steroid sulphokinases in adult human tissues. *Acta Endocr.* (Kobenhavn) (*Suppl.*) *100:*129, 1964.

32. Bradlow, H. L., Fukushima, D. K., Hellman, L., and Gallagher, T. F. Transformation of epimeric delta 5-pregnene-3-beta, 17, 20-triols in man. *J. Clin. Endocr. 24:*359, 1964.

33. Burger, H. G., Catt, K. J., and Brown, J. B. Relationship between plasma luteinizing hormone and urinary estrogen excretion during the menstrual cycle *J. Clin. Endocr. 28:*1508, 1968.

34. Burger, H. G., Kent, J. C., and Kellie, A. E. Determination of testosterone in human peripheral and adrenal venous plasma. *J. Clin. Endocr. 24:*432, 1964.

35. Burnstein, S., and Dorfman, R. I. Biosynthesis of C_{19} steroids from 4-^{14}C cholesterol and 7-^{3}H-pregnenolone *in vivo* consideration of new pathways. *Acta Endocr.* (Kobenhavn) *40:*188, 1962.

36. Calvin, H. I., and Lieberman, S. Evidence that steroid sulfates serve as biosynthetic intermediates. II. *In vitro* conversion of pregnenolone-^{3}H sulfate-^{35}S to 17α-hydroxypregnenolone-^{3}H sulfate-^{35}S. *Biochemistry 3:*259, 1964.

37. Calvin, H. I., Vande Wiele, R. L., and Lieberman, S. Evidence that steroid sulfates serve as biosynthetic intermediates: *in vivo* conversion of pregnenolone sulfate-S^{35} to dehydroisoandrosterone sulfate-S^{35}. *Biochemistry 2:*648, 1963.

38. Camacho, A. M., and Migeon, C. J. Isolation, identification and quantitation of testosterone in urine of normal adults and patients with endocrine disorders. *J. Clin. Endocr. 23:*301, 1963.

39. Camacho, A., and Migeon, C. J. Studies in origin of testosterone in urine of normal adult subjects and patients with various endocrine disorders. *J. Clin. Invest. 43:*1083, 1964.

40. Camacho, A. M., and Migeon, C. J. Testosterone excretion and production rate in normal adults and in patients with congenital adrenal hyperplasia. *J. Clin. Endocr. 26:*893, 1966.

41. Carnes, W. H. Androgenic assay of the human fetal adrenal. *Proc. Soc. Exp. Biol. Med. 45:*502, 1940.

42. CATT, K. J., NIALL, H. D., TREGEAR, G. W., and BURGER, H. G. Disc solid-phase radioimmunoassay of human luteinizing hormone. *J. Clin. Endocr. 28:*121, 1968.

43. CEDARD, L., ALSAT, E., EGO, C., and VARANGOT, J. Influence of luteinizing hormone on the aromatization of testosterone by human placenta perfused *in vitro. Steroids 11:*179, 1968.

44. CHANG, E., MITTLEMAN, A., and DAO, T. L. Metabolism of 4-C^{14}-testosterone in normal human adrenal homogenate. *J. Biol. Chem. 238:*913, 1963.

45. CHAPDELAINE, A., MACDONALD, P. C., GONZALEZ, O., GURPIDE, E., VANDE WIELE, R. L., and LIEBERMAN, S. Studies on the secretion and interconversion of the androgens. IV. Quantitative results in a normal man whose gonadal and adrenal functions were altered experimentally. *J. Clin. Endocr. 25:*1569, 1965.

46. CHARREAU, E., JUNG, W. T., LORING, J., and VILLEE, C. Biosynthesis of estrogens by perfused full term placentas. *Steroids 12:*29, 1968.

47. CHEATUM, S. G., DIEBOLD, J. C., and WARREN, J. C. Failure of placental microsomes to aromatize testosterone sulfate. *J. Clin. Endocr. 26:*916, 1968.

48. COHN, G. L., and MULROW, P. J. Androgen release and synthesis *in vitro* by human adult adrenal glands. *J. Clin. Invest. 42:*64, 1963.

49. COLÁS, A., and HEINRICHS, W. L. Pettenkofer chromogens in the maternal and fetal circulation: anencephalic pregnancies, cesarean sections and tentative identification of 3β, 17β-dihydroxyandrost-5-en-16-one in umbilical cord blood. *Steroids 5:*753, 1965.

50. COLÁS, A., HEINRICHS, W. L., and TATUM, H. J. Pettenkoffer chromogens in the maternal and fetal circulations: detection of 3β, 16α-dihydroxy-androst-5-en-17-one in umbilical cord blood. *Steroids 3:*417, 1964.

51. COPPAGE, W. S., and COONER, A. E. Testosterone in human plasma. *New Eng. J. Med. 273:*902, 1965.

52. DAVID, R., AUGUST, G., and GANDY, H. M. A virilizing adrenal adenoma with minimal elevation of 17-ketosteroids. *Pediatrics 42:*139, 1968.

53. DAVID, R. R., WIENER, M., ROSS, L., and LANDAU, R. L. Steroid metabolism in the syndrome of testicular feminization. *J. Clin. Endocr. 25:*1393, 1965.

54. DELL'ACQUA, S., MANCUSO, S., BENAGIANA, G., WIQVIST, N., and DICZFALUSY, E. Androgen metabolism in the human foeto-placental unit at midterm. *Excerpta Med. Int. Cong. Sr. 111:*60, 1966.

55. DEMISCH, K., GRANT, J. K., and BLACK, W. Plasma testosterone in women in late pregnancy and after delivery. *J. Endocr. 42:*477, 1968.

56. DEMOOR, P., and HEYNS, W. Gas chromatographic determination of some urinary steroids by comparison with spectrophotometric methods. *Excerpta Med Int. Cong. Sr. 101:*54, 1966.

57. DENEVE, L., and VERMEULEN, A. The determination of 17-oxosteroid sulfates in human plasma. *J. Endocr. 32:*295, 1965.

58. DESHPANDE, N., JENSEN, V., BULBROOK, R. D., DOOUSS, T. W. *In vivo* steroidogenesis by the human adrenal gland. *Steroids 9:*393, 1967.

59. DESSPYRIS, A., DROSDOWSKY, M. A., MCNIVEN, N. L., and DORFMAN, R. I. Identification of testosterone sulfate in urine of normal adult subjects. *Proc. Soc. Exp. Biol. Med. 121:*1128, 1966.

60. Diczfalusy, E. Chorionic gonadotropin and oestrogens in the human placenta. *Acta Endocr.* (Kobenhavn) *Suppl. 12:*1, 1953.

61. Diczfalusy, E. Endocrine functions of the human placental unit. *Fed. Proc. 23:*791, 1964.

62. Diczfalusy, E., and Troen, P. Endocrine functions of the human placenta. *Vitamins Hormones* (*N.Y.*) *19:*229, 1961.

63. Dignam, W. J., Pion, R. J., Lamb, E. J., and Simmer, H. H. Plasma androgens in women. II. Patients with polycystic ovaries and hirsutism. *Acta Endocr.* (Kobenhavn) *45:*254, 1964.

64. Dixon, R., Vincent, V., and Kase, N. Biosynthesis of steroid sulfates by normal human testes. *Steroids 6:*757, 1965.

65. Dominguez, O. V. Biosynthesis of steroids by testicular tumors complicating congenital adrenocortical hyperplasia. *J. Clin. Endocr. 21:*663, 1961.

66. Donovan, B. T. "The Regulation of Secretion of Follicle-Stimulating Hormone." In *The Pituitary Gland,* G. W. Harris and B. T. Donovan (Eds.), University of California Press, Berkeley, 1966, p. 49.

67. Dorfman, R. I. "Androgens and Anabolic Agents." In *Methods in Hormone Research,* R. I. Dorfman (Ed.), Academic Press, New York, 1962, p. 275.

68. Dorfman, R. I. "Androgens." In *Methods in Hormone Research,* Vol. 5, Part C, R. I. Dorfman (Ed.), Academic Press, New York, 1966, p. 235.

69. Dorfman, R. I., and Shipley, R. A. *Androgens,* Wiley, New York, 1956, p. 218.

70. Dorfman, R. I., and Ungar, F. *Metabolism of Steroid Hormones.* Academic Press, New York, 1966, p. 22.

71. Dufau, M. L., Villee, D. B., and Kliman, B. Pregnenolone metabolism in an aldosterone secreting tumor of the adrenal and its adjacent adrenal tissue. *J. Clin. Endocr. 28:*983, 1968.

72. Dupre, J., Brooks, R. V., Hyde, R., London, D. R., Prunty, F. T. G., and Self, J. B. Preliminary observations on testosterone in testicular vein blood from abnormal human testes. *J. Endocr. 29:*VII, 1964.

73. Easterling, W. E., Simmer, H. H., Dignam, W. J., Frankland, M. V., and Naftolin, F. Neutral C_{19} steroids and steroid sulfates in human pregnancy. II. Dehydroepiandrosterone sulfate, 16α-hydroxy-dehydroepiandrosterone sulfate in maternal and fetal blood of pregnancies with anencephalic and normal fetuses. *Steroids 8:*157, 1966.

74. Eberlein, W. R., Winter, J., and Rosenfield, R. L. "The Androgens." In *Hormones in Blood,* C. H. Gray and A. L. Bacharach (Eds.), Academic Press, New York, 1967, p. 187.

75. Eik-Nes, K. B. Effects of gonadotropins on secretion of steroids by the testis and ovary. *Physiol. Rev. 44:*609, 1964.

76. Everett, J. W. Central neural control of reproductive function of the adenophypophysis. *Physiol. Rev. 44:*373, 1964.

77. Faiman, C., and Ryan, R. J. Radioimmunoassay for human follicle stimulating hormone. *J. Clin. Endocr. 27:*444, 1967.

78. Faiman, C., Ryan, R. J., and Albert, A. FSH and LH activity in urinary extracts: a comparison of radioimmunoassay and bioassay methods. *J. Clin. Endocr. 28:*1076, 1968.

79. FAIMAN, C., RYAN, R. J., ZWIREK, S. J., and RUBIN, M. E. Serum FSH and HCG during human pregnancy and puerperium. *J. Clin Endocr. 28:*1323, 1968.

80. FINKELSTEIN, M., FORCHIELLI, E., and DORFMAN, R. I. Estimation of testosterone in human plasma. *J. Clin. Endocr. 21:*98, 1961.

81. FLICKINGER, G. L., WU, C. H., and TOUCHSTONE, J. C. Neutral steroid metabolites of dehydroepiandrosterone 7α-^{3}H in human ovarian tissue. *Steroids 11:*389, 1968.

82. FORCHIELLI, E., RAO, G. S., SARDA, I. R., GILBREE, N. B., POCHI, P. E., STRAUSS, J. S., and DORFMAN, R. I. Effect of ethinyl oestradiol on plasma testosterone levels and urinary testosterone excretion in man. *Acta Endocr.* (Kobenhavn) *50:*51, 1965.

83. FORCHIELLI, E., SORCINI, G., NIGHTINGALE, M. B., BRUST, N., DORFMAN, R. I., PERLOFF, W. H., and JACOBSON, G. Testosterone in human plasma. *Anal. Biochem. 5:*416, 1963.

84. FOREST, M. G., RIVAROLA, M. A., and MIGEON, C. J. Percentage binding of testosterone, androstenedione and dehydroisoandrosterone in human plasma. *Steroids 12:*323, 1968.

85. FORLEO, R., and INGIULLA, W. A time study of steroid transformations *in vitro* in the testis of a patient with the feminine type of male pseudohermaphroditism. *Steroids 10:*347, 1967.

86. FRANDSEN, V. A., and STAKEMANN, G. The site of production of oestrogenic hormones in human pregnancy. *Acta Endocr.* (Kobenhavn) *38:*383, 1961.

87. FRASIER, S. D., and HORTON, R. Androgens in the peripheral plasma of prepubertal children and adults. *Steroids 8:*777, 1966.

88. FRENCH, F. S., BAGGETT, B., VAN WYK, J. J., TALBERT, L. M., HUBBARD, W. R., JOHNSTON, F. R., WEAVER, R. P., FORCHIELLI, E., RAO, G. S., and SARDA, I. R. Testicular feminization: clinical, morphological and biochemical studies. *J. Clin. Endocr. 25:*661, 1965.

89. FRENCH, F. S., SPOONER, I., and BAGGETT, B. Metabolism of 17-hydroxyprogesterone in testicular tissue from a patient with the syndrome of testicular feminization. *J. Clin. Endocr. 27:*437, 1967.

90. FRENCH, A. P., and WARREN, J. C. Steroid 3β-sulfatase in fetal placental tissues. *Steroids 6:*865, 1965.

91. FRENCH, A. P., and WARREN, J. C. Sulfatase activity in the human placenta. *Steroids 8:*79, 1966.

92. FUKUSHIMA, M., STEVENS, V. C., GANTT, C. L., and VORYS, N. Urinary FSH and LH excretion during the normal menstrual cycle. *J. Clin. Endocr. 24:*205, 1964.

93. GALLAGHER, T. F., FUKUSHIMA, D., BERRY, M., and DOBRINER, K. Studies with isotopic steroid hormones. *Recent Prog. Hormone Res. 6:*131, 1951.

94. GALLEGOS, A. J., and BERLINER, D. L. Transformation and conjugation of dehydroepiandrosterone by human skin. *J. Clin. Endocr. 27:*1214, 1967.

95. GANDY, H. M. Concentration of testosterone, androstenedione, dehydroepiandrosterone, dehydroepiandrosterone sulfate, pregnenolone, pregnenolone sulfate and progesterone in maternal venous and umbilical venous and arterial plasma. *Excerpta Med. Int. Cong. Sr. 157:*172, 1968.

96. GANDY, H. M. Unpublished data.

97. GANDY, H. M., MOODY, C. B., and PETERSON, R. E. Androgen levels in ovarian and adrenal venous plasma. *Excerpta Med. Int. Cong. Sr. 112:*223, 1965.

98. GANDY, H. M., and PETERSON, R. E. Measurement of testosterone and 17-ketosteroids in plasma by the double isotope dilution derivative technique. *J. Clin. Endocr. 28:*949, 1968.

99. GARDNER, W. U., and PFEIFFER, C. A. Influence of estrogens and androgens on skeletal system. *Physiol. Rev. 23:*139, 1943.

100. GEMZELL, C. Induction of ovulation with human gonadotropins. *Recent Prog. Hormone Res. 21:*179, 1965.

101. GILLMAN, J. The development of gonads in man, with a consideration of the role of foetal endocrines and the histogenesis of ovarian tumors. *Carneg. Inst. Wash. Contrib. Embryol. 210:*81, 1948.

102. GOLDFIEN, A., JONES, J., YANNONE, M. E., and WHITE, B. "The Estimation of Plasma Androgens by Gas-liquid Chromatography." In *Gas Chromatography of Steroids in Biological Fluids,* M. B. Lipsett (Ed.), Plenium Press, New York, 1965, p. 35.

103. GRIFFITHS, K., CUNNINGHAM, D., and CAMERON, E. H. D. A comparison of the conversion *in vitro* of pregnenolone sulphate and pregnenolone to steroid hormones by tissue from a clear cell adenoma of the adrenal gland. *J. Endocr. 40:*49, 1948.

104. GUAL, C., SANCHEZ, J., DORFMAN, R. I., and ROSENTHAL, I. M. Androgen biosynthesis in an interstitial cell tumor of the testes. *J. Clin. Endocr. 22:*1040, 1962.

105. GUILLEMIN, R. Hypothalamic factors releasing pituitary hormones. *Recent Prog. Hormone Res. 20:*89, 1964.

106. GURPIDE, E., MACDONALD, P. C., VANDE WIELE, R., and LIEBERMAN, S. Measurement of the rates of secretion of peripheral metabolism of two interconvertible compounds: dehydroisoandrosterone and dehydroisoandrosterone sulfate. *J. Clin. Endocr. 23:*346, 1963.

107. HARRIS, G. W., and CAMPBELL, H. J. "The Regulation of Secretion of Luteinizing Hormone and Ovulation." In *The Pituitary Gland,* G. W. Harris and B. T. Donovan (Eds.), University of California Press, Berkeley, 1966, p. 99.

108. HARRIS, G. W., MITCHELL, R. P., and SCOTT, P. P. "Neurological Site of Action of Stilbesterol in Eliciting Sexual Behavior." In *Ciba Foundation Symposium on the Neurological Basis of Behaviour,* G. E. W. Wolstenholme and C. M. O'Connor (Eds.), Little, Brown, Boston, 1958, p. 236.

109. HAYANO, M., LONGCHAMPT, J., KELLY, W., GUAL, C., and DORFMAN, R. I. Studies on the biosynthesis of estrogens by human placental microsomes. *Acta Endocr.* (Kobenhavn) *Suppl. 51:*699, 1960.

110. HECHTER, O., and HALKERSTON, I. D. K. "On the Action of Mammalian Hormones." In *The Hormones,* Vol. 5, G. Pincus, K. V. Thimann, and E. B. Astwood (Eds.), Academic Press, New York, 1964, p. 697.

111. HELLMAN, L., BRADLOW, H. L., ZUMOFF, B., FUKUSHIMA, D. K., and GAL-

LAGHER, T. F. Thyroid-androgen interrelations and the hypercholesteremic effect of androsterone. *J. Clin. Endocr. 19:*936, 1959.

112. HIRSCHMANN, H., DE COURCY, C., LEVY, R. P., and MILLER, K. L. Adrenal precursors of urinary 17-ketosteroids. *J. Biol. Chem. 235:*pc 48, 1960.

113. HOLLANDER, N., and HOLLANDER, V. P. Microdetermination of testosterone in human spermatic vein blood. *J. Clin. Endocr. 18:*966, 1958.

114. HORTON, R. Estimation of androstenedione in human peripheral blood with ^{35}S-thiosemicabazide. *J. Clin. Endocr. 25:*1237, 1965.

115. HORTON, R., ROMANOFF, E., and WALKER, J. Androstenedione and testosterone in ovarian venous and peripheral plasma during ovariectomy for breast cancer. *J. Clin. Endocr. 26:*1267, 1966.

116. HORTON, R., SHINSAKO, J., and FORSHAM, P. H. Testosterone production and metabolic clearance with volumes of distribution in normal adult men and women. *Acta Endocr.* (Kobenhavn) *48:*446, 1965.

117. HORTON, R., and TAIT, J. F. Androstenedione production and interconversion in peripheral blood and studies on the possible sites of its conversion to testosterone. *J. Clin. Invest. 45:*301, 1966.

118. HORTON, R., and TAIT, J. F. *In vivo* conversion of dehydroepiandrosterone to androstenedione and testosterone in man. *J. Clin. Endocr. 27:*79, 1967.

119. HOWARD, E. Steroids and bone formation in infant mice: relative activities of dehydroepiandrosterone and testosterone. *Endocrinology 70:*131, 1962.

120. HUANG, W. Y. Studies on the hydroxylation and metabolism of Δ^4-androstene-3, 17-dione-7-H^3 in the human corpus luteum tissue. *Steroids 9:*485, 1967.

121. HUANG, W. Y., and PEARLMAN, W. H. The corpus luteum and steroid formation. *J. Biol. Chem. 238:*1308, 1963.

122. HUDSON, B., COGHLAN, J. P., and DULMANIS, A. "Testicular Function in Man." In *Endocrinology of the Testis,* G. E. Wolstenholme and M. O'Connor (Eds.), Little, Brown, Boston, 1967, p. 140.

123. HUDSON, B., COGHLAN, J. P., DULMANIS, A., and WINTOUR, M. The measurement of testosterone in biological fluids in the evaluation of androgen activity. *Excerpta Med. Int. Cong. Sr. 83:*1127, 1965.

124. HUDSON, B., DULMANIS, A., COGHLAN, J. B., and WINTOUR, M. The measurement of androgen production in normal subjects. *Aust. Ann. Med. 15:*236, 1966.

125. HUDSON, B., COGHLAN, J., DULMANIS, A., WINTOUR, M., and EKKEL, I. Estimation of testosterone in biological fluid. *Aust. J. Exp. Biol. Med. Sci. 41:*235, 1963.

126. HUTCHINSON, H. T., SIITERI, P. K., MACDONALD, P. C. Studies on the metabolic clearance of dehydroisoandrosterone sulfate (DS) in pregnancy. Soc. for Gynecologic Investigation, 16th Annual Meeting, March 20, 1969 (Abstract, p. 12).

127. ISCHII, S., FORCHIELLI, E., CASSIDY, C. E., ROSOFF, C. B., and DORFMAN, R. I. Biosynthesis of androgens by homogenates of normal and abnormal human adrenal glands. *Biochem, Biophys. Res. Comman. 9:*344, 1962.

128. Jaffe, R. B., Pérez-Palacios, G., and Lamont, K. G. *De novo* steroid sulfate biosynthesis. *J. Clin. Endocr. 28:*1671, 1968.

129. Johnsen, S. G. Studies on the testicular-hypophyseal feed-back mechanism in man. *Acta Endocr.* (Kobenhavn) *Suppl. 90:*99, 1964.

130. Jost, A., Jacquot, R., and Cohen, A. "The Pituitary Control of the Foetal Adrenal Cortex." In *The Human Adrenal Cortex,* A. R. Currie, J. Symington and J. K. Grant (Eds.), E. & S. Livingstone, Edinburgh, 1962, p. 569.

131. Jungmann, R. A., and Schweppe, J. S. Biosynthesis and metabolism of neutral steroids by human midterm placenta and fetal liver. *J. Clin. Endocr. 27:*1151, 1967.

132. Kaplan, N. M. Successful pregnancy following hypophysectomy during the twelfth week of gestation. *J. Clin. Endocr. 21:*1139, 1961.

133. Kappas, A., Hellman, L., Fukushima, D. K., and Gallagher, T. F. The thermogenic effect and metabolic fate of etiocholanolone. *J. Clin. Endocr. 18:*1043, 1958.

134. Kase, N., Forchielli, E., and Dorfman, R. I. *In vitro* production of testosterone and androst-4-ene-3,17-dione in a human ovarian homogenate. *Acta Endocr.* (Kobenhavn) *37:*19, 1961.

135. Kase, N., and Korwal. *In vitro* production of testosterone in a human adrenal homogenate. *Steroids 22:*925, 1962.

136. Kato, T., and Horton, R. Studies of testosterone binding globulin. *J. Clin. Endocr. 28:*1160, 1968.

137. Keller, P. J. Studies on pituitary gonadotropins in plasma. I. Normal values in men and women of all ages. *Acta Endocr.* (Kobenhavn) *52:*348, 1966.

138. Kent, J. R. and Acone, A. B. Plasma testosterone levels and aging in males. *Excerpta Med. Int. Cong. Sr. 101:*31, 1966.

139. Kim, M. H., and Herrmann, W. L. *In vitro* metabolism of dehydroepiandrosterone sulfate in foreskin, abdominal skin and vaginal mucosa. *J. Clin. Endocr. 28:*187, 1968.

140. Kirschner, M., Lipsett, M., and Collins, D. Plasma ketosteroids and testosterone in man: a study of the pituitary-testicular axis. *J. Clin. Invest. 44:*657, 1965.

141. Klein, G. P., and Giroud, C. J. P. Incorporation of 7-H^3-pregnenolone and 4-^{14}C-progesterone into corticosteroids and some of their ester sulfates by human newborn adrenal slices. *Steroids 9:*113, 1967.

142. Knapstein, V. P., Wendlberger, F., Menzel, P., and Oertel, G. W. *In vivo* Perfusion eines menschlichen Testis mit (4-^{14}C) Androstenolon und (7α-^3H) Androstenolone (^{35}S) sulfate. *Hoppe Seyler Z. Physiol. Chem. 348:*990, 1967.

143. Knapstein, P., Wendlberger, F., Menzel, P., Oertel, G., and Touchstone, J. C. Biosynthesis of steroid hormones in human gonads. VI. *In vivo* perfusion of the testes with 1-^{14}C-acetate with 7-^3H-cholesterol. *Steroids 12:*191, 1968.

144. Knapstein, V. P., Wendlberger, F., Menzel, P., Treiber, L., and Oertel,

G. W. *In-vivo*-perfusion eines Testis mit (7α-^{3}H) Progesterone und (4-^{14}C) Androstenolon. *Hoppe Seyler Z. Physiol. Chem. 348:*1066, 1967.

145. Knowlton, K., Kenyon, A., Sandiford, L., Lotwin, G., and Fricker, R. Comparative study of metabolic effects of estradiol benzoate and testosterone proprionate in man. *J. Clin. Endocr. 2:*671, 1942.

146. Korenman, S. G., Kirschner, M. A., and Lipsett, M. P. Testosterone production in normal women and women with Stein-Leventhal syndrome or idiopathic hirsutism. *J. Clin. Endocr. 25:*798, 1965.

147. Korenman, S. G., and Lipsett, M. B. Is testosterone glucuroniside uniquely derived from plasma testosterone? *J. Clin. Invest. 43:*2125, 1964.

148. Korenman, S. G., Wilson, H., and Lipsett, M. B. Testosterone production rates in normal adults. *J. Clin. Invest. 42:*1753, 1963.

149. Kumari, L., and Goldzieher, J. W. *In vitro* steroidogenesis in normal human ovarian tissue. *Acta Endocr.* (Kobenhavn) *52:*455, 1966.

150. Lamb, E. J., Dignam, W., Pion, and Simmer, H. Plasma androgens in women. I. Normal and non hirsute females, oophorectomized and adrenalectomized patients. *Acta Endocr.* (Kobenhavn) *45:*243, 1964.

151. Lamb, E., Mancuso, S., Dell'Acqua, S., Wiqvist, N., and Diczfalusy, E. Studies on the metabolism of C_{19} steroids in the human foeto-placental unit. I. Neutral metabolites formed from dehydroepiandrosterone and dehydroepiandrosterone sulphate by the placenta at midterm pregnancy. *Acta Endocr.* (Kobenhavn) *55:*263, 1967.

152. Lanman, J. T. The fetal zone of the adrenal gland. *Medicine 32:*389, 1953.

153. Lanman, J. T. "An Interpretation of Human Foetal Adrenal Structure and Function." In *The Human Adrenal Cortex,* A. R. Currie, J. Symington, and J. K. Grant (Eds.), E. & S. Livingstone, Edinburgh, 1962, p. 381.

154. Lebeau, M. C., Alberga, A., and Baulieu, E. E. Adrenal biosynthesis of dehydroisoandrosterone sulfate. *Biochem. Biophys. Res. Commun. 17:*570, 1964.

155. Leon, N., Castro, M. N., and Dorfman, R. I. Biosynthesis of testosterone by a Stein-Leventhal ovary. *Acta Endocr.* (Kobenhavn) *39:*411, 1962.

156. Leusden, van H., and Villee, C. A. The *de novo* synthesis of steroids and steroids from acetate by preparations of human term placenta. *Steroids 6:*31, 1965.

157. Levitz, M., Emerman, S., and Dancis, J. Sterol synthesis in perfused human placenta. *Excerpta Med. Int. Cong. Sr. 51:*266, 1962.

158. Lieberman, S., and Gurpide, E. "Isotopic Dilution Methods for the Estimation of Rates of Secretion of the Steroid Hormones." In *Steroid Dynamics,* G. Pincus, T. Nakao, and J. F. Tait (Eds.), Academic Press, New York, 1966, p. 531.

159. Lipsett, M. B., Coffman, G. D., and Nixon, W. E. Lack of activity of dehydroepiandrosterone sulfate in metabolic balance studies. *J. Clin. Endocr. 25:*993, 1965.

160. Lipsett, M. B., Wilson, H., Kirschner, M. A., Korenman, S. G., Fishman, L. M., Sarfarty, G. A., and Bardin, W. Studies on Leydig cell physiology

and pathology: secretion and metabolism of testosterone. *Recent Prog. Hormone Res. 22:*245, 1966.

161. LITTLE, B., SHAW, A., and PURDY, R. The conversion of progesterone to 16α-hydroxy-pregn-ene-3, 20-dione and androst-4-ene-3, 17-dione by human placenta *in vitro. Acta Endocr.* (Kobenhavn) *43:*510, 1963.

162. LITTLE, B., SMITH, O. W., JESSIMAN, A. G., SELENKOW, H. A., VAN'T HOFF, W., EGLIN, J. M., and MOORE, F. D. Hypophysectomy during pregnancy in a patient with cancer of the breast: case report with hormone studies. *J. Clin. Endocr. 18:*425, 1958.

163. LLOYD, C. W., LOBOTSKY, J., SEGRE, E. J., KOBAYASHI, T., TAYMOR, M. L., and BATT, R. E. Plasma testosterone and urinary 17-ketosteroids in women with hirsutism and polycystic ovaries. *J. Clin. Endocr. 26:*314, 1966.

164. LOBOTSKY, J., WYSS, H. I., SEGRE, E., and LLOYD, C. Plasma testosterone in normal women. *J. Clin. Endocr. 24:*1261, 1964.

165. LOMBARDO, M. E., MCMORRIS, C., and HUDSON, P. B. The isolation of steroidal substances from human adrenal vein blood. *Endocrinology 65:*426, 1959.

166. LONGCHAMPT, J. E., GUAL, C., EHRENSTEIN, M., and DORFMAN, R. I. 19-hydroxy-Δ^4-androstene-3, 17-dione, an intermediate in estrogen biosynthesis. *Endocrinology 66:*416, 1960.

167. LUCIS, O. J., RAHEJA, M. C., MILLARD, O., and MORSE, W. I. Utilization of circulating precursors for the synthesis of testosterone by human testis *in vivo. Canad. J. Biochem. 45:*1213, 1967.

168. MACAULAY, M. A., and WELSKY, I. Metabolism of pregnenolone-7α-H^3 and progesterone-4-C^{14} in human granulosa cell tumor slices. *J. Clin. Endocr. 28:*819, 1968.

169. MACDONALD, P. C., CHAPDELAINE, A., GONZALES, O., GURPIDE, E., VANDE WIELE, R. L., and LIEBERMAN, S. Studies on the secretion and interconversion of the androgens III. Results obtained after the injection of several radioactive C_{19} steroids, singly or as mixtures. *J. Clin. Endocr. 25:*1557, 1965.

170. MACDONALD, P. C., ROMBAUT, R. P., and SIITERI, P. K. Plasma precursors of estrogen. I. Extent of conversion of plasma Δ^4-androstenedione to estrone in normal males and nonpregnant normal, castrate and adrenalectomized females. *J. Clin. Endocr. 27:*1103, 1967.

171. MAGENDANTZ, H. G., and RYAN, K. J. Isolation of an estriol precursor, 16α-hydroxy-dehydroepiandrosterone from human umbilical sera. *J. Clin. Endocr. 24:*1155, 1964.

172. MAHESH, V. B., and GREENBLATT, R. B. The *in vivo* conversion of dehydroepiandrosterone and androstenedione to testosterone in the human. *Acta Endocr.* (Kobenhavn) *41:*400, 1962.

173. MANCUSO, S., DELL'ACQUA, S., BENAGIANO, G., WIQVIST, N., and DICZFALUSY, E. Metabolism of testosterone and androstenedione in the human foetus. *Acta Endocr.* (Kobenhavn) (*Suppl.*) *100:*45, 1965.

174. Mancuso, S., Mancuso, F. P., Tillinger, K. G., and Diczfalusy, E. Lack of aromatisation of circulating dehydroepiandrosterone and dehydroepiandrosterone sulfate in amenorrhoeic women stimulated with human gonadotropins. *Acta Endocr.* (Kobenhavn) *49:*248, 1965.

175. Marota, S., Shikita, M., and Tamaoki, B. Androgen formation in testicular tissue of patients with prostatic CA. *Biochim. Biophys. Acta. 117:*241, 1966.

176. McArthur, J. W., Worcester, J., and Ingersoll, F. M. The urinary excretion of interstitial cell and follicle-stimulating hormone activity during the normal menstrual cycle. *J. Clin. Endocr. 18:*1186, 1958.

177. McCann, S. M., and Ramirez, V. D. The neuroendocrine regulation of hypophyseal luteinizing hormone secretion. *Recent Prog. Hormone Res. 20:*131, 1964.

178. McCullagh, E. P., and Schaffenberg, C. A. The role of the seminiferous tubules in the production of hormones. *Ann. N.Y. Acad. Sci. 55:*674, 1952.

179. McSwiney, R. R., Bold, A. M., Brooks, R. V., London, D. R., Middleton, J. E., Mills, I. H., and Prunty, F. T. G. Lack of anabolic effects of C_{19} 17-oxosteroid administered to humans, and some observations on their metabolism. *J. Endocr. 29:*X, 1964.

180. Meeker, C. I. Plasma testosterone levels in pregnancy. *Excerpta Med. Int. Cong. Sr. 111:*174, 1966.

181. Midgley, A. R., Jr. Radioimmunoassay for human follicle-stimulating hormone. *J. Clin. Endocr. 27:*295, 1967.

182. Midgley, A. R., Jr., and Jaffe, R. B. Regulation of human gonadotropins. IV. Correlation of serum concentration of follicle stimulating and luteinizing hormones during the menstrual cycle. *J. Clin. Endocr. 28:*1699, 1968.

183. Midgley, A. R., Jr., and Jaffe, R. B. Regulation of human gonadotropins. II. Disappearance of human chorionic gonadotropin following delivery. *J. Clin. Endocr. 28:*1712, 1968.

184. Migeon, C. J., Keller, A. R., and Holmstrom, E. G. Dehydroepiandrosterone, androsterone and 17-hydroxycorticosteroid levels in maternal and cord plasma in cases of vaginal delivery. *Bull. Hopkins Hosp. 97:*415, 1955.

185. Migeon, C. J., Keller, A. R., Lawrence, B., and Shepard, T. H. Dehydroepiandrosterone and androsterone levels in human plasma. Effect of age and sex: day to day and diurnal variation. *J. Clin. Endocr. 17:*1051, 1957.

186. Mitchell, F. L. "Steroid Metabolism in the Fetoplacental Unit and in Early Childhood." In *Vitamins and Hormones,* R. S. Harris, I. G. Wool, and J. A. Loraine (Eds.), Academic Press, New York, 1967, p. 191.

187. Mizuno, M., Lobotsky, J., Lloyd, C. W., Kobayashi, T., and Murasawa, Y. Plasma androstenedione and testosterone during pregnancy and in the newborn. *J. Clin. Endocr. 82:*1133, 1968.

188. Morato, T., Lemus, A. E., and Gual, C. Efficiency of dehydroepiandrosterone as estrogen precursor. *Steroids* (*Suppl. 1*) *5:*59, 1965.

189. Neher, R., Kahnt, F. W., Roversi, G. D., and Bompiani, A. Steroid transformations *in vitro* by testicular tissue from 2 cases of testicular feminization. *Acta Endocr.* (Kobenhavn) *49:*177, 1965.

190. Neville, M. A., and Webb, J. L. The *in vitro* formation of 3β-hydroxyandrost-5-ene-7, 17-dione by human adrenal glands. *Steroids 6:*421, 1965.

191. Niemi, M., Ikonen, M., and Hervonen, A. "Histochemistry and Fine Structure of the Interstitial Tissue in the Human Foetal Testis." In *Endocrinology of the Testis,* G. E. Wolstenholme and M. O'Connor (Eds.), Little Brown, Boston, 1967, p. 31.

192. Noall, M. W., Alexander, F., and Allen, W. M. Dehydroisoandrosterone synthesis by the human ovary. *Biochim. Biophys. Acta 59:*520, 1962.

193. Odell, W. D., Parlow, A. F., Cargille, C. M., and Ross, G. T. Radioimmunoassay for human follicle-stimulating hormone: physiological studies. *J. Clin. Invest. 47:*2551, 1968.

194. Odell, W. D., Ross, G. T., and Rayford, P. L. Radioimmunoassay for luteinizing hormone in human plasma or serum: physiological studies. *J. Clin. Invest. 46:*248, 1967.

195. Oertel, G. W., and Kaiser, E. Determination of dehydroepiandrosterone, androsterone, etiocholanolone, and 11β-hydroxyetiocholanolone in plasma. *Clin. Chem. Acta 7:*221, 1962.

196. Paulsen, C. A., Gordon, D. L., Carpenter, R. W., Gandy, H. M., and Drucker, W. D. Klinefelter's syndrome and its variant: a hormonal and chromosomal study. *Recent Prog. Hormone Res. 24:*321, 1968.

197. Pearlman, W. H., Cerceo, E., and Thomas, M. Conversion of Δ^5-pregnen-3β-ol-20-one to progesterone by homogenates of human placental tissue. *J. Biol. Chem. 208:*231, 1954.

198. Pearlman, W. H., Crépy, O., and Murphy, M. Testosterone binding levels in the serum of women during the normal menstrual cycle, pregnancy, and the post partum period. *J. Clin. Endocr. 27:*1012, 1967.

199. Pérez-Palacios, G., Pérez, A. E., and Jaffe, R. B. Conversion of pregnenolone-7α-^{3}H-sulfate to other Δ^5-3β-hydroxysteroid sulfates by the human fetal adrenal *in vitro. J. Clin. Endocr. 28:*19, 1968.

200. Peterson, N. T., Midgley, J. R., and Jaffe, R. B. Regulation of human gonadotropins. III. Luteinizing hormone and follicle stimulating hormone in sera from adult males. *J. Clin. Endocr. 28:*1473, 1968.

201. Pierrepoint, C. G., Griffiths, K., Grant, J. K., and Stewart, J. S. S. Neutral steroid sulfation and estrogen biosynthesis *in vitro* by a feminizing Leydig cell tumor of testis. *J. Endocr. 35:*409, 1966.

202. Pincus, G., and Romanoff, E. B. "The Synthesis of Corticosteroids by the Human Adrenal Cortex," In *Ciba Foundation Colloquia on Endocrinology,* Vol. 8, G. E. Wolstenholme (Ed.), Little, Brown, Boston, 1955, p. 97.

203. Pulkkinen, M. O. Arylsulphatase and the hydrolysis of some steroid sulphates in developing organism and placenta. *Acta Physiol. Scand. 52, Suppl. 180:*1, 1961.

204. Raiti, S., and Blizzard, R. M. Measurement of immunologically reactive follicle stimulating hormone in human urine by radioimmunoassay. *J. Clin. Endocr. 28:*1719, 1968.

205. Resko, J. A., and Eik-Nes, K. B. Diurnal testosterone levels in peripheral plasma of human male subjects. *J. Clin. Endocr. 26:*573, 1966.

206. Rice, B. F., Cleveland, W. W., Sandberg, D. H., Ahmad, N., Politano, V. T., and Savard, K. Steroid hormone fromation by testes of a male pseudohermaphrodite. *J. Clin. Endocr. 27:*29, 1967.

207. Rice, B. F., Hammerstein, J., and Savard, K. Steroid hormone formation in the human ovary: III. Action of gonadotropins on testosterone synthesis by normal ovarian stromal tissue. *Steroids 4:*199, 1964.

208. Rice, B. F., Johanson, C. A., Sternberger, W. H. Formation of steroid hormone from acetate-1-^{14}C by a human fetal testes preparation grown in organ culture. *Steroids 7:*79, 1966.

209. Rice, B. F., and Savard, K. Steroid hormone formation in the human ovary: IV. Ovarian stromal compartment; formation of radioactive steroids from acetate-1-C^{14} and action of gonadotropins. *J. Clin. Endocr. 26:*593, 1966.

210. Riondel, A., Tait, J. F., Gut, M., Tait, S. A. S., Joachim, E., and Little, B. Estimation of testosterone in human peripheral blood using ^{35}S thiosemicarbazide. *J. Clin. Endocr. 23:*620, 1963.

211. Rivarola, M. A., Forest, M. G., and Migeon, C. J. Testosterone, androstenedione and dehydroepiandrosterone in plasma during pregnancy and at delivery: concentration and binding. *J. Clin. Endocr. 28:*34, 1968.

212. Rivarola, M. A., and Migeon, C. J. Determination of testosterone and androst-4-ene-3, 17-dione concentration in human plasma. *Steroids 7:*103, 1966.

213. Rivarola, M. A., Saez, J. M., Jones, H. W., Jones, G. S., and Migeon, C. J. The secretion of androgens by the normal, polycystic and neoplastic ovaries. *Johns Hopkins Med. J. 121:*82, 1967.

214. Rivarola, M. A., Saez, J. M., Meyer, W. J., Jenkins, M. E., and Migeon, C. J. Metabolic clearance rate and blood production. Rate of testosterone and androst-4-ene-3, 17-dione under basal conditions. ACTH and HCG stimulation. Comparison with urinary production rate of testosterone. *J. Clin. Endocr. 26:*1208, 1966.

215. Rivarola, M. A., Saez, J. M., Meyer, W. J., Kenny, F. M., Migeon, C. J. Studies of androgens in the syndrome of male psuedohermaphroditism with testicular feminization. *J. Clin. Endocr. 27:*371, 1967.

216. Robel, P., Emiliozzi, R., and Baulieu, E. E. Studies on testosterone metabolism. III. The selective "5β-metabolism of testosterone glucuronide." *J. Biol. Chem. 241:*20, 1966.

217. Roberts, K. D., Bandi, L., Calvin, H. I., Drucker, W. D., and Lieberman, S. Evidence that cholesterol sulfate is a precursor of steroid hormones. *J. Amer. Chem. Soc. 86:*958, 1964.

218. Rosenfeld, R. S., Fukushima, D. K., and Gallagher, T. F. "Metabolism

of Adrenal Cortical Hormones." In *The Adrenal Cortex,* A. B. Eisenstein (Ed.), Little, Brown, Boston, 1967, p. 103.

219. Ryan, G. M., Goss, D. A., and Reid, D. E. Pituitary gonadotropins during long term Enovid therapy. *Amer. J. Obstet. Gynecol. 94:*515, 1966.

220. Ryan, K. J. Conversion of androstenedione to estrone by placental microsomes. *Biochim. Biophys. Acta 27:*658, 1958.

221. Ryan, K. J. Biological aromatization o fsteroids. *J. Biol. Chem. 234:*268, 1959.

222. Ryan, K. J., and Petro, Z. Steroid biosynthesis by human ovarian granulosa and thecal cells. *J. Clin. Endocr. 26:*46, 1966.

223. Ryan, K. J., Petro, Z., and Kaiser, J. Steroid formation of isolated and recombined ovarian granulosa and theca cells. *J. Clin. Endocr. 28:*355, 1968.

224. Ryan, K. J., and Smith, O. W. Biogenesis of estrogens by human ovary. IV. Formation of neutral steroid intermediates. *J. Biol. Chem. 236:*2207, 1961.

225. Ryan, K. J., and Smith, O. W. Biogenesis of steroid hormones in the human ovary. *Recent Prog. Hormone Res. 21:*367, 1965.

226. Saez, J. M., and Bertrand, J. Studies on testicular function in children; plasma concentration of testosterone, dehydroepiandrosterone and its sulfate before and after stimulation with human chorionic gonadotropin. *Steroids 12:*749, 1968.

227. Samuels, L. T., and Uchikawa, T. "Biosynthesis of Adrenal Steroids." In *Adrenal Cortex,* B. Eisenstein (Ed.), Little, Brown, Boston, 1967, p. 61.

228. Sandberg, A. A., Slaunwhite, W. R., Jackson, J. E., and Frawley, T. F. Androgen biosynthesis by ovarian lipoid cell tumor. *J. Clin. Endocr. 22:*929, 1962.

229. Sandberg, E. C., Jenkins, C. R., and Trifon, H. M. Biosynthetic studies of human ovarian arrhenoblastomatous tissue *in vitro.* II. Formation of androgens from dehydroisoandrosterone sulfate. *Steroids 8:*249, 1966.

230. Saroff, J., Keenan, R. E., Sandberg, A. A., and Slaunwhite, W. R. Determination of testosterone, androstenedione and dehydroepiandrosterone in human plasma using bromine[82] *Steroids 10:*15, 1967.

231. Savard, K., Dorfman, R. I., Baggett, B., Fielding, L. L., Engel, L. L., McPherson, H. T., Lister, L. M., Johnson, D. D., Hamblen, E. C., and Engel, F. L. Clinical, morphological and biochemical studies of a virilizing tumor in the testes. *J. Clin. Invest. 39:*534, 1960.

232. Savard, K., Dorfman, R. I., and Poutasse, E. Biogenesis of androgens in the human testes. *J. Clin. Endocr. 12:*935, 1952.

233. Savard, K., Gut, M., Dorfman, R. I., Gabrilove, J. L., and Soffer, L. J. Formation of androgens by human arrhenoblastoma tissue *in vitro. J. Clin. Endocr. 21:*165, 1961.

234. Savard, K., Marsh, J. M., and Rice, B. F. Gonadotropins and ovarian steroidogenesis. *Recent Prog. Hormone Res. 21:*285, 1965.

235. Saxena, B. B., Demura, H., Gandy, H. M., and Peterson, R. E. Radioim-

munoassay of human follicle stimulating and luteinizing hormones in plasma. *J. Clin. Endocr. 28:*519, 1968.

236. Saxena, B. B., Gandy, H. M., and Peterson, R. E. "Radioimmuno-assay of FSH and LH in Body Fluids." In *Gonadotropins 1968,* E. Rosemberg (Ed.), Geron-X, Inc., Los Altos, California, 1968, p. 339.
237. Schalch, D. S., Parlow, A. F., Boon, R. C., and Reichlin, S. Measurement of human luteinizing hormone in plasma by radioimmunoassay. *J. Clin. Invest. 47:*665, 1968.
238. Schindler, A. E., and Ratanasopa, V. Profile of steroids in amniotic fluid of normal and complicated pregnancies. *Acta Endocr.* (Kobenhavn) *59:*239, 1968.
239. Schindler, A. E., and Siiteri, P. K. Isolation and quantitation of steroids from normal human amniotic fluid. *J. Clin. Endocr. 28:*1189, 1968.
240. Schneider, J. J., and Lewbart, M. L. Enzymatic synthesis of steroid sulfates. *J. Biol. Chem. 222:*787, 1956.
241. Schonfeld, W. A. Primary and secondary sexual characteristics: study of their development in males from birth through maturity, with biometric study of penis and testis. *Amer. J. Dis. Child. 65:*535, 1943.
242. Schubert, K., Wehrberger, K., and Frankenberg, G. 6β-hydroxytestosterone and 11β-hydroxytestosterone in human urine. *Steroids 3:*579, 1964.
243. Schwers, J., Govaerts-Videtsky, M., Wiqvist, N., and Diczfalusy, E. Metabolism of estrone sulfate by the previable human foetus. *Acta Endocr.* (Kobenhavn) *50:*597, 1965.
244. Segaloff, A., and Gabbard, R. B. Steroid structure and androgenicity. *Endocrinology 71:*949, 1962.
245. Segaloff, A., Gordon, D. L., Bowers, C. Y., Schlosser, J. V., and Murison, P. H. Hormonal therapy in cancer of the breast. XI. The effect of dehydroepiandrosterone on clinical course and hormonal excretion. *Cancer 10:*1114, 1957.
246. Shimizu, K. Conversion of 20α-hydroxycholesterol *in vitro* to pregnenolone sulfate. *J. Biochem. 59:*430, 1966.
247. Shimizu, K., Shimao, S., and Tanaka, M. Conversion *in vitro* of 20α-hydroxycholesterol to 17α, 20α-dihydroxy cholesterol by human fetal adrenals. *Steroids* (*Suppl. 1*) *5:*85, 1965.
248. Short, R. V. The secretion of sex hormones by the adrenal glands. *Biochem. Soc. Symp. 18:*59, 1960.
249. Siiteri, P. K., and MacDonald, P. C. The utilization of circulating dehydroisoandrosterone sulfate for estrogen synthesis during human pregnancy. *Steroids 2:*713, 1963.
250. Siiteri, P. K., and MacDonald, P. C. Placental estrogen biosynthesis during human pregnancy. *J. Clin. Endocr. 26:*750, 1966.
251. Simmer, H. H., Dignam, W. J., Easterling, W. E., Frankland, M. V., and Naftolin, F. Neutral C_{19} steroids and steroid sulfates in human pregnancy. III. Dehydroepiandrosterone sulfate, 16α-hydroxydehydroepian-

drosterone and 16α-hydroxy-dehydroepiandrosterone sulfate in cord blood and blood of pregnant women with and without treatment with corticoids. *Steroids 8:*179, 1966.

252. Simmer, H. H., Easterling, W. E., Pion, R. J., and Dignam, W. J. Neutral C_{19} steroids and steroid sulfates in human pregnancy. I. Identification of dehydroepiandrosterone sulfate in fetal blood and quantification of this hormone in cord arterial, cord venous and maternal peripheral blood in normal pregnancies. *Steroids 4:*125, 1964.
253. Slaunwhite, W. R., Karsay, M. A., Hollmer, A., Sandberg, A. A., and Niswander, K. Fetal liver as an endocrine tissue. *Steroids* (*Suppl. 2*) *6:*211, 1965.
254. Slaunwhite, W. R., Sandberg, A. A., Jackson, J. E., and Staubitz, W. J. Effects of estrogen and HCG on androgen synthesis by human testes. *J. Clin. Endocr. 22:*992, 1962.
255. Slaunwhite, W. R., Sandberg, A. A., Staubitz, W. J., Jackson, J. E., and Koepf, G. F. Synthesis of testosterone by subjects with gonadal dysgenesis and XXY chromosome constitution. *J. Clin. Endocr. 22:*989, 1968.
256. Smith, E. R., Breuer, H., and Schriefers, H. A study of the steroid metabolism of an interstitial cell tumor of the testis. *Biochem. J. 93:*583, 1964.
257. Smith, O. W., and Ryan, K. J. Estrogen in the human ovary. *Amer. J. Obstet. Gynec. 84:*141, 1962.
258. Solomon, S. Formation and metabolism of neutral steroids in the human placenta and fetus. *J. Clin. Endocr. 26:*762, 1966.
259. Solomon, S., Carter, A. C., and Lieberman, S. The conversion *in vivo* of 17α-hydroxy-pregnenolone to dehydroisoandrosterone and other 17-ketosteroids. *J. Biol. Chem. 235:*351, 1960.
260. Solomon, S., Lanman, J. T., Lind, J., and Lieberman, S. The biosynthesis of Δ^4-androstenedione and 17α-hydroxy-progesterone from progesterone by surviving human fetal adrenals. *J. Biol. Chem. 233:*1084, 1958.
261. Southern, A. L., Gordon, G. G., and Tochimoto, S. Further study of factors affecting the metabolic clearance of testosterone in man. *J. Clin. Endocr. 28:*1105, 1968.
262. Southern, A. L., Ross, H., Sharma, D. C., Gordon, G., Weingold, A. B., and Dorfman, R. I. Plasma concentration and biosynthesis of testosterone in the syndrome of feminizing testes. *J. Clin. Endocr. 25:*518, 1965.
263. Southern, A. L., Tochimoto, S., Carmody, N. C., and Isurugi, K. Plasma production rates of testosterone in normal adult men and women and in patients with the syndrome of feminizing testes. *J. Clin. Endocr. 25:*1441, 1965.
264. Tait, J. F., and Horton, R. "The *in vivo* Estimation of Blood Production and Interconversion Rates of Androstenedione and the Calculation of Their Secretion Rates." In *Steroid Dynamics,* G. Pincus, T. Nakao, and J. F. Tait (Eds.), Academic Press, New York, 1966. p. 393.

265. TAYMOR, M. L. Effect of synthetic progestins on pituitary gonadotropin excretion. *J. Clin. Endocr. 24:*803, 1964.

266. TAYMOR, M. L., AONO, T., and PHETEPLACE, C. "Serum Levels of FSH and LH by radioimmunoassay." In *Gonadotropins 1968,* E. Rosemberg (Ed.), Geron-X, Inc., Los Altos, California, 1968, p. 349.

267. UNGAR, F., and DORFMAN, R. I. Incorporation of C^{14} in the urinary steroids. *J. Biol. Chem. 205:*125, 1953.

268. VANDE WIELE, R. L., DYRENFURTH, I., and GURPIDE, E. "Estimation of the Rates of Secretion of the Ovarian Hormones by Isotope Dilution Methods." In *Clinical Endocrinology,* Vol. 2, E. B. Astwood and C. E. Cassidy (Eds.), Grune & Stratton, New York, 1968, p. 603.

269. VANDE WIELE, R. L., MACDONALD, P. C., GURPIDE, E., and LIEBERMAN, S. Studies on the secretion and interconversion of the androgens. *Recent Prog. Hormone Res. 19:*275, 1963.

270. VIHKO, R. Gas chromatographic mass spectrometric studies of solvolyzable steroids in human plasma. *Acta Endocr.* (Kobenhavn) (*Suppl.*) *109:*1, 1966.

271. VILLEE, D. B., and DRISCOLL, S. G. Pregnenolone and progesterone metabolism in human adrenals from twin female fetuses. *Endocrinology 77:*602, 1965.

272. VILLEE, C. A., and LORING, J. M. Synthesis of steroids in the newborn human adrenals *in vitro. J. Clin. Endocr. 25:*307, 1965.

273. VILLEE, C. A., LORING, J. M., and VILLEE, D. B. Synthesis of dehydroepiandrosterone and 16-hydroxy-pregnenolone. *Excerpta Med. Int. Cong. Sr. 51:*143, 1962.

274. VILLEE, D. B., ROTMER, H., KLIMAN, B., BRIEFER, C., and FEDERMAN, D. D. Androgen synthesis in a patient with virilizing adrenocortical carcinoma. *J. Clin. Endocr. 27:*1112, 1968.

275. VILLEE, D. B., and VILLEE, C. A. Synthesis of corticosteroids in the fetal-placental unit. *Excerpta Med. Int. Cong. Sr. 83:*709, 1964.

276. WARREN, J. C., and CHEATUM, S. G. Demonstration of a steroid 17-20 demolase in the human placenta. *Canad. J. Biochem. 42:*143, 1964.

277. WARREN, J. C., and FRENCH, A. P. Distribution of steroid sulfatase in human tissues. *J. Clin. Endocr. 25:*278, 1965.

278. WARREN, J. C., and SALHANICK, H. A. Steroid biosynthesis in the human ovary. *J. Clin. Endocr. 21:*1218, 1961.

279. WARREN, J. C., and TIMBERLAKE, C. E. Steroid sulfatase in human placenta. *J. Clin. Endocr. 22:*1148, 1962.

280. WARREN, J. C., and TIMBERLAKE, C. E. Biosynthesis of estrogens in pregnancy: precursor role of plasma dehydroisoandrosterone. *Obstet. Gynecol. 23:*689, 1964.

281. WEINHEIMER, B., OERTEL, G. W., LEPPLA, W., BLAISE, H., and BETTE, L. Plasma concentrations of adrenal venous blood from women with and without hirsutism. *Excerpta Med. Int. Cong. Sr. 111:*309, 1966.

282. WENGLE, B. Distribution of some steroid sulphokinases in foetal human tissues. *Acta Endocr.* (Kobenhavn) *52:*607, 1966.

283. WIELAND, R. C., DE COURCY, C., LEVY, P. R., ZALA, A. P., and HIRSCHMANN, H. $C_{19}O_2$ steroids and some of their precursors in blood from normal human adrenals. *J. Clin. Invest. 44:*159, 1965.

284. WIEST, W. G., ZANDER, J., and HOLMSTROM, E. G. Metabolism of progesterone-4-C^{14} by an arrhenoblastoma. *J. Clin. Endocr. 19:*297, 1959.

285. WILSON, R., BIRD, C. E., WIQVIST, N., SOLOMON, S., and DICZFALUSY, E. Metabolism of progesterone by the perfused adrenalectomized human fetus. *J. Clin. Endocr. 26:*1155, 1966.

Chapter Six

Cortisol

Ralph E. Peterson

The adrenal cortex secretes corticoids (C_{21} steroids with three or more oxygen atoms), progestins (C_{21} steroids with two or more oxygen atoms), androgens (C_{19} steroids with two or more oxygen atoms), and estrogens (C_{18} steroids with a phenolic A ring).

The major biological activities of the adrenal cortical steroids may be classified into: (1) those influencing the intermediary metabolism of carbohydrate, protein, and lipids and suppressing certain inflammatory processes; (2) those effecting electrolyte transport; (3) those with androgenic action; and (4) those with estrogenic action. The first group are the glucocorticoids. In man, cortisol and corticosterone make up the major fraction of glucocorticoids, although cortisol accounts for most of the activity. The second group includes aldosterone and desoxycorticosterone; the former accounts for most of the mineralocorticoid activity. The adrenal cortex also synthesizes the three classes of sex steroids—estrogens, androgens, and progestins—although the functional significance of their adrenal secretion is unclear. The estrogens and progestins are not normally secreted in amounts that significantly influence biological activity. It is not certain whether the adrenal cortex secretes the estrogens or forms precursors which are converted to estrogens within the adrenals or in other tissues. In females, adrenal secretion accounts for most of the androgen production, whereas in males, even though the adrenal secretes neutral C_{19} steroids, the testes account for most of the androgenic activity. The adrenals are the only endocrine glands in which all of these five groups of steroid hormones have been detected with certainty.

METABOLISM OF CORTISOL

Emphasis is placed on cortisol metabolism because this steroid constitutes the major glucocorticoid secreted by the human adrenal cortex and is the major glucocorticoid in the peripheral blood. In the normal adult, 8–25 mg of cortisol are produced per day,[53] and this figure probably closely approximates the daily rate of adrenal secretion of cortisol. Cortisol exists in the plasma in three different physical-chemical states: (1) free or unbound in aqueous solution, (2) albumin-bound, and (3) globulin glycoprotein-bound (transcortin).[7,11,12,19,40,61,70] In normal subjects with a normal plasma cortisol level, about 90 per cent of the cortisol is protein-bound; approximately 10 per cent is bound to albumin, and 80 per cent to transcortin.[64] The 7–9 A.M. plasma cortisol level as measured by a modified Porter-Silber method[49] is 6–25 μg/100 ml (mean: 13 μg/100 ml); however, the level as measured with a selective isotope dilution procedure, is 5–20 μg/100 ml (mean: 11.5 μg/100 ml).[47] At concentrations exceeding 20 μg/100 ml, transcortin is completely saturated, and 70–80 per cent of the excess cortisol binds to serum albumin. The importance of the steroid protein-binding resides in the effects that this may have on the distribution, transport, excretion, and biotransformation of the steroid.[18] The extravascular or tissue concentration of cortisol will depend as much upon the concentration and properties of the plasma protein or proteins with which it is bound as upon the concentrations of the steroid. This is because at lower transcortin concentrations within the extracellular fluid the total concentration of cortisol is lower. If the transcortin-bound steroid represents an inactive transport complex, then it is likely that only the non-transcortin-bound steroid is biologically active, and the transcortin would normally be expected to protect the tissues from abnormally high levels of cortisol.

The secretion of cortisol is determined by the rate of release of adrenocorticotropin (ACTH) by the adenohypophysis. The rate of release of ACTH represents the balance between the excitatory influence of the central nervous system and the inhibitory influence of the cortisol on pituitary or hypothalamic centers.[71] A fall in plasma non-protein-bound cortisol leads to increased ACTH secretion, and a rise inhibits such secretion. This negative feedback control of ACTH secretion maintains the circulating plasma level within rather narrow limits.

The basal rate of secretion of ACTH in man is estimated to be about one unit per day,[16] and the 8 A.M. plasma concentration is estimated at 0.25 mU/100 ml.[44] The plasma ACTH and cortisol concentrations show a constant pattern of cyclic variation within an approximate 24-hour period in normal persons not subjected to stress.[44] The plasma levels are highest between the hours of 7–9 A.M. and decline slowly thereafter to the lowest values at midnight. This circadian rhythm is dependent on the sleep-wake pattern and independent of food intake, exercise, or light.[46]

Cortisol is distributed in an intra- and extra-vascular miscible pool of 10–15 liters[53] which contains 1–2 mg of cortisol. The fractional turnover is 0.5 pools per hour, or a turnover of approximately 10 pools per day. The metabolic clearance rate is about 200 liters per day[64] and the maximum hepatic plasma extraction is about 20 liters per day. Following rapid intravenous administration of cortisol, the steroid disappears promptly from the plasma; when infused at different concentrations, it disappears from the plasma at rates approximately proportional to its concentration.[54] This results in linear concentration-time relationships when plotted on a semilogarithmic scale; the biological half-life of the steroid can be calculated from such considerations. If the plasma and tissue levels have equilibrated, the half-time of disappearance of the steroid from the plasma (pool) is equivalent to the time required for the plasma concentration to fall from some initial value to half that value, and is inversely related to the factional turnover rate. Following the rapid infusion of 50–400 mg of cortisol, the half-time of disappearance of steroid from the plasma is 1.5–2 hours; however, the rapid infusion of a trace amount of radioactive labeled cortisol yields a more rapid disappearance rate (90 minutes).

EXCRETION

Neither the quantitative nor the qualitative aspects of urinary excretion of the steroids depend wholly upon the rate of secretion of the steroids by the adrenal; many non-endocrine factors influence the amount and nature of the urinary steroid metabolites. During metabolism, certain of the structural differences between the various steroid hormones tend to be eliminated, and thus may obscure the nature of the true precursor or precursors of any given urinary metabolite. There is little information to suggest that the catabolic fate of the steroids is related to their physiological or biochemical functions as hormones. However, the rate of metabolism and the nature of the metabolites, both quantitative and qualitative, afford significant information regarding the in vivo rate of production and peripheral interconversion of various steroids.

The major route of excretion of cortisol and its metabolites is via the urine. Normal subjects excrete over 90 per cent of intravenously administered radioactive labeled hormone as urinary metabolites within 72 hours. [10, 20, 22, 26, 27, 39, 54, 60] By far the largest fraction of radioactivity appears within the first 12 hours and about 70 per cent within 24 hours. Only a small fraction is excreted as labeled metabolites extracted directly with dichloromethane, and less than 0.5 per cent of an injected tracer quantity is recovered as unaltered cortisol. Approximately 3 per cent is recovered in the feces, and since this is only slightly less than the quantity present in the bile, it indicates that the bile is probably the major source of the fecal products.[27,39,54]

Trace amounts of cortisol may be eliminated by urinary and biliary excretion and enzymatic inactivation in various tissues of the body. Enzymatic transformation by the liver, however, is the major means of disposal.

The enzymatic mechanisms that contribute to the disposal of cortisol may be deduced from the nature of the urinary metabolites. From such studies, the major metabolites of cortisol have been identified, and these account for 80–90 per cent of the metabolized steroid.[22] About 4 per cent of an administered dose of labeled steroid appears in the urine as unconjugated products, and 60–70 per cent appears as metabolites which can be hydrolyzed by β-glucuronidase. Only about 0.5 per cent of the administered steroid escapes transformation and is excreted unchanged. An equivalent amount is also excreted as cortisone. These metabolites represent about 75 per cent of the total urinary radioactivity, and thus 25 per cent remains as labeled products not extracted by dichloromethane after glucuronidase hydrolysis. Thus, approximately two-thirds of the metabolites can be accounted for as known compounds. Cortisol is converted in small amounts to at least seven different 17-ketosteroids of the 11-oxygenated type.[5,6,56] If the fraction metabolized as C_{19}, 17-ketosteroids is subtracted, about 60 per cent remains as known C_{21} steroids. All of these are ketogenic and are estimated with the urinary 17-ketogenic steroid assays,[1] whereas approximately 40 per cent retain the dihydroxyacetone side chain, and are estimated as Porter-Silber chromagens.[54] Thus, the urinary 17-ketogenic steroid assay accounts for slightly more than one-half of the total daily production of cortisol, and the Porter-Silber assay accounts for approximately one-third of the total cortisol production.

CORTISOL METABOLISM DURING PREGNANCY

Marked changes in steroid metabolism take place during pregnancy. These effects result from the appearance of a new endocrine organ, the placenta and fetus. The alterations may be attributed to: (1) the effects of altered levels of certain steroids on both the biosynthesis of adrenal steroids and the hepatic and extrahepatic catabolism of these steroids;

(2) changes in rate of secretion of various steroids by the maternal adrenal and ovaries; (3) the influence of the fetal adrenal on steroid hormone production and metabolism; and (4) the influence of the placenta on steroid metabolism. The fetus and the placenta function as a physiological unit with regard to steroid metabolism and elimination of one significantly alters the function of the other.

Cortisol metabolism is significantly altered during pregnancy, and the plasma cortisol level rises progressively throughout pregnancy,[9, 23, 34] but the normal circadian rhythm persists.[9] The plasma level of transcortin also rises progressively, from about 3 to 7 mg/100 ml throughout pregnancy.[17]

There is either no change or only a slight increase in the urinary levels of cortisol metabolites.[2, 9, 34, 65] A more recent study shows that subjects in mid- and late pregnancy have decreased urinary 17-hydroxysteroids and a decreased rate of cortisol secretion.[37] There is, however, a small but progressive increase in the urinary excretion of the unconjugated polar metabolites of cortisol during pregnancy.[43]

The normal (or high normal) levels of urinary free cortisol during the latter half of pregnancy lend support to the thesis that there is little or no increase in plasma free cortisol.[28] Attention has centered around unbound cortisol as the biologically active steroid because of its correlation with the clinical status of the patient and in vitro studies.[58, 62] In addition, pregnant women do not manifest the signs and symptoms of hypercorticism (Cushing's syndrome). Controversy persists, however, regarding the amount of unbound cortisol in either estrogen-treated subjects or in pregnant women.[15, 57]

Following infusion of labeled or unlabeled cortisol, especially near term, there is a significant prolongation of the plasma half-time.[8, 9, 34, 36] The calculated metabolic clearance rate of the free and albumin-bound cortisol is thus reduced,[71] but without alteration in hepatic blood flow.[42] This may be interpreted as due to either increased protein-binding of the cortisol or some hormonally induced effect on the liver enzymes that transform the cortisol.[31] Either or both of these effects are most likely due to the high plasma levels of estrogen, especially in late pregnancy. Many of these alterations in cortisol metabolism can be induced by administration of estrogens to normal adult males or females.[50]

Radioactive labeled cortisol administered to mothers prior to delivery can be recovered in the infants at birth, and the ratio of free labeled cortisol in maternal blood to that in cord blood is approximately 3:1.[36] This is similar to the ratio of the free endogenous plasma cortisol in the maternal and cord plasma.[38] The fetal plasma contains a lower concentration of transcortin than the plasma of nonpregnant females,[59] but the cortisol-binding affinity is the same.[14] Thus, there would appear to be no need for cortisol synthesis by the fetus, although in vitro incubations of the fetal adrenals reveal that the fetus is capable of synthesizing all of the important corticosteroids, especially cortisol.[3,67,68] The plasma cortisol level in the cord blood of the anencephalic fetus is similar to that of the normal fetus,[45] and since the adrenal cortex of the anencephalic infant is atrophic, it can be inferred that fetal cortisol is largely of maternal origin. The placenta does not synthesize cortisol. The concentration of cortisol metabolites conjugated as glucuronides is higher in the cord plasma, and thus the fetus has the capacity for metabolic transformation of cortisol.[35]

EFFECT OF ESTROGENS ON CORTISOL METABOLISM

Estrogen treatment of men and women produces changes in cortisol metabolism similar to those seen in pregnancy. After the second month of pregnancy, there is a marked progressive rise in estrogen production, and therefore it seems reasonable to attribute the alteration in cortisol metabolism during pregnancy to high plasma estrogen levels.

The administration of synthetic estrogens (i.e., stilbestrol, 5–10 mg/day, or ethinyl estradiol, 0.1 or 0.5 mg/day) to normal males or females produces an elevation in the level of plasma cortisol.[24,32,41,50,55,69] Following chronic administration, the effect persists for 3–4 weeks after discontinuing the estrogens. The urinary 17-hydroxycorticosteriod excretion may be decreased by as much as 50 per cent; however, this effect may not be apparent for 10 days to 2 weeks following administration of the estrogens.[24,32,50,55] The urinary free cortisol concentration has been reported to decline[50] or remain unchanged[24] after estrogen treatment. Long continued administration of the estrogens produces little or no effect on urinary excretion of the 17-ketosteroids.[25,50]

Estrogen therapy does not abolish the diurnal changes in plasma cortisol concentration.[24,55] Following injection of ACTH into subjects treated with estrogen, the plasma cortisol and corticosterone concentrations show a further two- to four-fold increase.[50] After administration of labeled cortisol[41,50,55,69] or corticosterone[50] there is a marked prolongation of the biological half-time of the labeled steroid. However, after administration of cortisone, dihydrocortisol, or tetrahydrocortisol, there is little alteration in the clearance of these from the plasma.[50]

There is no significant change in the fraction of radioactive cortisol or corticosterone excreted in the urine after estrogen therapy, and no significant differences in the fraction of administered steroid excreted as the tetrahydrosteroid metabolite conjugated with glucuronic acid.[32,50] The estrogens markedly reduce the metabolic clearance rate of cortisol and the fractional removal by the liver. Estrogen-treated subjects show an increase in the size of the miscible cortisol pool with a decrease in the fraction of the pool turned over per hour,[50] and a 30–35 per cent decrease in the rate of turnover of cortisol.[24,29,32,41,50,55] Similar changes are noted for the rate of turnover of corticosterone.[51]

Estrogen treatment causes a marked increase in the concentration of plasma transcortin and therefore the binding capacity of the plasma for cortisol and corticosterone.[13,29,32,41,50,53] This is not associated with any change in the affinity of cortisol for transcortin.[14,63] It has been proposed that the increase in plasma protein-binding of cortisol explains the decreased rate of hepatic extraction of plasma cortisol. However, estrogen treatment is not associated with a decrease in the free, or albumin-bound cortisol, and thus it seems more likely that estrogens in some way influence the hepatic enzymatic reactions involved in the inactivation of cortisol. This view is supported by the evidence that estrogens inhibit cortisol metabolism in vitro.[31] It would not seem reasonable to postulate a competitive inhibition between cortisol and the estrogens at an enzymatic level, since the defect in biotransformation persists for weeks after the estrogen is discontinued. The estrogen therapy in some manner may alter the level of one of the hepatic coenzymes or NAPH-linked steroid dehydrogenases required for the enzymatic inactivation of steroid. It seems most likely that the estrogens alter the activity of the Δ^4 reductases, particularly the specific cortisol Δ^4 reductase, as evidenced by the failure of the estrogens to alter cortisone metabolism.[52] Also, the estrogens do not seem to influence the level of activity of the 3α-hydroxysteroid dehydrogenase or the rate of glucuronide conjugation of tetrahydrocortisol.[32,50] With very small doses of estrogen, it is possible to demonstrate a delay in the plasma clearance of cortisol in the presence of normal levels of plasma transcortin and cortisol.[32] This would lend support to the concept that the decreased removal rate is not related to the increased plasma protein binding, but rather to an effect of the estrogen upon hepatic enzyme systems.

The absence of any sign of hypercorticism (Cushing's syndrome) has been explained as due to the protective effect of the increased protein-binding to transcortin which makes the cortisol less available for catabolic or physiologic sites.[60,62] Kinetic studies of the disposition of labeled cortisol have demonstrated that estrogens cause a marked increase in the intravascular cortisol pool, but little change in the larger extravascular pool.[4] ACTH increases both pools. Free urinary cortisol reflects the level of unbound plasma cortisol, and thus the absence of increased urinary free cortisol during estrogen therapy[24] supports the concept that there is little or no increase in the plasma level of free cortisol, but rather a decrease in the fraction of unbound plasma cortisol.[41,50,59] Also the concentration of unbound cortisol, as measured by ultra-filtration in vivo (dialysis) in patients with renal insufficiency, does not change during estrogen treatment.[15] This undoubtedly explains the absence of signs and symptoms of hypercorticism in estrogen-treated subjects and in pregnancy. The decrease in rate of secretion of cortisol may suggest that there may be a small increase in unbound cortisol during treatment with estrogens, although a possible inhibitory effect of the estrogens on adrenal biosynthesis of cortisol has not been excluded. Subjects receiving estrogens respond normally to small suppressive doses of the synthetic glucocorticoid, dexamethasone.[24] It is of interest that 19-nor-17α-ethyl testosterone delays the disappearance of infused cortisol from the plasma but does not affect the plasma cortisol level.[32]

Estrogens increase the urinary excretion of 6β-hydroxycortisol. This probably indicates utilization of an alternate pathway for cortisol metabolism secondary to a possible suppression of the normal pathway for inactivation of cortisol through the Δ^4 steroid reductases.[30] Part of the increase in 6β-hydroxylation of cortisol following estrogen therapy may be due to an estrogen-induced activation of the 6β-hydroxylase, rather than an increase in 6β-hydroxylation secondary to utilization of an alternate pathway for metabolic disposal. It is also of interest that the normal urinary 6β-hydroxycortisol excretion is slightly higher in the female than in the male.[30] Other situations in which hepatic removal of cortisol is decreased, e.g., pregnancy,[21] cirrhosis,[48] and in the neonate,[66] are also associated with increased urinary excretion of 6β-hydroxycortisol. The in vitro conversion of labeled cortisol to tetrahydrocortisol and tetrahydrocortisone is depressed by estrogens while 6β-hydroxylation is increased.[33]

The 19-nor steroids used for contraceptive purposes are progestational steroids which may also possess slight intrinsic estrogenic activity and are combined with small amounts of synthetic estrogen. Enovid contains norethynodrel (98.5 per cent) and ethinyl estradiol, 3-methyl ether (1.5 per cent), and each of the steroids included in this preparation have a marked estrogenic effect on cortisol metabolism, i.e., increased plasma levels and increased plasma protein binding of cortisol, with a decreased excretion of urinary 17-hydroxycorticosteroids.[32] Both steroids produce a decrease in the rate of secretion of cortisol; however, progesterone alone does not alter the rate of cortisol secretion.[32]

REFERENCES

1. Appleby, J. I., Gibson, G., Norymberski, J. K., and Stubbs, R. D. Indirect analysis of Corticosteroids I. The Determination of 17-Hydroxy-corticosteroids. *Biochem. J. 60:*453, 1955.

2. Appleby, J. I., and Norymberski, J. K. The urinary excretion of 17-hydroxycorticosteroids in human pregnancy. *J. Endocr. 15:*310, 1957.

3. Bloch, E., and Benirschke, K. Synthesis in vitro of steroids by human fetal adrenal gland slices. *J. Biol. Chem. 234:*1085, 1959.

4. Bradley, E. M., and Waterhouse, C. Effect of estrogen administration on extra-vascular cortisol. *J. Clin. Endocr. 26:*705, 1966.

5. Burstein, S., Savard, K., and Dorfman, R. I. The vivo metabolism of hydrocortisone. *Endocrinology 53:*88, 1953.

6. Burstein, S., Savard, K., and Dorfman, R. I. The vivo metabolism of cortisone. *Endocrinology 52:*448, 1953.

7. Bush, I. E. The physicochemical state of cortisol in blood. In Hormones in Blood. *Ciba Found. Colloq. Endocr. 11:*263, 1957.

8. Christy, N. P., Wallace, E. Z., Gordon, W. E. L., and Jailer, J. W. On the rate of hydrocortisone clearance from plasma in pregnant women and in patients with Laennec's cirrhosis. *J. Clin. Invest. 38:*299, 1959.

9. Cohen, M., Stiefel, M., Reddy, W. J., and Laidlaw, J. C. The secretion and disposition of cortisol during pregnancy. *J. Clin. Endocr. 78:*1076, 1958.

10. Cope, C. L., and Black, E. G. The behavior of C^{14}-cortisol and estimation of cortisol production rate in man. *Clin. Sci. 17:*147, 1958.

11. Daughaday, W. H. Evidence for two corticosteroid binding systems in human plasma. *J. Lab. Clin. Med. 48:*799, 1956.

12. Daughaday, W. H. Steroid protein interactions. *Physiol. Rev. 39:*885, 1959.

13. Daughaday, W. H., Holloszy, J., and Mariz, I. K. Binding of corticosteroids by plasma proteins. VI. The binding of cortisol and aldosterone by corticosteroid-binding globulin and by the estrogen-induced binding system of plasma. *J. Clin. Endocr. 21:*53, 1961.

14. DeMoor, P., and Heyns, W. Cortisol binding affinity of plasma transcortin (CBA) as studied by competitive absorption. *J. Clin. Endocr. 28:*1281, 1968.

15. DeMoor, P., Verbenckmoes, R., and Heyns, W. Unbound plasma cortisol measured by ultrafiltration in vivo: effect of estrogen treatment. *J. Clin. Endocr. 28:*313, 1968.

16. DiRaimondo, V., and Island, D. Studies of the kinetics of the adrenocortical response to corticotropin. *J. Clin. Endocr. 15:*856, 1955.

17. Doe, R. P., Fernandex, R., and Seal, V. S. Measurement of corticosteroid-binding globulin in man. *J. Clin. Endocr. 24:*1029, 1964.

18. Doe, R. P., Zinneman, H. H., Flink, E. B., and Ulstrom, R. A. Significance of the concentration of non protein-bound plasma cortisol in normal subjects, Cushing's syndrome, pregnancy and during estrogen therapy. *J. Clin. Endocr. 20:*1484, 1960.

19. Eik-Nes, K., Schellman, J. A., Lumry, R., and Samuels, L. T. The binding of steroids to protein. I. Solubility determinations. *J. Biol. Chem. 206:*411, 1954.

20. Flood, C., Layne, D. S., Ramcharan, S., Rossipal, E., Tait, J. F., and Tait, S. A. S. An investigation of the urinary metabolites and secretion

rates of aldosterone and cortisol in man and a description of methods for their measurement. *Acta Endocr.* (Kobenhavn) *36:*237, 1961.

21. Franz, A. G., Katz, F. H., and Jailer, J. W. 6-β-hydroxy-cortisol: High levels in human urine in pregnancy and toxemia. *Proc. Soc. Exp. Biol. Med. 105:*41, 1960.
22. Fukushima, D. K., Bradlow, H. L., Hellman, L., Zumoff, B., and Gallagher, T. F. Metabolic transformation of hydrocortisone-4-C^{14} in normal men. *J. Biol. Chem. 235:*2246, 1960.
23. Gemzell, C. A. Blood levels of 17-hydroxycorticosteroids in normal pregnancy. *J. Clin. Endocr. 13:*898, 1953.
24. Grant, S. D., Pavlatos, F. C., and Forsham, P. H. Effect of estrogen therapy on cortisol metabolism. *J. Clin. Endocr. 25:*1057, 1965.
25. Halkerston, I. D. K., Hillman, J., Palmer, D., and Rimdca, A. Changes in the excretion pattern of neutral 17-ketosteroids during oestrogen administration to male subjects. *J. Endocr. 13:*433, 1956.
26. Hellman, L., Bradlow, H. L., Adesman, J., Fukushima, D. K., Kulp, J. L., and Gallagher, T. F. The fate of hydrocortison-4-C-14 in man. *J. Clin. Invest. 33:*1106, 1954.
27. Hellman, L., Bradlow, H. L., Frazell, E. I., and Gallagher, T. F. Tracer studies of the absorption and fate of steroid hormones in man. *J. Clin. Invest. 35:*1033, 1956.
28. Jones, K. M., Lloyd-Jones, R., Riondel, A., Tait, J. F., Tait, S. A. S., Bulbrook R. D., and Greenwood, F. C. Aldosterone secretion and metabolism in normal men and women and in pregnancy. *Acta Endocr.* (Kobenhavn) *30:*321, 1959.
29. Katz, F. H., and Kappas, A. The effect of estradiol and estriol on plasma levels of cortisol and thyroid hormone-binding globulins and on aldosterone and cortisol secretion rates in man. *J. Clin. Invest. 46:*1768, 1967.
30. Katz, F. H., Lipman, M. M., Frantz, A. G., and Jailer, J. W. The physiological significance of 6-β hydroxycortisol in human corticoid metabolism. *J. Clin. Endocr. 22:*71, 1962.
31. Kumagai, A., Otomo, M., Yano, S., Takuchi, N., Nishino, K., Ueda, H., Ko, S., and Kitamura, M. Inhibition of cortisol metabolism in the liver by other steroids. *Endocrin. Jap.* (Tokyo) *6:*85, 1959.
32. Layne, D. S., Meyer, C. J., Vaishwanar, P. S., and Pincus, G. The secretion and metabolism of cortisol and aldosterone in normal and in steroid treated women. *J. Clin. Endocr. 22:*107, 1962.
33. Lipman, M. M., Katz, F. H., and Jailer, J. W. An alternate pathway for cortisol metabolism; 6-β hydroxycortisol production by human tissue slices. *J. Clin. Endocr. 22:*268, 1962.
34. Martin, J. D., and Mills, I. H. The effects of pregnancy on adrenal steroid metabolism. *Clin. Sci. 17:*137, 1958.
35. Migeon, C. J., Bertrand, J., and Gemzell, C. A. The transplacental passage of various steroid hormones in mid-pregnancy. *Recent Prog. Hormone Res. 17:*207, 1961.
36. Migeon, C. J., Bertrand, J., and Wall, P. E. Physiological disposition of 4-C-14 cortisol during late pregnancy. *J. Clin. Invest. 36:*1350, 1957.

37. Migeon, C. J., Kenny, F. M., and Taylor, F. H. Cortisol production rate. VIII. Pregnancy. *J. Clin. Endocr. 28:*661, 1968.

38. Migeon, C. J., Prystowsky, H., Grumbach, M., and Byron, M. C. Placental passage of 17-hydroxycorticosteroids: comparison of the levels in maternal and fetal plasma and effect of ACTH and hydrocortisone administration. *J. Clin. Invest. 35:*488, 1956.

39. Migeon, C. J., Sandberg, A. A., Deckern, H. A., Smith, D. F., Paul, A. C., and Samuels, L. T. Metabolism of 4-C-14 cortisol in man: body distribution and rates of conjugation. *J. Clin. Endocr. 16:*1137, 1956.

40. Mills, I. H. Transport and metabolism of steroids. *Brit. Med. Bull. 18:*127, 1962.

41. Mills, I. H., Schedl, H. P., Chen, P. S., Jr., and Bartter, F. C. The effect of estrogen administration on the metabolism and protein binding of hydrocortisone. *J. Clin. Endocr. 20:*515, 1960.

42. Munnell, G. W., and Taylor, H. C. Liver blood flow in pregnancy—hepatic vein catherization. *J. Clin. Invest. 26:*952, 1947.

43. Nadel, E. M., Young, B. G., Hilgarn, A. G., and Burstein, S. Urinary excretion of free polar corticosteroid. *J. Lab. Clin. Med. 63:*44, 1964.

44. Ney, R. L., Shimizu, N., Nicholson, W. E., Island, D. P., and Liddle, G. W. Correlation of plasma ACTH concentration with adrenocortical response in normal human subjects, surgical patients and patients with Cushing's disease. *J. Clin. Invest. 42:*1669, 1963.

45. Nichols, J., Lescure, O. L., and Migeon, C. J. Levels of 17-hydroxycorticosteroid and 17-ketosteroids in maternal and cord plasma in term anencephaly. *J. Clin. Endocr. 18:*144, 1958.

46. Orth, D. N., Island, D. P., and Liddle, G. W. Experimental alteration of circadian rhythm in plasma cortisol (17-OHCS) concentration in man. *J. Clin. Endocr. 27:*549, 1967.

47. Peterson, R. E. Metabolism of adrenocorticosteroids in man. *Ann. N.Y. Acad. Sci. 82:*846, 1959.

48. Peterson, R. E. Adrenocortical steroid metabolism and adrenal cortical function in liver disease. *J. Clin. Invest. 39:*320, 1960.

49. Peterson, R. E., Karrer, A., and Guerra, S. I. Evaluation of the Silber-Porter procedure for the determination of plasma hydrocortisone. *Anal. Chem. 29:*144, 1957.

50. Peterson, R. E., Nokes, G., Chen, P. S., Jr., and Black, R. L. Estrogens and adrenocortical function in man. *J. Clin. Endocr. 20:*495, 1960.

51. Peterson, R. E., and Pierce, C. E. The metabolism of corticosterone in man. *J. Clin. Invest. 39:*741, 1960.

52. Peterson, R. E., Pierce, C. E., Wyngaarden, J. B. Bunim, J. J., and Brodie, B. B. The physiological disposition and metabolic fate of cortisone in man. *J. Clin. Invest. 36:*1301, 1957.

53. Peterson, R. E., and Wyngaarden, J. B. The miscible pool and turnover rate of hydrocortisone in man. *J. Clin. Invest. 35:*552, 1956.

54. Peterson, R. E., Wyngaarden, J. B., Guerra, S. L., Brodie, B. B., and Bunim, J. J. The physiological disposition and metabolic fate of hydrocortisone in man. *J. Clin. Invest. 34:*1779, 1955.

55. Robertson, M. E., Stiefel, M., and Laidlaw, J. C. The influence of estrogen on the secretion disposition and biologic activity of cortisol. *J. Clin. Endocr. 19:*1381, 1959.

56. Sandberg, A. A., Chang, E., and Slaunwhite, W. R., Jr. The conversion of 4-C^{14} cortisol to C^{14}-17-ketosteroids. *J. Clin. Endocr. 17:*437, 1957.

57. Sandberg, A. A., Rosenthal, H., Schneider, S. L., and Slaunwhite, W. R., Jr. In *Steroid Dynamics,* G. Pincus, T. Nakoa, and J. F. Tait (Eds.), Academic Press, New York, 1966, p. 1.

58. Sandberg, A. A., and Slaunwhite, W. R., Jr. Differences in metabolism of prednisolone-C^{14} and cortisol-C^{14}. *J. Clin. Endocr. 17:*1040, 1957.

59. Sandberg, A. A., and Slaunwhite, W. R., Jr. Transcortin: A corticosteroid binding protein of plasma. II. Levels in various conditions and effects of estrogens. *J. Clin. Invest. 38:*1290, 1959.

60. Sandberg, A. A., and Slaunwhite, W. R., Jr. Transcortin: A corticosteroid binding protein of plasma. V. In vitro inhibition of cortisol metabolism. *J. Clin. Invest. 42:*51, 1963.

61. Sandberg, A. A., Slaunwhite, W. R., Jr., and Antoniades, H. N. The binding of steroids and steroid conjugates to human plasma proteins. *Recent. Prog. Hormone Res. 13:*209, 1957.

62. Slaunwhite, W. R., Jr., Lockie, G. N., Beck, N., and Sandberg, A. A. Transcortin: A corticosteroid-binding protein of plasma. IV. Inactivity in vivo of transcortin bound cortisol. *Science 135:*1062, 1962.

63. Seal, U. S., and Doe, R. P. Corticosteroid-binding globulin. I. Isolation from the plasma of diethylstilbestrol-treated men. *J. Biol. Chem. 237:*3136, 1962.

64. Tait, J. F., and Burstein, S. "In Vivo Studies of Steroid Dynamics in Man." In *The Hormones,* Vol. 5, C. Pincus and K. V. Thimann (Eds.), Academic Press, New York, 1964, p. 441.

65. Thomas, J. P., and Flynn, T. G. Adrenal function in normal pregnancy and toxaemia. *Clin. Sci. 26:*69, 1964.

66. Ulstrom, R. A., Colle, E., Burley, J., and Gunville, R. Adrenocortical steroid metabolism in newborn infants. I. Urinary excretion of free and conjugated 17-hydroxy-corticosteroids in normal full term infants. *J. Clin. Endocr. 20:*1066, 1960.

67. Villee, D. B., Engel, L. L., and Villee, C. A. Steroids hydroxylation in human fetal adrenals. *Endocrinology 65:*465, 1959.

68. Villee, D. B., and Villee, C. A. Synthesis of corticosteroids in the fetal-placental unit. Proc. Second Internat. Congr. Endocr. London 1964. *Excerpta Med. Int. Cong. Sr. 83:*709, 1965.

69. Wallace, E. Z., Silverberg, H. I., and Carter, A. C. Effect of ethinyl estradiol on plasma 17-hydroxycorticosteroids, ACTH responsiveness, and hydrocortisone clearance in man. *Proc. Soc. Exp. Biol. Med. 95:*805, 1957.

70. Westphal, U., and Ashley, B. D. Steroid-protein interactions. IV. Influence of functional groups in D4-3-ketosteroids in interaction with serum albumin and β-lactoglobulin. *J. Biol. Chem. 233:*57, 1958.

71. Yates, F. E., and Urquhart, J. Control of plasma concentration of adrenocortical hormones. *J. Physiol. Rev. 42:*359, 1962.

Chapter Seven

Renin-Angiotensin-Aldosterone and Toxemia of Pregnancy

Patrick J. Mulrow

The renin-angiotensin-aldosterone system has received considerable attention in toxemia of pregnancy. The studies of aldosterone production are more extensive, since only recently have renin measurements been widely employed.

ALDOSTERONE

Aldosterone is the most important mineralocorticoid synthesized by the adrenal gland. It is synthesized in its outer zone—the zona glomerulosa. The main site of action of aldosterone is the distal tubule of the kidney where it stimulates the reabsorption of sodium and the secretion of potassium. The normal secretion rate in nonpregnant women varies between 50 and 250 μg/day. The secretion rate is increased by sodium depletion, potassium loading, or acute administration of ACTH; the rate is decreased by sodium loading or potassium depletion.

The formula of aldosterone and its metabolism in the body is illustrated in Figure 7-1. There are two major classes of metabolites: the acid-labile conjugate and the tetrahydroaldosterone-glucuronide metabolites.

There is a controversy over whether aldosterone metabolism is altered during pregnancy.[15] Most studies of aldosterone excreted during pregnancy have measured the acid-labile conjugate. If metabolism should alter during the different stages of pregnancy or in toxemia, excretion

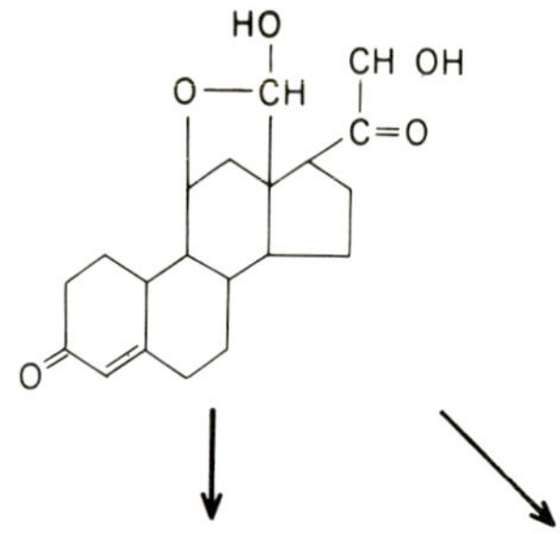

	FREE	pH-1	β-GLUCURONIDASE
NORMAL ♀	1.7	19 (8.3)	54 (20)
PREGNANT ♀	1.2	24 (9.5)	46 (21)

Fig. 7-1. The chemical formula of aldosterone. At bottom is shown the percentage of a dose of radioactive aldosterone excreted as three urinary metabolites: free alcohol, acid-labile conjugate, and β-glucuronidase hydrolyzable fractions. Numbers in parenthesis indicate per cent of PH-1 hydrolyzable radioactivity that was actually aldosterone and per cent of β-glucuronidase radioactivity that was tetrahydroaldosterone. (These data were reported by Watanabe *et al. J. Clin. Invest.* *42*:1619, 1963.)

rates of a single metabolite might change and yet not reflect changes in secretion rate. The aldosterone is produced by the maternal adrenal gland with little or no contribution from the placenta or fetal adrenal.

Some of the best published studies on the secretion rates of aldosterone during pregnancy have been performed by Sims, Solomon, and their colleagues.[19, 21] They have paid special attention to electrolyte balance, so that their studies have been performed under controlled conditions. These workers have shown that aldosterone secretion is already elevated by the 15th week of pregnancy, the earliest stage they studied, and that the secretion rate responds to alteration in sodium balance, increasing during sodium depletion and decreasing during sodium loading. A similar response occurs in the nonpregnant state except that the basal level is much lower (Table 7-1). Figure 7-2 illustrates the aldosterone secretion rates in the nonpregnant state, in normal pregnancy, and in mild and severe toxemia. The vertical lines indicate the range of aldosterone rates, the horizontal lines the mean. The week of gestation is shown at the bottom. Figure 7-2 shows that there is a considerable increase in the aldosterone secretion rate in pregnancy which becomes more marked with advancing gestation. There is, of course, considerable fluctuation even in a single patient when followed consecutively throughout pregnancy. Of special importance is the decrease in secretion rate when toxemia supervenes. During mild toxemia the secretion rate falls but is still higher than in the nonpregnant state. In severe toxemia the secretion rate falls to the levels found in the nonpregnant state or even lower than this. These secretion rate results are similar to the earlier findings measuring the excretion rate of the acid labile conjugate of aldosterone. It does not appear that toxemia of pregnancy is associated with a sudden increase of aldosterone production.

TABLE 7-1
EFFECT OF ALTERATIONS IN DIETARY SODIUM ON THE ALDOSTERONE SECRETION RATE OVER A PERIOD OF FOUR WEEKS*

Subject	Weeks of gestation	Dietary sodium (meq/d)		Aldosterone secretory rate (μg/d)		
Determination	1	1	2	1	2	%
Added salt						
M3	27	110	170	1000	1208	+ 21
J3	32	180	220	710	596	− 16
N1	32	170	210	1210	635	− 47
P2	32	90	160	1505	549	− 64
Restricted Salt						
S2	37	150	10	960	9220	+860
G1	31	150	10	2470	4060	+ 64
M4	35	150	10	1300	10250	+690

* From Sims, Meeker, Gray, Watanabe, and Solomon. In *Aldosterone—A Symposium*, Baulieu and Robel (Eds.), Blackwell, Oxford, 1964, p. 499.

There are certain puzzling questions about aldosterone in pregnancy. Why do not pregnant women develop potassium depletion from such high secretion rates? Why are they not potassium depleted like patients with primary aldosteronism? Pregnant women are similar to patients with nephrosis, cirrhosis, and those on a low-sodium diet, all of whom have high aldosterone secretion rates but do not waste potassium. These latter patients probably have one thing in common—marked proximal tubular reabsorption of sodium—hence little sodium is delivered to the distal ion exchange site for exchange with potassium in the kidney. Indeed, a low-sodium diet will prevent potassium wasting even when large doses of aldosterone are administered. This cannot be the explanation in pregnancy, since plenty of sodium is excreted. Perhaps the best explanation is that an antagonist to aldosterone, progesterone, is present during pregnancy. This inhibition must occur in the distal ion exchange site where aldosterone stimulates loss of potassium for sodium.

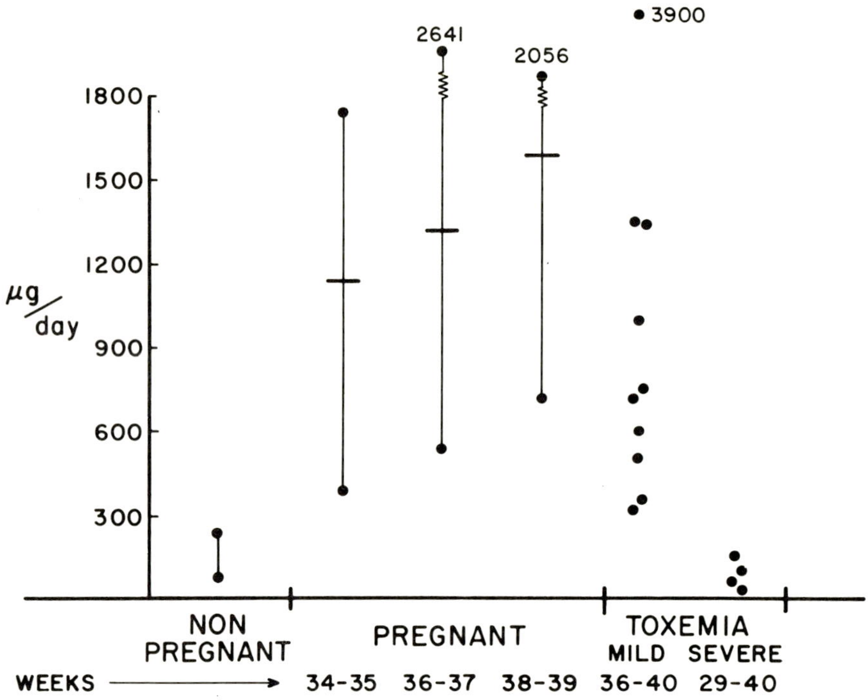

Fig. 7-2. Aldosterone secretion rates in nonpregnant, pregnant, and toxemic women. Circles connected by lines indicate the range of secretion rates in each time period; the bars indicate the mean. Individual secretion rates for the toxemic patients are shown. (Data from Sims *et al.* In *Aldosterone—A Symposium,* Baulieu and Robel (Eds.), Blackwell, Oxford, 1964, p. 499.)

Why is there such an increase in secretion rate during pregnancy? One explanation has just been given; the marked increase in progesterone inhibits the effect of aldosterone, a transient sodium loss ensues, and the aldosterone secretion increases in response to sodium depletion. Indeed, aldosterone secretion does appear to have the same time course as progesterone production, it increases early in pregnancy and continues to increase throughout pregnancy.

Another explanation is that the placenta and fetus behave like an arteriovenous fistula and, although the blood volume is increased, the arterial tree remains poorly filled and undistended, resulting in a compensatory increase in aldosterone secretion. Regardless of the cause, the renin-angiotensin system appears to be the major mechanism regulating the secretion of aldosterone.

RENIN-ANGIOTENSIN SYSTEM

Renin is an enzyme which is synthesized chiefly in the juxtaglomerular cells of the afferent arteriole of the kidney. Figure 7-3 is a diagram of a glomerulus and the juxtaglomerular apparatus. In the juxtaglomerular cells of the afferent arteriole are the granules which contain renin. One widely held hypothesis claims that the juxtaglomerular cells act like baroreceptors, that is, hypovolemia or constriction of the renal artery leads to decreased stretch of the vessel and increased renin production, while hypervolemia or increased pressure inhibits renin production.

Renin is liberated into the blood where it acts upon a substrate in the alpha-2-globulin fraction to form angiotensin I, a decapeptide which is

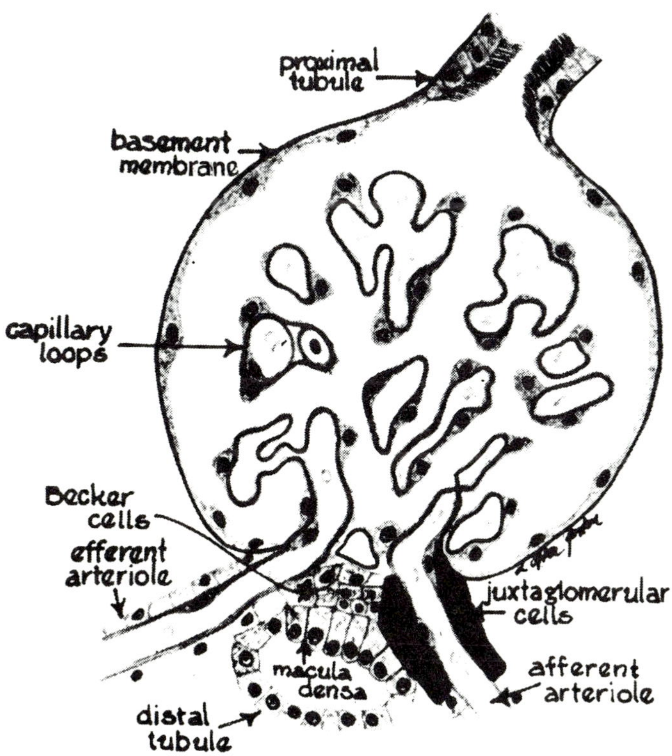

Fig. 7-3. Diagram of a glomerulus and juxtaglomerular apparatus. (Modified from Ham. *Histology,* Lippincott, Philadelphia, 1953, p. 666.)

rapidly converted by converting enzyme in plasma to angiotensin II, an octapeptide (Fig. 7-4). An authoritative account of the system which leads to the active principle, angiotensin II was given by Page and Bumpus.[18] Angiotensin II is not only a potent pressor agent but is also a major physiological regulator of aldosterone secretion. Also present in blood and in many tissues are peptidases called "angiotensinases" which rapidly destroy angiotensin. Indeed, the biological half-life of angiotensin is very short—a few minutes or less. In pregnancy, renin, renin substrate, and plasma angiotensinases are increased.

The site of action of renin on renin substrate is at a leucyl-leucyl bond. The renin splits off the decapeptide which is converted to the octapeptide by a converting enzyme (Fig. 7-5). Figure 7-6 illustrates the structure of the octapeptide angiotensin II.

As early as 1944, Dexter and Haynes reported elevated plasma renin concentration in toxemia of pregnancy,[8] but the methods of measuring renin were even poorer than they are today. In 1960, Hunter and Howard reported finding a pressor substance in extracts of decidual tissue and in the amniotic fluid of patients with toxemia but not in patients

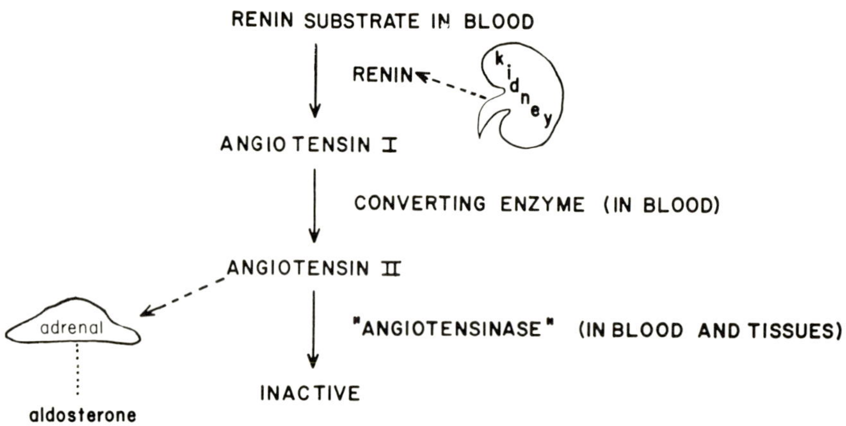

Fig. 7-4. Diagram of the renin-angiotensin system.

with normal pregnancies.[14] They called the pressor substance hysterotonin. Although others could not confirm these results,[10] it did appear from their data that they were dealing with a renin-like substance in the placenta or uterus of pregnant animals, but it was Gross *et al.* in 1964 who pointed out the large quantities of renin in the uterus of pregnant rabbits.[12] This observation gave credence to reports that constriction of

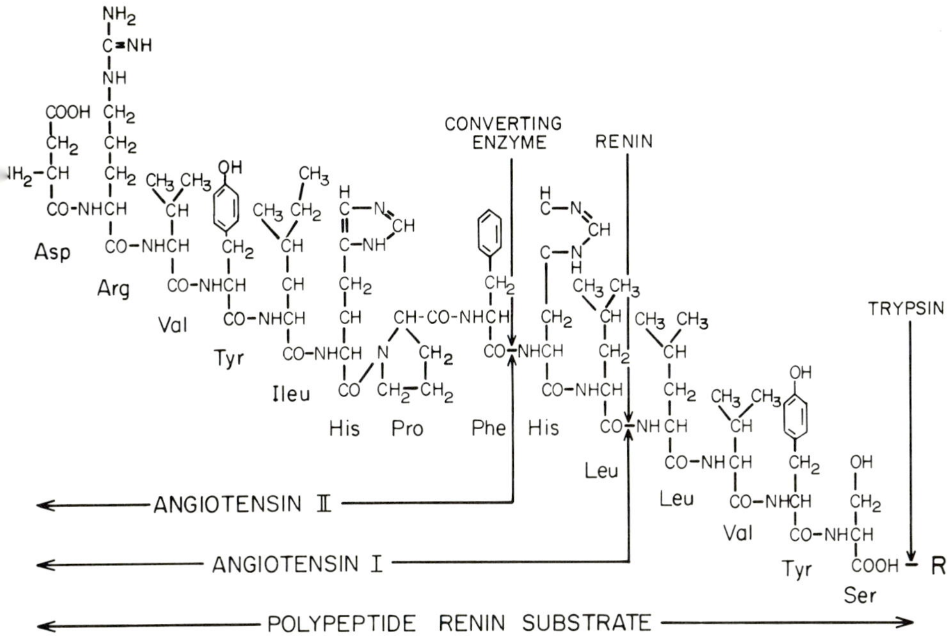

Fig. 7-5. The hydrolytic steps leading from renin substrate to angiotensin II.

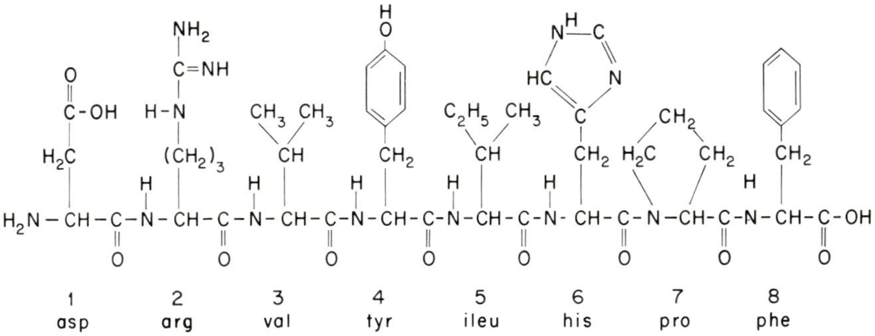

Fig. 7-6. Structure of angiotensin II.

the uterine arteries could lead to hypertension in pregnancy, presumably through the release of a pressor substance.[1,2]

Some of the best studies on renin in pregnancy have been done by Brown *et al.*[3,4,5,6,7] Their method involves the separation of renin in plasma by chromatography. The renin is incubated with a semipurified substrate, and the initial velocity is measured by estimating the rate of formation of angiotensin, which is quantified by bioassay. The scatter of values in nonpregnant and pregnant subjects is shown in Figure 7-7. Figure 7-8 shows the serial measurements of plasma renin concentration in five women throughout pregnancy. There are similarities with aldosterone secretion. Renin is elevated early in pregnancy, remains elevated throughout, and tends to increase in the last few weeks. There is, however, considerable fluctuation. The concentration of renin is still elevated 24 hours after delivery and returns toward the normal range by 96 hours (Fig. 7-9). It appears that neither the fetus nor the placenta is necessary for the raised concentration. A finding of special note is that the renin concentration in amniotic fluid is several times higher than in maternal plasma, raising the possibility of a uterine or placental source of this renin (Fig. 7-10). These data raised certain important questions:

1. What is the source of the elevated circulating renin in pregnancy?
2. What is the source of the elevated concentration of renin in the human amniotic fluid and the uterus of some animals?
3. Can this extrarenal renin re-enter the maternal circulation?
4. Are the levels of renin elevated in toxemia?

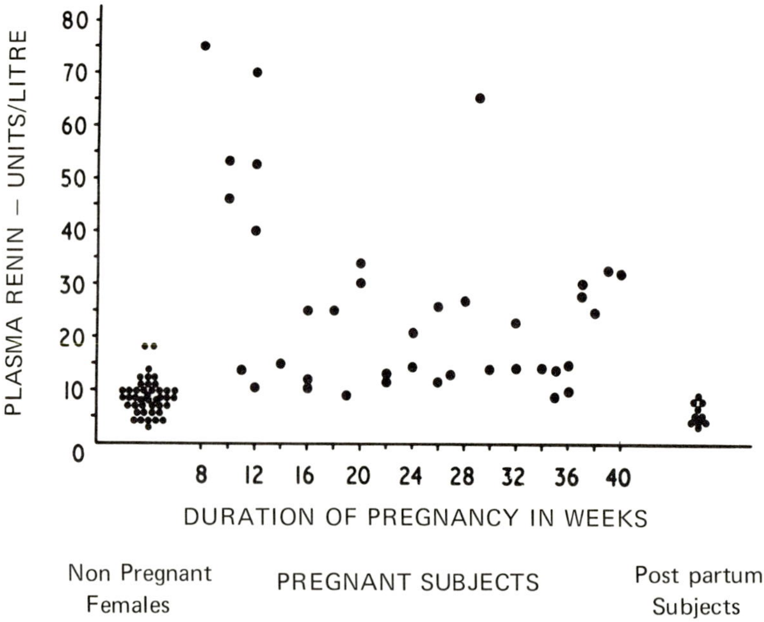

Fig. 7-7. Plasma renin concentrations in pregnant and nonpregnant subjects. (From Brown *et al. Lancet 2:* 900, 1963.)

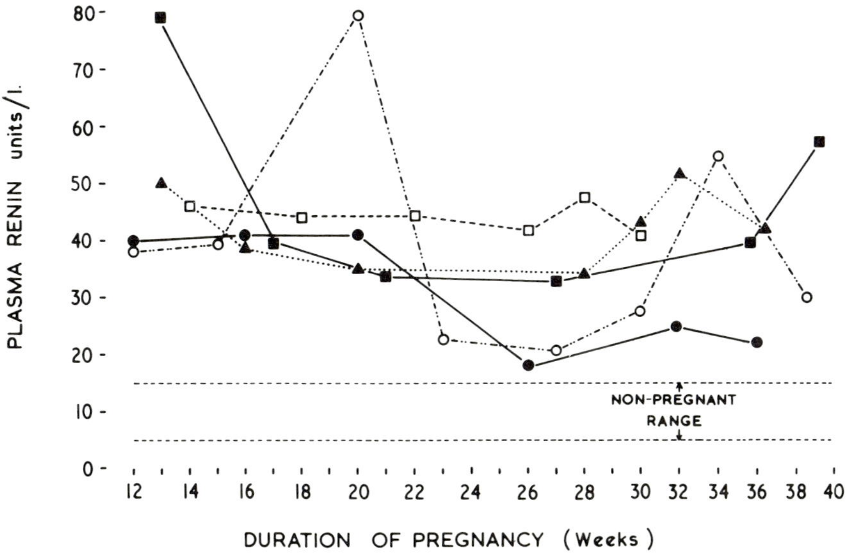

Fig. 7-8. Serial plasma renin concentrations in 5 pregnant women. (Reproduced by courtesy of Dr. A. F. Lever.)

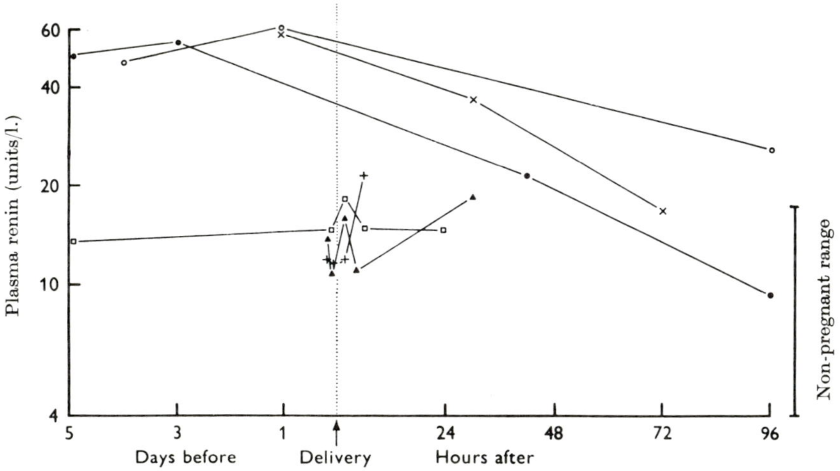

Fig. 7-9. Changes of plasma renin concentration in 6 pregnant women before and after delivery. (From Brown *et al. J. Endocr.* 35:373, 1966.)

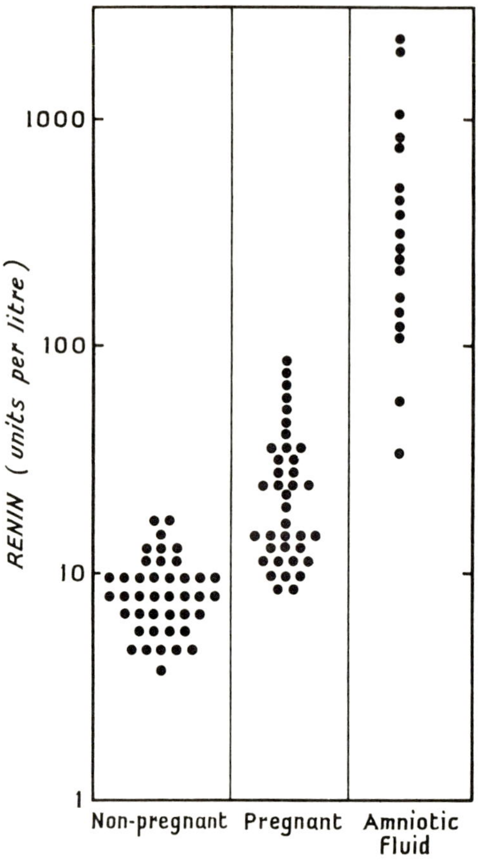

Fig. 7-10. Comparison of renin concentration in amniotic fluid with that in peripheral venous plasma of pregnant and nonpregnant women. (Reprinted from Brown *et al. Lancet* 2:64, 1964.)

In order to obtain information about the first three questions, Ferris, Gorden, and Mulrow[9,11] turned to an animal model, the rabbit, since the pregnant rabbit has a high concentration of renin in its uterus.

We confirmed Gross' work and found large quantities of renin-like pressor substance in the pregnant rabbit uterus, but very little in the placenta. The properties of this uterine renin are:

1. Non dialyzable, acid resistant, precipitated by 1.2M $(NH_4)_2SO_4$, heat labile
2. Inactivated by antirenin antibodies
3. Molecular weight by Sephadex G-100 approximately 45,000
4. Pressor curve similar to kidney renin in rat, rabbit, dog, and cat
5. Incubation with substrate forms angiotensin

These studies, therefore, suggested that this pressor substance was very similar to renin. In order to see if uterine renin was mainly kidney renin that was absorbed from the plasma, an attempt was made to suppress kidney renin and hence plasma renin by sodium loading pregnant rabbits by means of isotonic saline in the drinking water and intramuscular injection of desoxycorticosterone acetate. In the nonpregnant animal, this treatment diminishes kidney renin and plasma renin.

In Figure 7-11 the concentrations of renin in the rabbit kidney and pregnant rabbit uterus are shown. The renin was extracted by a method described previously[9] and assayed by injecting an aliquot into an anesthetized rabbit and recording the increase in blood pressure. Each extract was assayed in three separate rabbits. Each point is the mean of three assays for a tissue extract. As can be seen, the pregnant rabbit uterus had a renin concentration equal to or greater than the kidney. Desoxycorticosterone plus saline significantly decreased the concentration of the renin in the kidney, while the concentration in the uterus was unchanged. The plasma renin activity was measured[11] and reflected the

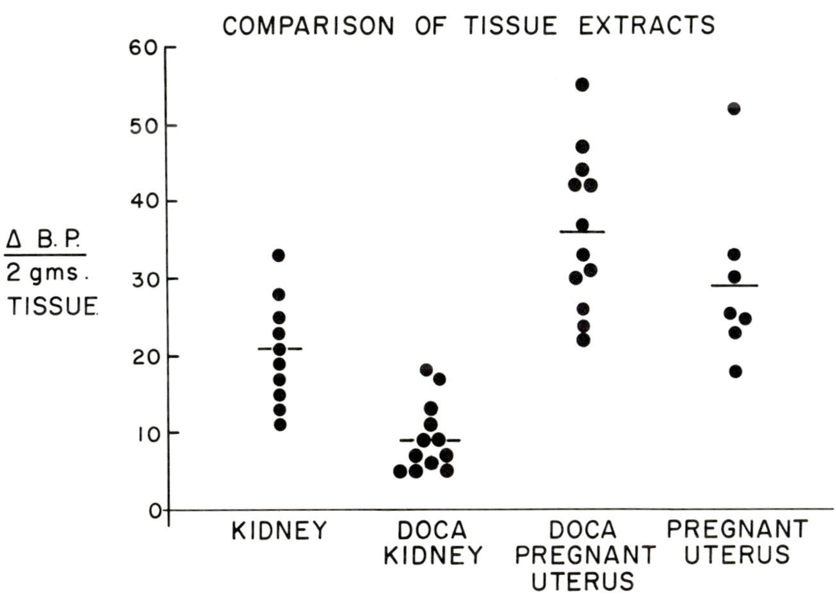

Fig. 7-11. A comparison of renin concentrations in the kidney and pregnant uterus of normal rabbits and of those treated with DOCA. Each point is the mean of three assays. (From Gorden, Ferris, and Mulrow. *Amer. J. Physiol. 212*:703, 1967.)

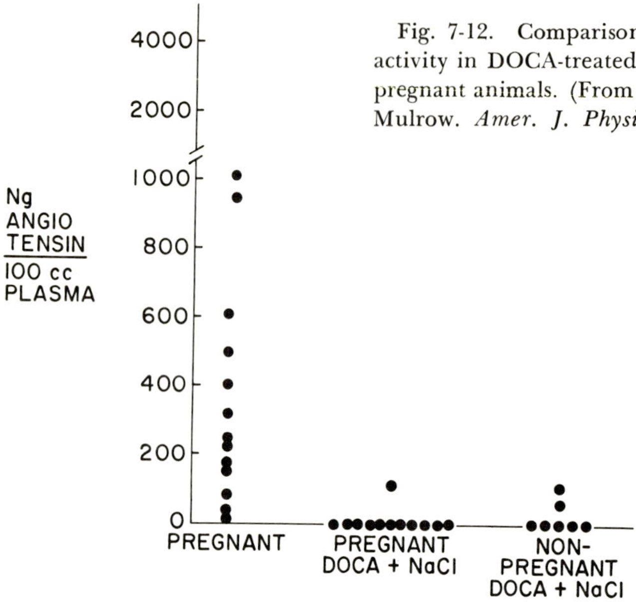

Fig. 7-12. Comparison of plasma renin activity in DOCA-treated pregnant and nonpregnant animals. (From Gorden, Ferris, and Mulrow. *Amer. J. Physiol. 212:*703, 1967.)

decrease in kidney renin. It is evident in Figure 7-12 that there is little detectable renin circulating following desoxycorticosterone and saline treatment. These data suggest that the increased circulating renin during pregnancy originates in the kidney and also suggest that the renin present in the uterus does not come from the circulation. Nevertheless, it was still possible that low concentrations of renin were circulating which were undetected by the method employed.

In order to study this possibility, we removed the kidneys of a pregnant rabbit and measured the concentration of renin in the uterus 24, 48, and 72 hours after nephrectomy. The uterine renin concentration did not change, despite the absence of the kidneys, for as long as 72 hours (Fig. 7-13). The plasma renin activity was most interesting. In Fig. 7-14 it is evident that the plasma renin concentrations are undetectable after nephrectomy in nonpregnant rabbits. However, 48 hours post nephrectomy in the pregnant rabbits, the plasma renin activity remains high, suggesting that under one circumstance, uremia, renin may enter the circulation from the uterus.

In addition to these animal experiments, Ferris and Gorden have extracted a substance from postpartum human uteri which, upon incubation with renin-free human plasma, produces an angiotensin-like substance. The concentration of this renin-like substance, however, is

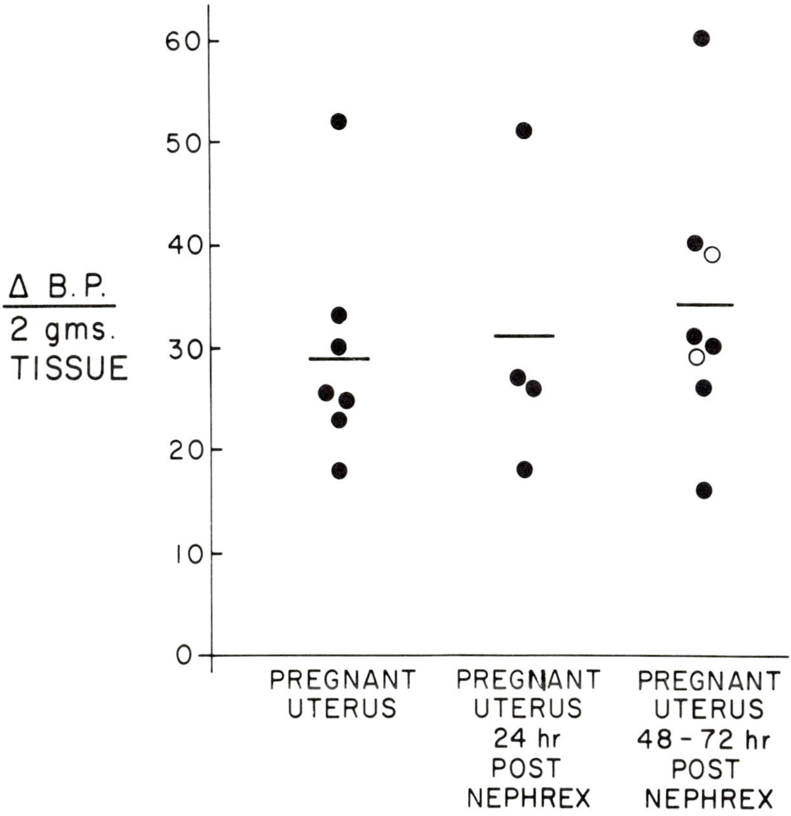

Fig. 7-13. The effect of nephrectomy on uterine renin concentration. The open circles represent extracts obtained from animals 72 hours post nephrectomy. (From Gorden, Ferris, and Mulrow. *Amer. J. Physiol. 212*:703, 1967.)

much smaller than in the pregnant rabbit uterus, but it must be remembered that the renin concentration in the human kidney is much smaller than in the pregnant rabbit uterus. More recently, Symonds, Stanley, and Skinner have grown human uterine tissue in tissue culture and have demonstrated the continued release of renin by these cells after several subcultures.[20]

The important question, however, is what happens to the plasma renin concentration during toxemia of pregnancy. From the aldosterone data, it can be predicted that plasma renin falls in toxemia. In Figure 7-15 are shown the results of Brown *et al.* In the presence of hypertension, with or without edema, the renin concentrations decrease.

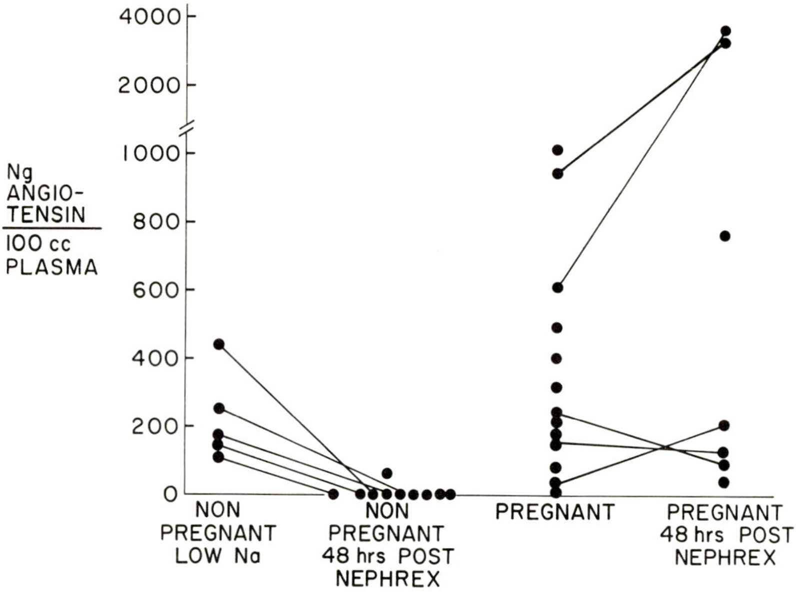

Fig. 7-14. Effect of nephrectomy on plasma renin activity in the nonpregnant and pregnant animal. The lines connect values obtained from the same animal. (From Gorden, Ferris, and Mulrow. *Amer. J. Physiol. 212:*703, 1967.)

It is evident that the renin-angiotensin-aldosterone system is quite active during pregnancy but becomes much less active during toxemia. Clearly, toxemia is not caused by a sudden and persistent excess of renin and aldosterone. The cause of the fall in the renin concentration and aldosterone secretion rate is a mystery. Possibly it is the result of the fluid retention that often accompanies toxemia. Possibly it is secondary to the fall in progesterone production that occurs. In any event, more work is needed to define the physiological role of this complex system in normal and toxemic pregnancy.

More recently, reports of the effects of oral contraceptive agents on the renin-angiotensin system have shown that these compounds may have a bearing on the pathophysiology of this system in pregnancy. In some patients, these agents increase renin activity, renin substrate concentration, and aldosterone secretion. In a few patients, hypertension appears to result from their use.[13, 17, 22]

The data from a patient that was studied by Kotchen, Morrow, and Mulrow (unpublished observations) are shown in Figure 7-16. While

Fig. 7-15. Plasma-renin concentration in hypertensive disease of pregnancy. (From Brown *et al. Lancet 2*:1219, 1965.)

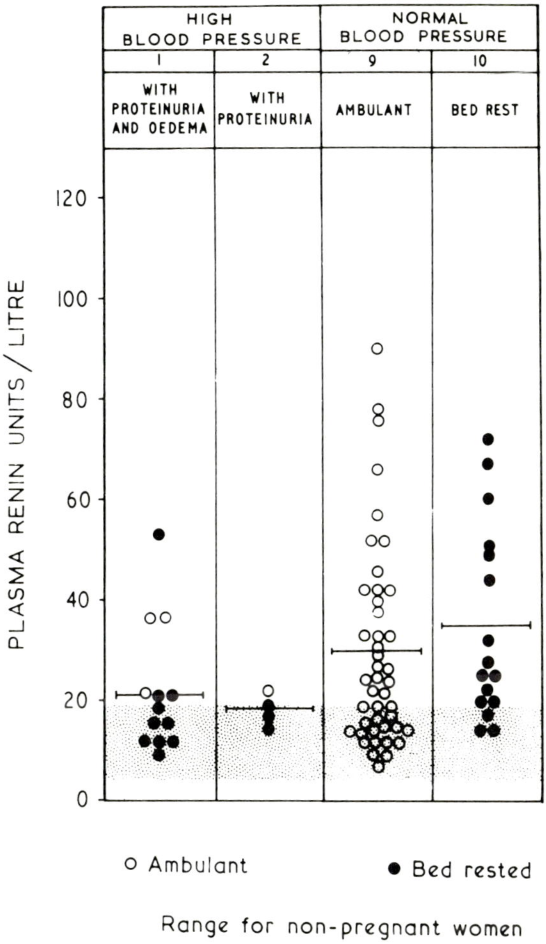

on oral contraceptive agents aldosterone secretion and excretion were elevated, but, as in normal pregnancy, there was a further increase in aldosterone secretion following sodium depletion. After stopping the oral contraceptive agent, aldosterone levels returned to normal but her hypertension persisted. The plasma renin levels followed a similar pattern; they were elevated despite a high-sodium diet but responded to sodium depletion and returned to the normal range after discontinuing the drug. The relationship of the contraceptive drug to the hypertension is not clear, but it is clear that the hyperaldosteronism was caused by the oral contraceptive agents.

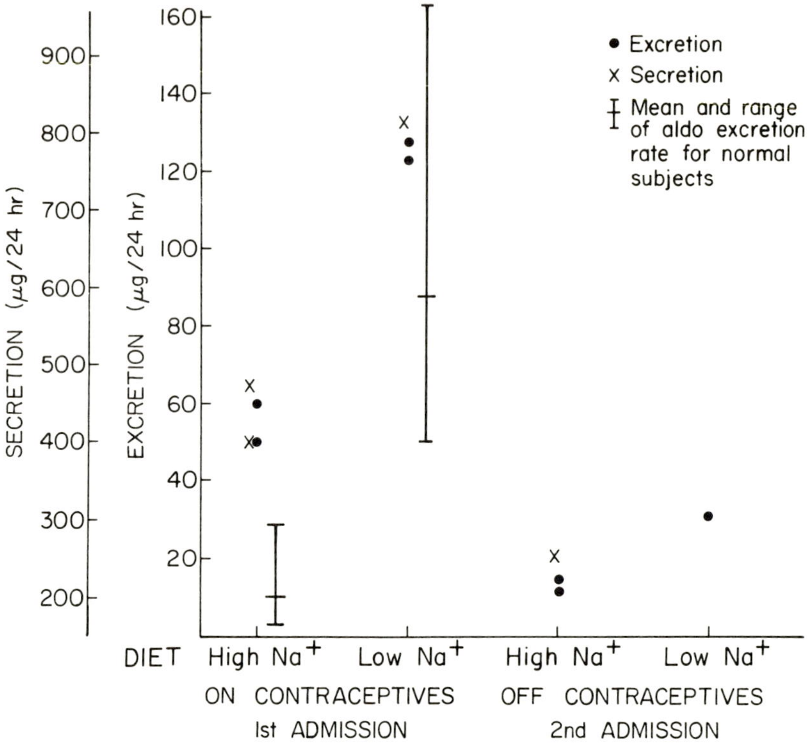

Fig. 7-16. Aldosterone secretion and excretion rates on high- and low-salt diets, during and after contraceptive therapy. (Kotchen, Morrow, and Mulrow. Unpublished observations.)

REFERENCES

1. Berger, M., and Boueck, R. J. Irreversible uterine and renal changes induced by placental ischemia (rabbit). *Amer. J. Obstet. Gynec. 89*:230, 1964.
2. Berger, M., and Cavanagh, D. Toxemia of pregnancy. *Amer. J. Obstet. Gynec. 87*:293, 1963.
3. Brown, J. J., Davies, D. L., Doak, P. B., Lever, A. F., and Robertson, J. I. S. Plasma renin in normal pregnancy. *Lancet 2*:900, 1963.
4. Brown, J. J., Davies, D. L., Doak, P. B., Lever, A. F., and Robertson, J. I. S. The presence of renin in human amniotic fluid. *Lancet 2*:64, 1964.
5. Brown, J. J., Davies, D. L., Doak, P. B., Lever, A. F., Robertson, J. I. S., and Trust, P. Plasma-renin concentration in hypertensive disease of pregnancy. *Lancet 2*:1219, 1965.
6. Brown, J. J., Davies, D. L., Doak, P. B., Lever, A. F., and Robertson,

J. I. S. Serial estimation of plasma renin concentration during pregnancy and after parturition. *J. Endocr. 35:*373, 1966.

7. Brown, J. J., Davies, D. L., Doak, P. B., Lever, A. F., Robertson, J. I. S. Plasma renin concentration in the hypertensive diseases of pregnancy. *J. Obstet. Gynaec. Brit. Comm. 73:*410, 1966.
8. Dexter, L., and Haynes, F. W. Relation of renin to human hypertension with particular reference to eclampsia, preeclampsia and acute glomerulonephritis. *Proc. Soc. Exp. Biol. 55:*288, 1944.
9. Ferris, T. F., Gorden, P., and Mulrow, P. J. Rabbit uterus as a source of renin. *Amer. J. Physiol. 212:*698, 1967.
10. Gomel, V., and Hardwick, D. F. Search for a pressor substance in toxemia of pregnancy. *Amer. J. Obstet. Gynec. 94:*308, 1966.
11. Gorden, P., Ferris, T. F., and Mulrow, P. J. Rabbit uterus as a possible site of renin synthesis. *Amer. J. Physiol. 212:*703, 1967.
12. Gross, F., Schaechtelin, G., Ziegler, M., and Berger, M. A renin-like substance in the placenta and uterus of the rabbit. *Lancet 1:*914, 1964.
13. Helmer, O. M., and Judson, W. E. Influence of high renin substrate levels on renin angiotensin system in pregnancy. *Amer. J. Obstet. Gynec. 99:*9, 1967.
14. Hunter, C. A., and Howard, W. F. A pressor substance (hysterotonin) occurring in toxemia. *Amer. J. Obstet. Gynec. 79:*838, 1960.
15. Jones, K. M., Lloyd-Jones, R., Riondel, A., Tait, J. F., Tait, S. A., Bulbrook, R. D., Greenwood, F. C. Aldosterone secretion and metabolism in normal men and women in pregnancy. *Acta Endocr.* (Kobenhavn) *30:*321, 1959.
16. Kotchen, T., Morrow, L., and Mulrow, P. J. Unpublished observations.
17. Laragh, J. H., Sealey, J. E., Ledingham, J. G. G., and Newton, M. A. Oral contraceptives: renin, aldosterone, and high blood pressure. *J.A.M.A. 201:*918, 1967.
18. Page, I. H., and Bumpus, F. M. Angiotensin. *Physiol. Rev. 41:*331, 1961.
19. Sims, E. A. H., Meeker, C. I., Gray, M. J., Watanabe, M., and Solomon, S. "The Secretion of Aldosterone in Normal Pregnancy and in Preeclampsia." In *Aldosterone—A Symposium,* E. E. Baulieu and P. Robel (Eds.), Blackwell, Oxford, 1964, p. 499.
20. Symonds, E. M., Stanley, M. A., and Skinner, S. L. Production of renin by in vitro cultures of human chorion and uterine muscle. *Nature* (London) *217:*1152, 1968.
21. Watanabe, M., Meeker, C. I., Gray, M. J., Sims, E. A. H., and Solomon, S. Secretion rate of aldosterone in normal pregnancy. *J. Clin. Invest. 42:*1619, 1963.
22. Woods, J. W. Oral contraceptives and hypertension. *Lancet 2:*653, 1967.

Chapter Eight

Placental Lactogenic Hormone

John B. Josimovich

Eight years ago, at the Boston Lying-In Hospital, we began attempts to identify and isolate the growth hormone-like substance found in increased concentrations in the serum of pregnant women.[10] Pituitary growth hormone, among other substances, is known to be diabetogenic and to increase mobilization of free fatty acids from fat depots.[6] We hoped, therefore, that the increased resistance to insulin and ability to mobilize fatty acids seen in late pregnancy[3,4] might be explained by the increased somatotrophic activity found in pregnancy sera. We found that the serum of pregnant women does indeed contain large amounts of a substance secreted by the placenta which is immunologically and chemically similar to pituitary growth hormone; and which, because of its pre-eminent lactogenic properties, we called human placental lactogen, or HPL.[21] Further work in our laboratory and in that of Kaplan and Grumbach[17,23] (who employ the term "chorionic growth hormone-prolactin (CGP)") suggests that this placental hormone could play a role in nitrogen retention in mother and fetus, and in the sparing of maternal glucose for use by the infant. In addition to its possible somatotrophic properties, it was shown that the hormone might help prepare the breast for lactation.[9,17] It was also found to be transiently luteotrophic alone,[18] and appears to synergize with HCG in controlling the secretion of estrogen and progesterone in pseudopregnant rats.[19]

This work supported by N.I.H. Grant HD-01554.

CHEMICAL STUDIES

HPL is a polypeptide with a molecular weight between 19,000 and 30,000.[5,8] Its electrophoretic mobility in different gels is similar to that of portions of HGH.[8,18,23] Furthermore, it is immunologically closely related to, but distinct from HGH.[21] Amino acid analyses reveal a pattern of composition quite like that found after hydrolysis of pituitary HGH.[8] The solubility properties of HPL are also similar to those of HGH. Because of these similarities, it has been postulated that the chemical structure of HPL is quite similar to that of HGH.[5,34] Sherwood has found identity in the amino acid content of about 40 percent of tryptic digest fragments of the two hormones.[34]

The two-dimensional, chromatographic mobility of peptic digest fragments obtained from a preparation of human growth hormone containing three polypeptides of similar molecular weight and from an electrophoretically homogeneous preparation of placental lactogen, displayed similar mobility for over 40 percent of about 45 fragments.[20] Figure 8-1 is a statistical expression of the 95 percent limits of position of the mean mobility of such peptic digest fragments (in relation to a ^{14}C-leucine marker) of HPL and HGH, in two-dimensional, thin-layer chromatography. This study by Izenson in our laboratory shows that at least 50 percent of the digest fragments obtained from equal degrees of digestion of the inhomogeneous growth hormone and apparently homogeneous HPL preparation have significantly different mobilities. These data suggest that these two hormone preparations contain considerably different structural components. Final determination of the degree of similarity of the two hormones must await amino acid sequence determination of the entire HPL molecule or of digest fragments obtained under identical conditions from homogeneous preparations of the two hormones in the same laboratory.

PRODUCTION SITES

Production of HPL in tissue culture conclusively demonstrates that the trophoblast is the site of production of this hormone;[12] immunofluorescent antibody histological studies, moreover, strongly suggest the syncytial trophoblast as the cellular site of origin.[32] A variety of studies have shown that the fetus and the maternal pituitary are not sites of hormone production.[17] Furthermore, the hormone has been found in the blood of males suffering from metastatic testicular choriocarcinoma.[7,30]

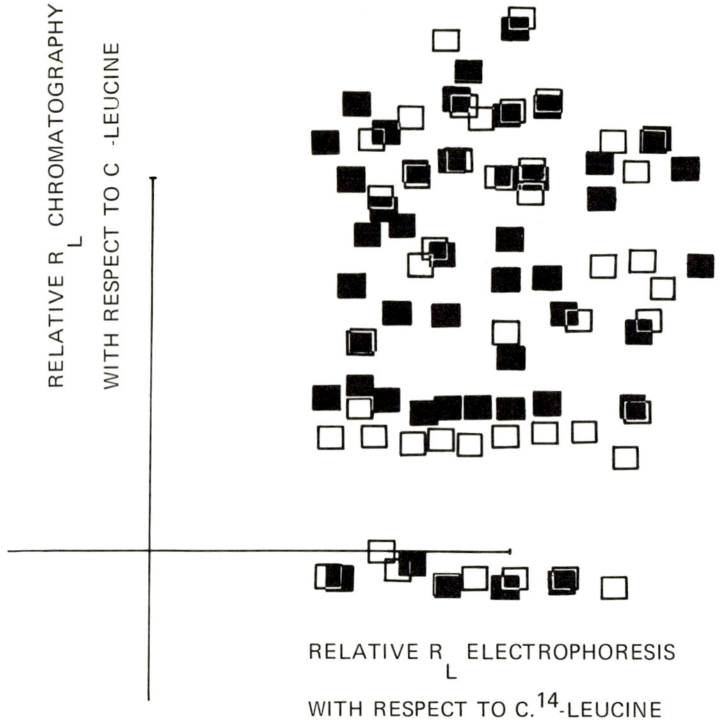

Fig. 8-1. Mobility of peptic digest fragments of HPL (clear rectangles) and human pituitary growth hormone (shaded rectangles). The mean mobility of the centers of ninhydrin-stained peptic fragments on thin layer chromatographic plates relative to the migration of ^{14}C-leucine (R_1) was calculated. Each side of a rectangle represents plus and minus two standard deviations in the mobility of the fragments. Thus, failure of overlap of rectangles signifies a 95% likelihood that two rectangles do not have an identical mobility, suggesting different chemical substructure.

SECRETION RATE

Beck, Parker, and Daughaday measured the disappearance of HPL from the maternal blood stream after delivery of the placenta, and determined the half-life to be 21–23 minutes.[2] Samaan *et al.* derived a half-life of about 30 minutes.[30] Grumbach and colleagues, however, have questioned the linearity of this rate of disappearance.[11] Nevertheless, Beck and Daughaday found the half-life of HPL intravenously infused into nonpregnant subjects to be about 20 minutes.[1] Calculating a volume of distribution of 7.2 percent of body weight and a term plasma concentration of 1.15 μg/ml (in comparison with their own HPL standard), they calculated a daily secretion rate of 390 mg at term. This agrees with the 0.5–3.0 gm estimated by Kaplan and Grumbach[24] and ourselves employing different standard preparations of HPL.

Figures 8-2 and 8-3, derived from work performed by Mrs. B. Kosor in our laboratory in collaboration with Dr. D. Mintz, demonstrate that there is a correlation in the plasma concentration of HPL and placental tissue weight, although others were not able to demonstrate this previously.[35] Figure 8-2 shows the wide scattering of plasma concentrations at

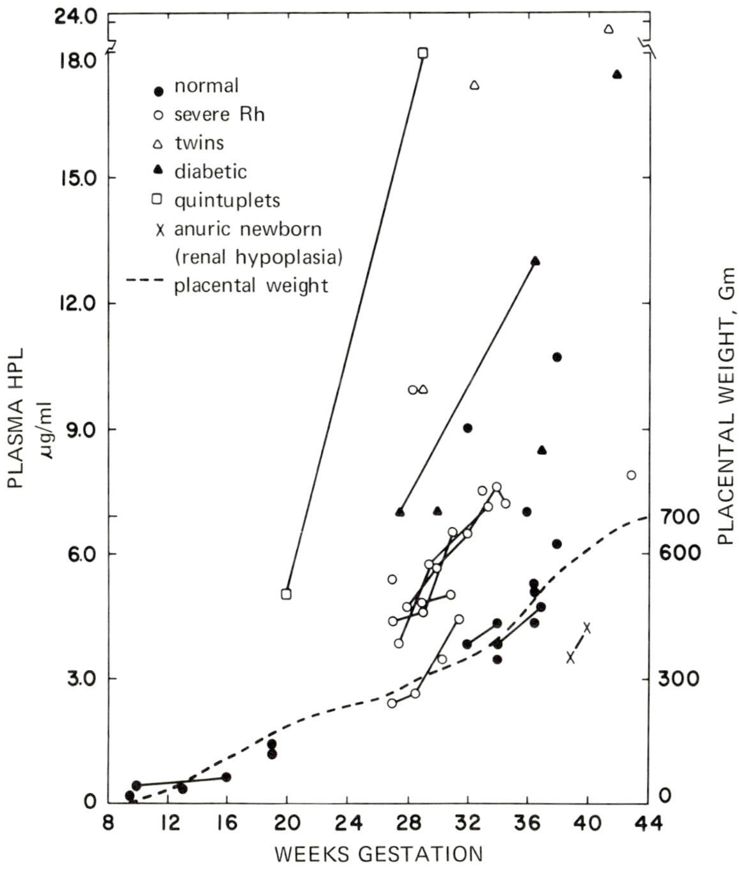

Fig. 8-2. Maternal plasma HPL concentration at different weeks gestation. Lines connect values obtained from the same patient. Dashed line represents the normal mean placental weight curve, based on data from Javert.[15] (From Josimovich in *Fetal Homeostasis,* vol. 4, Wynn (Ed.), New York, Appleton-Century-Crofts, 1969, pp. 110–111.)

different times of gestation in 34 patients, many of whom had twin pregnancies and various gestational disturbances which caused large variation in placental weight.

Figure 8-2 also displays the mean placental weight at various stages of gestation for normal pregnancies. At delivery of the patients depicted in Figure 8-2, the placental weights derived from the mean normal curve at that date of gestation were divided by the actual placental weight and the resultant fraction multiplied by the plasma HPL concentration shown in Figure 8-2.

Figure 8-3 displays these plasma HPL values thus normalized for placental weight. It can be seen that the maternal plasma HPL concentrations fall remarkably close to the mean normal placental growth curve, which represents an almost linear twelve-fold increase from 12 weeks to at least 37 weeks. Figure 8-3 can be interpreted to mean that,

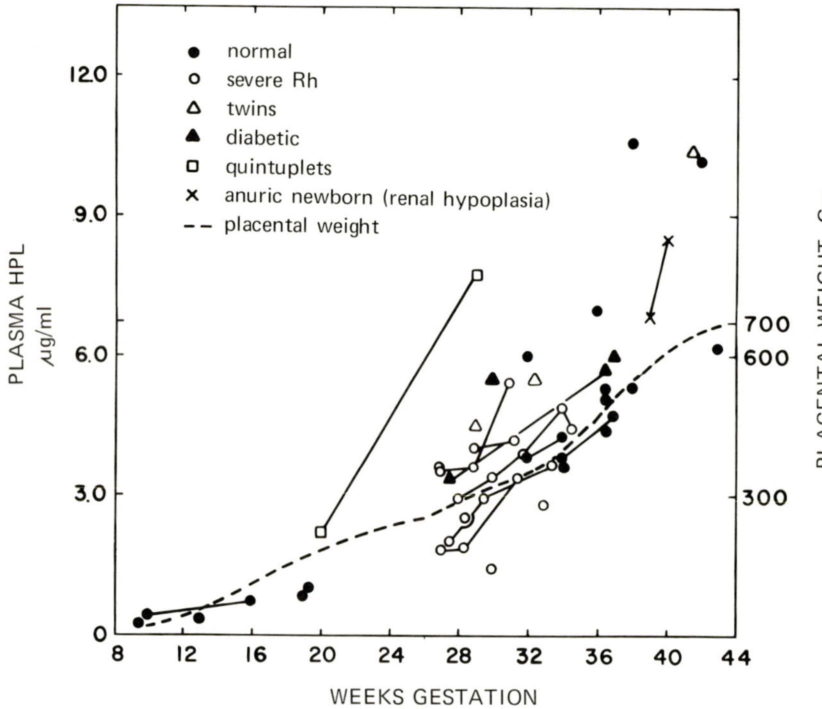

Fig. 8-3. Plasma HPL concentrations normalized for deviant placental weight (see text). Mean placental weight curve is signified by the dashed line, based on data from Javert.[15] (From Josimovich in *Fetal Homeostasis*, vol. 4, Wynn (Ed.), New York, Appleton-Century-Crofts, 1969, pp. 110–111.)

with few exceptions, secretion is maintained such that a concentration of 1μg/ml HPL/100 gm of placenta, in reference to our HPL standard, exists in the maternal plasma. This finding suggests that HPL secretion is closely related to placental weight and might be about 0.5 gm/100 gm/24 hours, or as high as 3 gm/24 hours at term.

METABOLISM AND CONCENTRATIONS

The total quantity of HPL found in the fetal circulation, amniotic fluid, and maternal urine is negligible (less than 0.5 mg) compared to the approximately 15–20 mg found in the maternal bloodstream at term and the 10–30 mg found in the placenta. The mode of metabolism of the 0.5–3 gm secreted daily is unknown, but is thought to be the same as that found for HGH, since the two hormones disappear from the bloodstream at a similar rate after administration to humans.

Table 8-1 lists concentrations of HPL found in various tissues and fluids at term. The values are expressed in terms of our standard preparation prepared by passage of Lederle Laboratories' 45 per cent electrophoretically pure HPL ("purified placental protein") through a Sephadex G-100 column.[20] The data were obtained by Mrs. Kosor. The values for term maternal serum and urine and fetal serum are comparable to those reported by other workers.[1,12,17,30,35] It is obvious that a considerable quantity of HPL is present in amniotic fluid (about 0.5 mg at term), while little exists in the fetal circulation (about 4 μg), and there is usually less than 1 ng/ml in the fetal urine collected within one-half hour of birth. The data in Table 8-1 suggest the hypothesis that HPL probably arrives in the amniotic fluid by passage through chorion and amnion from the placenta or maternal decidua rather than via the fetus. Figure 8-4 is derived from maternal plasma and amniotic fluid samples of Rh-negative mothers obtained by Drs. D. L. Hutchinson, Paul Taylor,

TABLE 8-1

CONCENTRATION OF HPL IN FETAL AND MATERNAL COMPARTMENTS

Source	Weeks gestation	HPL concentration
Maternal plasma	10–14	0.3 μg/ml
	36–42	5.4 ± 0.5* μg/ml
Maternal placenta	throughout	10–20 mg/100 gm
Maternal urine	36–40	200–500 μg/24 hr
Fetal cord serum	36–42	15.5 ± 3.1* mμg/ml
Newborn urine	36–42	Less than 0.8 mμg/ml in 14 cases; 3 cases: 1.2 mμg/ml
Amniotic fluid	36–41	0.55 ± .06* μg/ml

* Standard error of the mean.

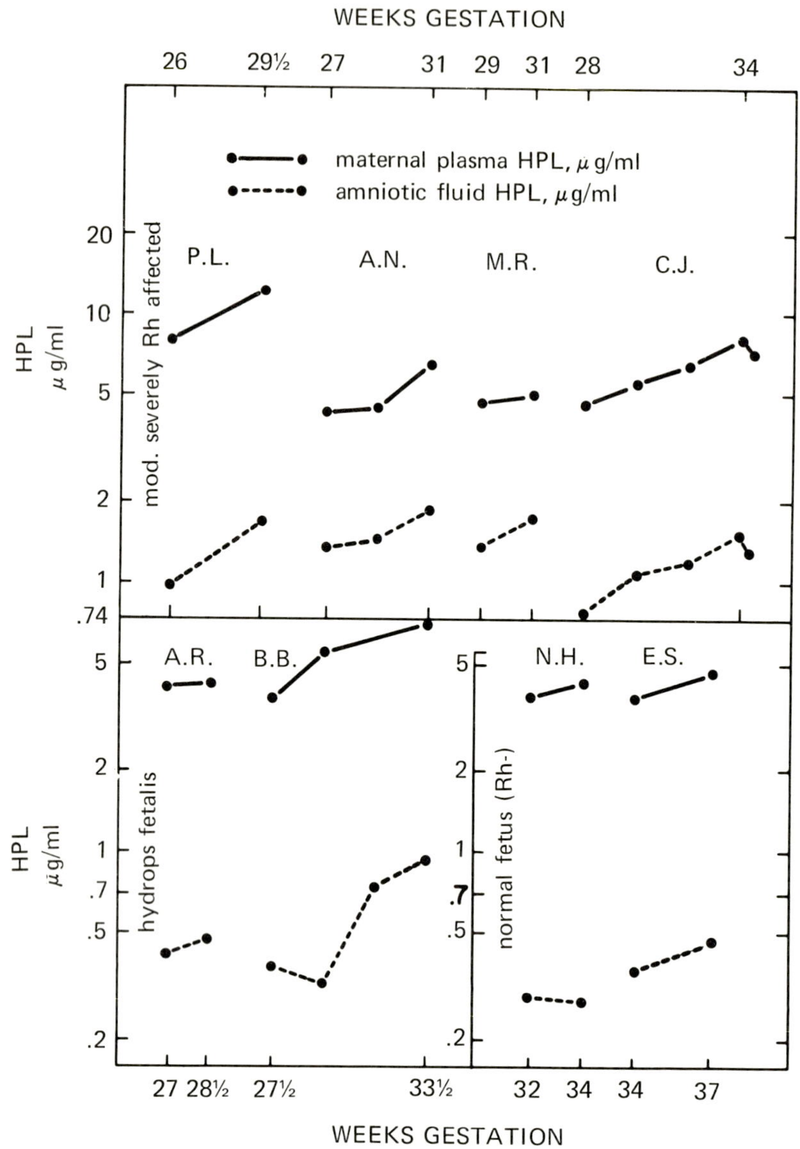

Fig. 8-4. Tendency for amniotic fluid HPL concentrations (dashed lines) to parallel maternal plasma values (solid lines) in eight Rh-negative patients of Dr. D. L. Hutchinson (see text for details).

and their colleagues of the University of Pittsburgh. In these eight patients, there is clearly a tendency for the amniotic fluid concentrations to parallel maternal plasma concentrations, although the absolute and relative values vary from patient to patient. In contrast to this probable parallelism of amniotic fluid concentrations to the gradually rising concentrations found in maternal plasma, umbilical vein or mixed cord arterial-venous plasma does not appear to vary in HPL content between 29 and 43 weeks from the mean for term fetuses given in Table 8-1. Thus, the placenta appears to secrete little HPL into the fetal circulation; at most it secretes the amount needed to maintain a concentration of about 0.3 percent of that found in the maternal plasma at term.

ASSAYS

No agreement has been reached on a biological standard for HPL. Therefore, one cannot state in absolute terms the amounts measured by the immunological assay techniques first introduced by Kaplan and Grumbach.[24] They employed a radioimmunoassay involving chromatoelectrophoresis of ^{131}I-labeled HPL in competition with cold HPL for antibody to HPL. Our laboratory has modified this by employing dextran-coated charcoal for separation of antibody-bound ^{131}I-HPL, in a manner similar to that used for assays of pituitary growth hormone.[29] Beck and colleagues have presented data on their assay using two species of antibodies which precipitate ^{131}I-HPL in competition with unknown amounts of unlabeled HPL.[1] Modifications have been made by Samaan *et al.*[30]

PLACENTAL TRANSFER

As stated above, the concentration of HPL in fetal cord plasma is only about 0.3 percent of that found in the maternal circulation at term. Thus, there appears to be even a greater barrier to passage of HPL than the barrier to passage of pituitary growth hormone (HGH) from fetus to mother:[24,30] Only a thirty-fold higher concentration of HGH was found in fetal serum compared to that found in maternal serum.

MECHANISM OF ACTION AND PHYSIOLOGICAL ROLES OF HPL IN PREGNANCY

Studies of the action of this hormone in the human being are only in preliminary stages, but many suppositions can be derived from animal experiments.

HPL is lactogenic in vivo when administered to rabbits and pigeons, as well as in vitro when added to cultures of mouse mammary tissue.[9,21,36] HPL may, therefore, play a preparatory role for successful lactation.

HPL is luteotrophic when administered alone or in conjunction with HCG in permitting balanced progesterone and estrogen secretion by the corpora lutea of pseudopregnant, hypophysectomized rats.[18,19] The hormone may, therefore, be synergistic with HCG in exerting control over some aspects of steroid production during pregnancy.

Indirect growth hormone-like effects may be in large part responsible for maternal glucose-sparing effects noted in late pregnancy.[17] Glucose-sparing appears to be required for meeting fetal energy requirements. The view that the fetus can utilize only glucose for energy needs, in a manner similar to that found in the adult brain, is supported by: (1) the finding that the respiratory quotient in newborn babies is near 1.0 (signifying sole use of glucose),[33] (2) the ready transport of glucose across the placenta,[28] (3) the large umbilical arterial-venous differences in glucose concentrations in the primate fetus,[27] (4) the limited passage of fatty acids across the placenta of many species,[26,37] and (5) the apparent inability of fetal or neonatal muscle to burn fatty acids efficiently.[38] An increased ability of pregnant animals and humans to mobilize free fatty acids from body fat depots[4,25] and the resistance to insulin and tolbutamide[3] are mechanisms by which the mother might spare glucose for fetal needs and increase her use of fatty acids for her own fuel requirements. HGH will produce such effects under certain conditions, so that it is naturally hoped that HPL might explain these phenomena during pregnancy.

Studies on the rabbit and rat have shown that HPL will not mobilize free fatty acid or protect against insulin-induced hypoglycemia, but will potentiate HGH in these actions.[8,16] Grumbach and colleagues were, however, able to demonstrate increased concentrations of serum free fatty acids and increased resistance to insulin-induced hypoglycemia in hypopituitary children given doses of HPL about 100 times the minimum effective dose of HGH.[11,13] Beck and Daughaday were also able to alter glucose tolerance and consequent insulin release after an overnight intravenous infusion of HPL.[1] Clearly, the hormone must be given chronically and in amounts sufficient to approximate the plasma concentrations of HPL found at term. Dr. Mintz and I have found lower doses to be insufficient.

The work of Kalkhoff carried out in nonpregnant females, has suggested that administration of HPL will provoke a diabetic glucose tolerance test in those patients showing such abnormal curves during gestation.[22]

In view of the finding of Schultz and Blizzard that HPL, given to hypopituitary children with or without HGH, failed to increase positive nitrogen balance[31] makes it appear doubtful that HPL, acting directly or in synergism with HGH, is responsible for the increased nitrogen retention seen in pregnant females.[14] Grumbach has shown, however, that chronic administration of higher doses of HPL will promote nitrogen retention.[11] Our laboratory has shown enhanced growth promotion in specific somatotrophic hormone assays performed in hypophysectomized rats when HPL is given in conjunction with HGH.[16,17]

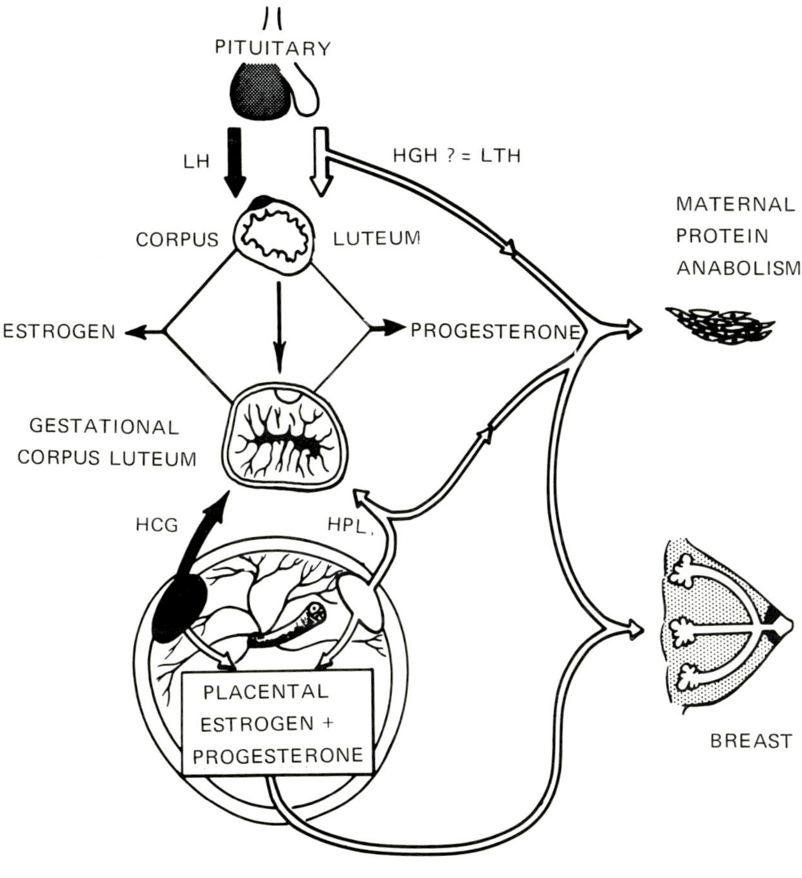

Fig. 8-5. Possible physiological roles of HPL. Solid arrows represent roles whose validity is supported by studies in primates; open-spaced arrows represent proposed functions supported by lower animal data. HCG = human chorionic gonadotrophin; HPL = human placental lactogen; HGH = human pituitary growth hormone; LTH = a postulated pituitary prolactin. (Modified from Josimovich and Atwood. *Amer. J. Obstet. Gynec. 88*:867, 1964.)

Clearly, HPL is not identical in its somatotrophic properties with HGH, although it may be partially responsible for the glucose-sparing and nitrogen-retaining phenomena observed in late human gestation. An important effect of this hormone may be the maintenance of progesterone and estrogen secretion through interaction with the effects of chorionic gonadotrophin. Figure 8-5, summarizes the proposed multiple synergistic roles of HPL.

REFERENCES

1. Beck, P., and Daughaday, W. H. Human placental lactogen: studies of its acute metabolic effects and disposition in normal man. *J. Clin. Invest. 46:*103, 1967.
2. Beck, P., Parker, M. L., and Daughaday, W. H. Radioimmunologic measurement of human placental lactogen in plasma by a double antibody method during normal and diabetic pregnancies. *J. Clin. Endocr. 25:*1457, 1965.
3. Burt, R. L. Peripheral utilization of glucose in pregnancy. III. Insulin tolerance. *Obstet. Gynec. 7:*658, 1956.
4. Burt, R. L. Plasma nonesterified fatty acids in normal pregnancy and the puerperium. *Obstet. Gynec. 15:*460, 1960.
5. Catt, K. J., Moffat, B., and Niall, H. D. Human growth hormone and placental lactogen: structural similarity. *Science 157:*321, 1967.
6. Evans, H. M., Briggs, J. H., and Dixon, J. S. "The Physiology and Chemistry of Growth Hormone." In *Pituitary Gland,* Vol. 1, G. W. Harris and B. T. Donovan (Eds.), University of California Press, Berkeley, 1966.
7. Frantz, A. G., Rabkin, M. T., and Friesen, H. Human placental lactogen in choriocarcinoma of the male. Measurement by radioimmunoassay. *J. Clin. Endocr. 25:*1136, 1965.
8. Friesen, H. Purification of a placental factor with immunological and chemical similarity to human growth hormone. *Endocrinology 76:*369, 1965.
9. Friesen, H. Lactation induced by human placental lactogen and cortisone acetate in rabbits. *Endocrinology 79:*212, 1966.
10. Gemzell, C. A., Heijkenskjöld, F., and Ström, L. A method for demonstrating growth hormone activity in human plasma. *J. Clin. Endocr. 15:*537, 1955.
11. Grumbach, M. M. Growth hormone-like activity of chorionic growth hormone-prolactin (CGP) and its postulated function in pregnancy. Summaries, *Int. Symp. Pharmacol. Hormonal Polypeptides,* Milan, Italy, 1967, p. 57.
12. Grumbach, M. M., and Kaplan, S. L. On the placental origin and purification of chorionic "growth hormone-prolactin" and its immunoassay in pregnancy. *Trans. N.Y. Acad. Sci. 27:*167, 1964.

13. Grumbach, M. M., Kaplan, S. L., Abrams, C. L., Bell, J. J., and Conte, F. A. Plasma free fatty acid response to the administration of chorionic "growth hormone-prolactin." *J. Clin. Endocr. 26:*478, 1966.

14. Hunscher, H. A., Hummel, F. C., Erickson, B. N., and Macy, I. G. Metabolism of women during the reproductive cycle. VI. A case study of the continuous nitrogen utilization of a multipara during pregnancy. *J. Nutr. 10:*579, 1935.

15. Javert, C. T. *Spontaneous and Habitual Abortion.* McGraw-Hill, New York, 1957.

16. Josimovich, J. B. Potentiation of somatotrophic and diabetogenic effects of growth hormone by human placental lactogen (HPL). *Endocrinology 78:*707, 1966.

17. Josimovich, J. B., and Atwood, B. L. Human placental lactogen (HPL), a trophoblastic hormone synergizing with chorionic gonadotropin and potentiating the anabolic effects of pituitary growth hormone. *Amer. J. Obstet. Gynec. 88:*867, 1964.

18. Josimovich, J. B., Atwood, B. D., and Goss, D. A. Luteotrophic, immunologic and electrophoretic properties of human placental lactogen. *Endocrinology 73:*410, 1963.

19. Josimovich, J. B., and Cato, L. Unique Luteotrophic Properties of Combinations of Human Placental Lactogen and Chorionic Gonadotrophin. In *Fertility and Sterility,* B. Westin and N. Wiqvist (Eds.), *Excerpta Med. Int. Cong. Sr. No. 133:*502, 1967.

20. Josimovich, J. B. Correlation of biological and immunochemical studies on human placental lactogen. International Symposium on Growth Hormone, Milan, Italy, 1967. *Excerpta Med. Int. Cong. Sr. No. 142:*7, 1967.

21. Josimovich, J. B., and MacLaren, J. A. Presence in the human placenta and term serum of a highly lactogenic substance immunologically related to pituitary growth hormone. *Endocrinology 71:*209, 1962.

22. Kalkhoff, R. K. Effects of placental lactogen and glucocorticoids on glucose tolerance in normal and diabetic subjects. *Clin. Res. 15:*321, 1967.

23. Kaplan, S. L., and Grumbach, M. M. Studies of a human and simian placental hormone with growth hormone-like and prolactin-like activities. *J. Clin. Endocr. 24:*80, 1964.

24. Kaplan, S. L., and Grumbach, M. M. Serum chorionic "growth hormone-prolactin" and serum pituitary growth hormone in mother and fetus at term. *J. Clin. Endocr. 25:*1370, 1965.

25. Knobil, E., and Josimovich, J. B. Fatty acid mobilization during pregnancy in the rat. *Fed. Proc. 19* (1) :223, 1960. (Abstract)

26. Koren, Z., and Shafrir, E. Placental transfer of free fatty acids in the pregnant rat. *Proc. Soc. Exp. Biol. Med. 116:*411, 1964.

27. MacRae, D. J., and Palavidji, D. Some aspects of the transfer of glucose to the foetus. *J. Obstet. Gynaec. Brit. Comm. 71:*954, 1964.

28. Milner, R. D. G., and Hales, C. N. Effect of intravenous glucose on concentration of insulin in maternal and venous cord plasma. *Brit. Med. J. 1:*284, 1965.

29. Mintz, D. H., Finster, J. L., and Josimovich, J. B. Effect of estrogen therapy on carbohydrate metabolism in acromegaly. *J. Clin. Endocr. 27:*1321, 1967.

30. Samaan, N., Yen, S. C. C., Friesen, H., and Pearson, O. H. Serum placental lactogen levels during pregnancy and in trophoblastic disease. *J. Clin. Endocr. 26:*1303, 1966.

31. Schultz, R. B., and Blizzard, R. M. A comparison of human placental lactogen (HPL) and human growth hormone (HGH) in hypopituitary patients. *J. Clin. Endocr. 26:*921, 1966.

32. Sciarra, J. J., Kaplan, S. L., and Grumbach, M. M. Localization of anti-human growth hormone serum within the human placenta: Evidence for a human chorionic "growth hormone-prolactin." *Nature* (London) *199:* 1005, 1963.

33. Shelley, H. J., and Neligan, G. A. Neonatal hypoglycaemia. *Brit. Med. Bull. 22:*34, 1966.

34. Sherwood, L. M. Similarities in the chemical structure of human placental lactogen and pituitary growth hormone. *Proc. Nat. Acad. Sci. 58:*2307, 1967.

35. Spellacy, W. N., Carlson, K. L., and Birk, S. A. Human placental lactogen levels as a variable of placental weight and infant weight. *Amer. J. Obstet. Gynec. 95:*118, 1966.

36. Turkington, R. W., and Topper, Y. J. Stimulation of casein synthesis and histological development of mammary gland by human placental lactogen *in vitro. Endocrinology 79:*175, 1966.

37. Van Duyne, C. M., and Havel, R. J. Plasma unesterified fatty acid in fetal and neonatal life. *Proc. Soc. Exp. Biol. Med. 102:*599, 1959.

38. Wittels, B., and Bressler, R. Lipid metabolism in the newborn heart. *J. Clin. Invest. 44:*1639, 1965.

Chapter Nine

Insulin

William N. Spellacy

It is only fifty years since the obstetricians first encountered the problem of the pregnant patient with diabetes mellitus with any frequency. Before the discovery of insulin by Banting and Best, most women with diabetes mellitus were infertile. In recent years the incidence of pregnant, diabetic patients has risen rapidly. This has been due to both the restoration of a normal fertility status with insulin treatment, and to better detection procedures being more widely applied to obstetrical populations so that the milder cases are now recognized. The management of these patients has also greatly improved. Physicians now strive for perfect maternal glucose control, prevention of salt and water retention, early deliveries based on fetal maturity and placental function tests, and careful observation of the newborn for hypoglycemia or respiratory distress problems. This therapy has resulted in maternal mortality rates not much different from those of women with uncomplicated pregnancies. But although the perinatal mortality is less than one-half of its pre-insulin level, it still remains at 15–20 percent in most large series. Many centers have poorer results. These figures do not reflect the additional complications of maternal morbidity, fetal congenital anomalies, or newborn morbidity.

It is clear that many medical problems remain unsolved. It is equally clear that progress in resolving these problems must come from a more basic understanding of carbohydrate metabolism in pregnancy. Research

This work was supported in part by Grant HD 01463 from the National Institute of Child Health and Human Development.

in any area is dependent upon the development of new tools. The introduction of the radioimmunoassay technique to protein hormone analysis was the tool that investigators needed in order to explore carbohydrate metabolism. Now measurements of blood insulin and of pituitary and placental growth hormones can be performed accurately and more easily than ever before. The determination of these hormone patterns in normal and abnormal pregnancy has begun to outline carbohydrate metabolism in pregnancy. The purpose of this chapter is to summarize some of the new findings and to attempt to show how this basic knowledge can aid in understanding and resolving the complicated cases of diabetes mellitus and pregnancy.

RESEARCH METHODS USED

All of the subjects described were studied with a fasting blood sample and blood samples after a glucose stimulation of the pancreatic beta cells. It has been previously shown by several investigators that the oral glucose tolerance test (GTT) measures both the absorption of glucose from the gastrointestinal tract and the utilization of that glucose by the body. Much attention has been given recently to the mechanism of insulin secretion. It is well recognized that insulin levels are higher after an oral glucose stimulus than after an intravenous stimulus, even if both produce similar blood glucose levels. Gastrointestinal motility and absorption may be erratic during pregnancy. The results of an intravenous test are dependent only upon glucose utilization. In Figure 9-1 the blood glucose levels from an oral and an intravenous GTT on the same term pregnant individual done four days apart are plotted. The difference is striking. Although the intravenous glucose stimulus may not be the maximum one for insulin release, nor the most physiological stimulus, nor perhaps the most sensitive one for detecting diabetes mellitus, it is a stimulus that can be consistently applied in a research situation where the emphasis is on determining plasma insulin patterns. For this reason the results expressed below are all based upon intravenous stimuli.

All of the tests were begun between eight and nine o'clock in the morning to minimize the effect of circadian variations. Each subject had fasted overnight. No patient was receiving thiazide diuretics and none had previously received exogenous insulin. There is evidence that the thiazide diuretics can alter carbohydrate metabolism, and previous insulin treatment interferes with immunoassay techniques. All of the subjects had an adequate dietary history. During the test procedure the physical activity of each subject was limited to sitting or lying down. All of these variables must be controlled to give reproducible and reliable

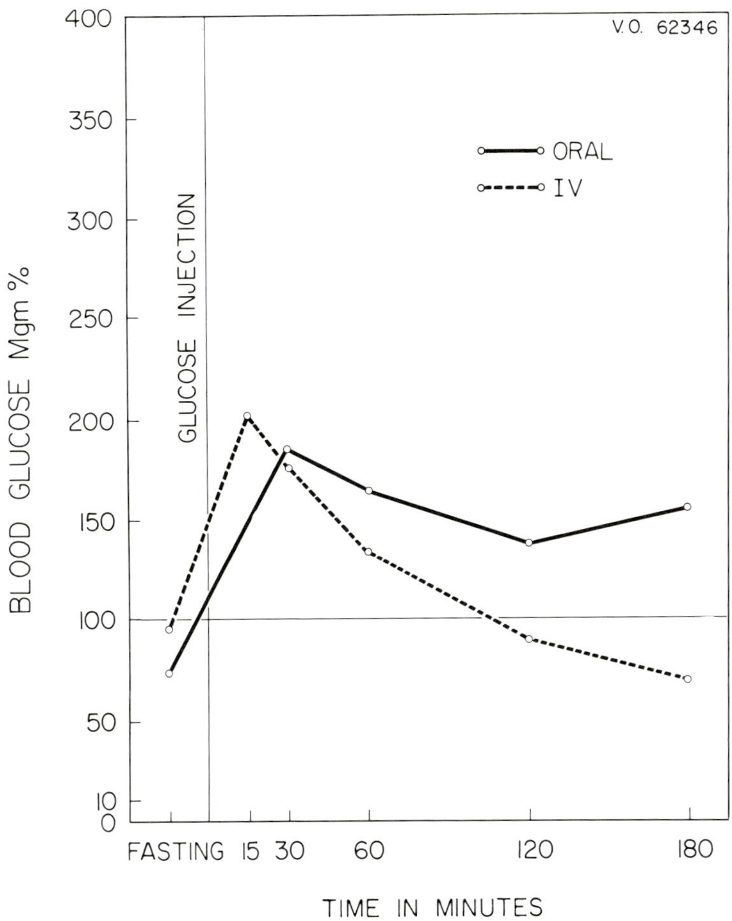

Fig. 9-1. Comparison of the blood glucose values in a term pregnant patient tested with both an oral and an intravenous glucose tolerance test.

results. A blood sample was drawn from the antecubital vein and then 25 gm of glucose as a 50% solution was injected intravenously over a period of less than 2 minutes. Repeat venous blood samples were then drawn at 15, 30, 60, 120, and occasionally 180 and 240 minutes after the glucose injection.

The blood for glucose determination was placed in tubes with potassium oxalate as anticoagulant and also containing sodium fluoride as an inhibitor of glycolysis. The blood and additions were mixed well and then frozen at −20° C. Later the blood was analyzed in duplicate for its glucose content by the method of Nelson and Somogyi.[15,17]

The blood for insulin determination was placed in tubes containing powdered heparin as an anticoagulant. They were mixed well and then centrifuged at 2000 r.p.m. for 10 minutes. The plasma was removed and frozen at −20° C. Later all the plasma samples from a given subject were analyzed in duplicate by a radioimmunoassay procedure similar to that described by Goetz *et al.*[9] The insulin levels are reported in microunits per milliliter of plasma as compared with a standard. The standard used was crystalline human insulin which was bioassayed for its insulin content per milligram weight.* The immunoassay seems to measure true total circulating insulin and agrees well with the hemidiaphragm bioassay insulin test.[14]

In every phase of this study the subjects were tested at least twice. This included one or more tests performed during pregnancy, and another test later than six weeks post partum. The latter test will be referred to as the control test. Studies from this laboratory have shown that the carbohydrate metabolism has reverted to its pre-pregnancy state by approximately two weeks post partum. The same glucose stimulus was given for each test, and thus, on a body weight basis, the individual received a larger dose when she was not pregnant. This type of research design allows for the comparison of each individual in a pregnant condition with herself as her own nonpregnant control. Since the results always compare correlated pairs which differ only by one factor, pregnancy, the data can be analyzed statistically by the determination of the differences, the means of the differences, the Student's t value for each mean, and the probability (p) values for each t. Only significant differences will be discussed.

NORMAL PREGNANCY

The first studies involved 60 normal pregnant subjects. They were divided into three groups and each group was tested twice as outlined above. The groups were at 13–15 weeks ("early"), 25–29 weeks ("mid"), and 36–40 weeks ("late") of gestation as calculated from the last menstrual period.[20, 22, 23] The mean blood glucose results are shown in Figure 9-2. It is clear that the blood glucose values are normal throughout pregnancy, and also that the absolute values are somewhat lower while the subjects are pregnant. The tests show no alteration in glucose metabolism during gestation.

The plasma insulin values are shown in Figure 9-3. It can be seen that there is an excess of circulating insulin in the fasting state during preg-

* The human insulin was kindly supplied by M. Root, Ph.D. and W. R. Kirtley, M.D. of the Eli Lilly Research Laboratories of Indianapolis, Indiana.

nancy. The excess of insulin released after intravenous glucose is even more pronounced. This becomes more marked as the groups approach the end of gestation.

Individual Serial Study

The patterns of insulin release following glucose stimulation clearly change with the progress of gestation. In order to be certain that these results were not due to variations among the three patient groups, several normal individuals were serially studied at similar periods of gestation. The blood glucose results were all normal, and, again, the pregnant values were slightly lower than the matched control values. Four insulin curves for four subjects are shown in Figure 9-4. These serial assays show the same change during pregnancy as that found in the group studies. The findings indicate that during pregnancy hyperfunction of the pancreatic beta cells starts toward the end of the first trimester and reaches its maximum by the time of delivery.

Tolbutamide Stimulation

As one more test of beta cell function during pregnancy, subjects were stimulated with an intravenous injection of 1 gm of tolbutamide.* The mean insulin values for 12 subjects in the last month of a normal pregnancy are shown in Figure 9-5. There was a smaller blood glucose fall during pregnancy but there is obviously a more marked insulin rise in the pregnant group.[24] Since one accepted action of tolbutamide is a direct stimulation of the pancreatic beta cell to release insulin, this is another piece of evidence that the hyperinsulinemia of pregnancy is due to a pancreatic hyperfunction. These data also indicate the normal pregnant patient's resistance to insulin of either endogenous or exogenous source as had previously been noted by Burt.[3]

Source of Hyperinsulinemia

The excess insulin present in the normal pregnant subject could be coming from either the fetus, the placenta, or her own pancreas. By measuring insulin on both sides of the placenta (maternal and cord venous blood) it was shown that natural insulin probably does not pass freely through the placental barrier and that the fetal insulin was lower than, and unrelated to, the maternal insulin level.[13] Many other studies have been conducted on the problem of placental permeability to insulin. For example, radioactive insulin studies by Buse, Roberts, and Buse indicated that the placenta was impermeable to insulin.[4] Gitlin,

* Tolbutamide was supplied as sodium salt by the Upjohn Company, Kalamazoo, Michigan.

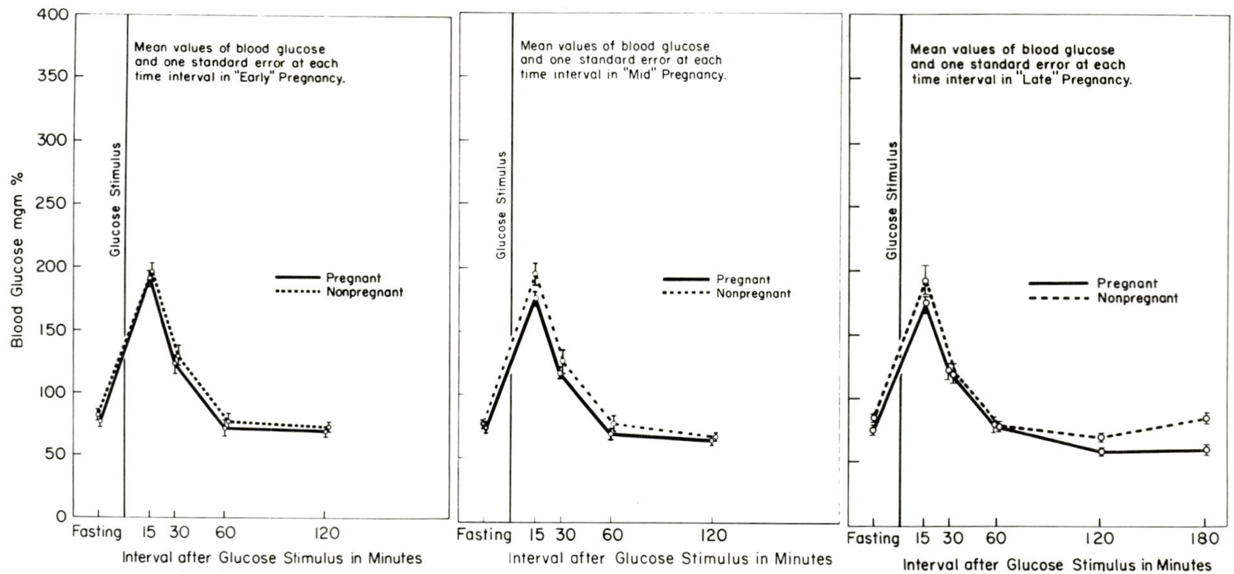

Fig. 9-2. Mean blood glucose values for three groups of 20 subjects each studied at the end of each trimester of a normal gestation and again in a control state more than 6 weeks post partum. (From Spellacy and Goetz. *New Eng. J. Med. 268*:988, 1963.)

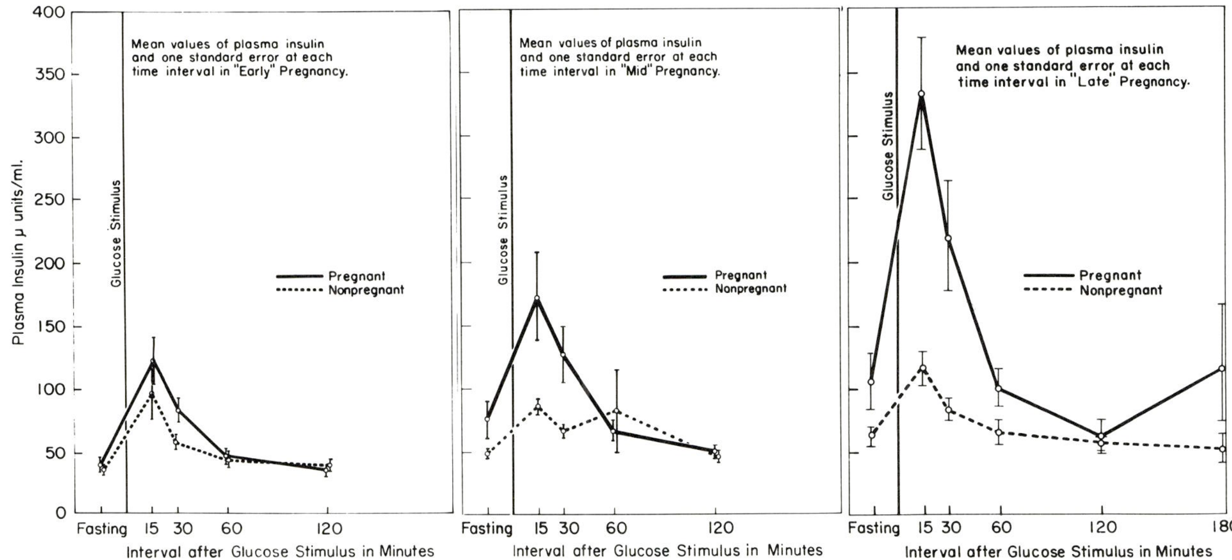

Fig. 9-3. **Mean plasma insulin values for three groups of 20 subjects each studied at the end of each trimester of a normal gestation and again in a control state more than 6 weeks post partum.** (From Spellacy and Goetz. *New Eng. J. Med. 268*:988, 1963.)

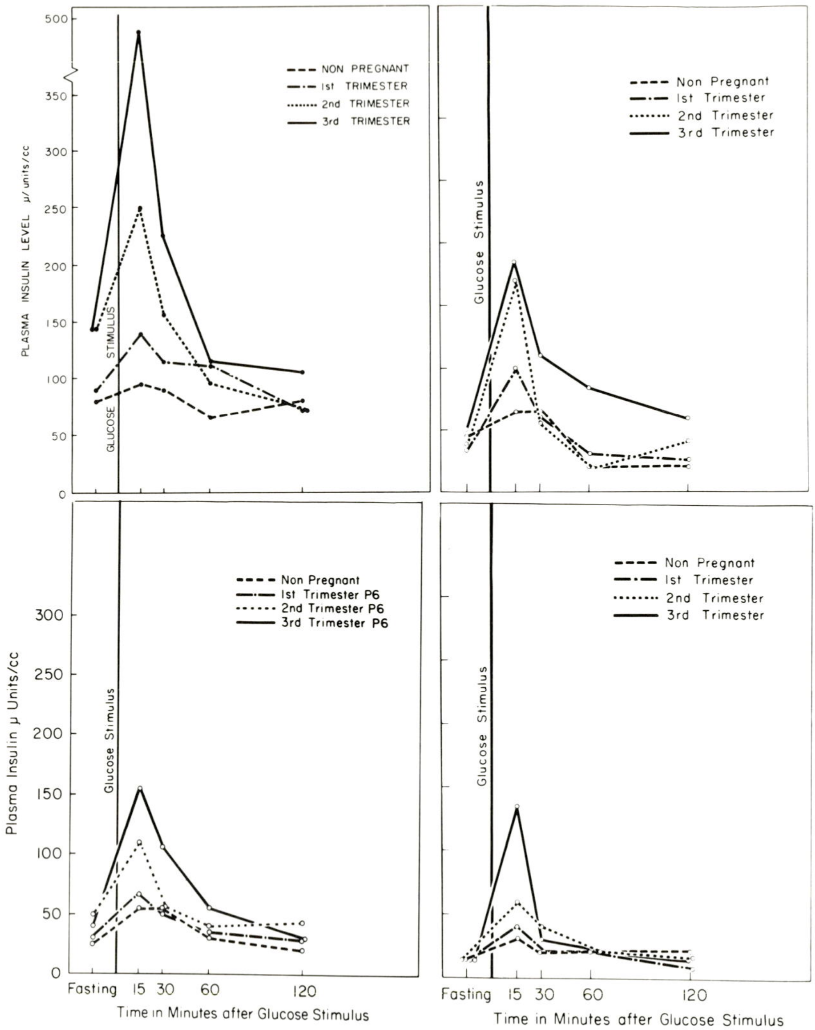

Fig. 9-4. Plasma insulin values following glucose load in four individuals during normal pregnancy. Insulin assays in each trimester and in the puerperium.

Kumate, and Morales, however, concluded that insulin passes the placenta in both directions.[8] It would appear that although this problem is not completely resolved, the placenta does impose a barrier to insulin transfer.

Additional investigations have been made in patients with a fetal death in utero and also in patients soon after a normal vaginal delivery of the infant and placenta. In both of these groups of subjects it was

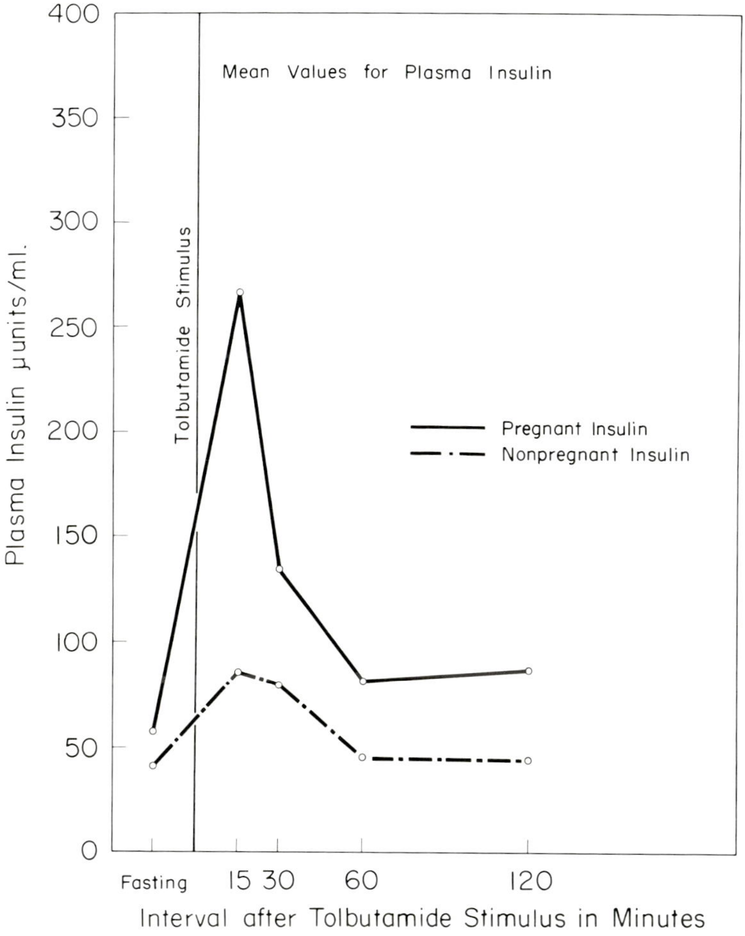

Fig. 9-5. Mean plasma insulin values for 12 subjects following tolbutamide stimulation. Pregnant values obtained during last month of pregnancy. (From Spellacy *et al. J. Clin. Endocr. 25:*1251, 1965.)

found that there is an excess of circulating insulin present during the pregnant state as compared to the nonpregnant state.[19] The excess insulin could obviously not be coming from either the placenta or the fetus. The conclusion from all of these studies is that the measured hyperinsulinemia in normal pregnant women is indeed from a hyperfunctioning maternal pancreatic beta cell mass.

These biochemical data are well correlated with the histological appearance of the pancreas during pregnancy. Hellman noted an increase in the number of beta cells in the pancreas of the pregnant rat,[10] and Rosenloecher had also noted an increase in both size and number of the islands of Langerhans in the human during pregnancy.[16]

Other studies of insulin levels in pregnancy have been reported. In 1959 Gestaldi and Crosignani, using the immunological method of Arquilla, found no difference between control and pregnant women's insulin levels.[7] Carrington and McWilliams, using a different immunological method, have reported similar results.[5] The finding of hyperinsulinemia at the end of a normal pregnancy has now been shown by many independent investigators using either bioassay or immunological methods.[2,11,13,25]

From these observations one can develop a concept of normal beta cell function during pregnancy. The area under the insulin curve is taken as an approximation of total insulin secretion during a fixed stimulus. Figure 9-6 shows the theoretical beta cell function in response to the "diabetogenic" stress of pregnancy. The maximum function is at the time of delivery.

"Stress Factor" to the Pancreas in Pregnancy

There are most probably several factors which cause the pancreas to produce more insulin in a normal pregnancy. Many of these factors seem to be related to the placenta.

Freinkel and Goodner have shown that the placenta contains an active proteolytic enzyme system that can degrade the insulin molecule.[6] Such destruction would necessitate the biosynthesis of more insulin in order to maintain a steady state. The magnitude of effect of this factor on insulin secretion is not known. Josimovich and MacLaren have demonstrated that the placenta produces a large protein hormone, human placental lactogen (HPL).[12] This protein is chemically, immunologically, and metabolically similar to pituitary growth hormone. Extracted and purified HPL has been given to human beings, and Beck and Daughaday have demonstrated that it can produce alterations in the blood glucose-insulin patterns similar to those demonstrated during pregnancy.[1] Finally, many recent studies have shown that the currently used oral contraceptive drugs containing estrogens and progestins can also change blood glucose and insulin levels. Thus, although it is not known which of the placental factors are responsible, it is clear that the "diabetogenic" stress of pregnancy is related at least in part to the placenta.

ABNORMAL PREGNANCY

In order to relate these normal data to clinical problems, subjects with abnormal blood glucose values have also been studied serially during

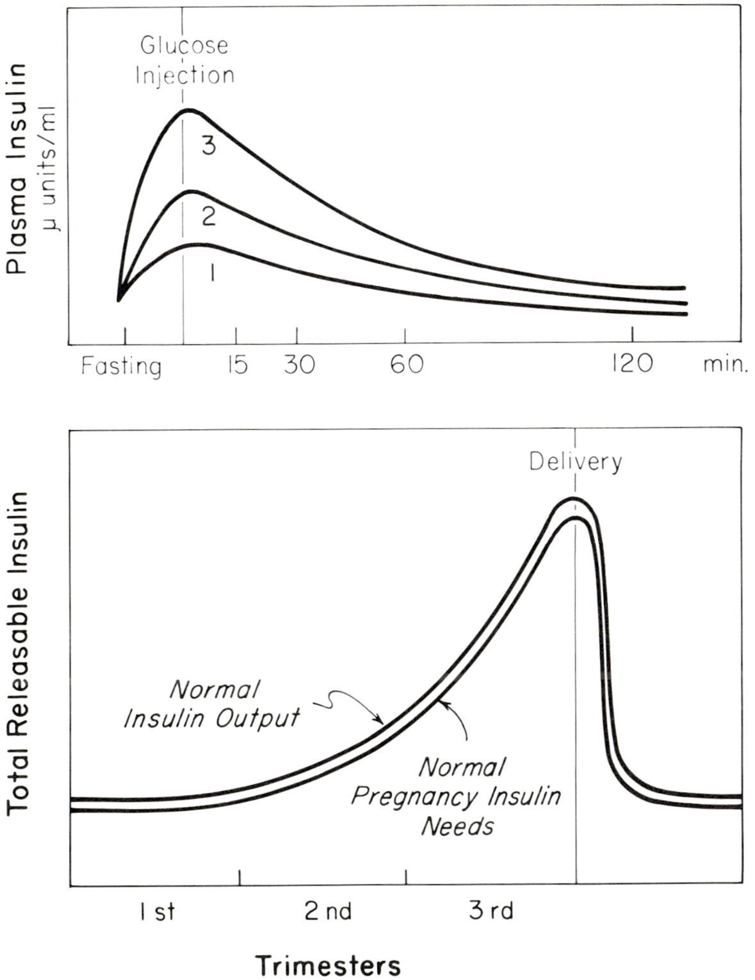

Fig. 9-6. Theoretical pattern of "total releasable insulin" in a normal pregnancy. The curves 1, 2 and 3 in the upper graph correspond to the first, second and third trimesters.

pregnancy. In Figure 9-7 the blood glucose and plasma insulin values of nine patients with chemical diabetes mellitus are shown. They were studied serially with three-hour glucose tolerance tests throughout pregnancy and not treated with exogenous insulin. The blood glucose values are all abnormally high. It can be seen that an entirely different pattern of insulin release is present. It is different in two respects. First, the peak insulin output does not occur in the last trimester. In fact, the third trimester insulin values are lower than the second trimester values in

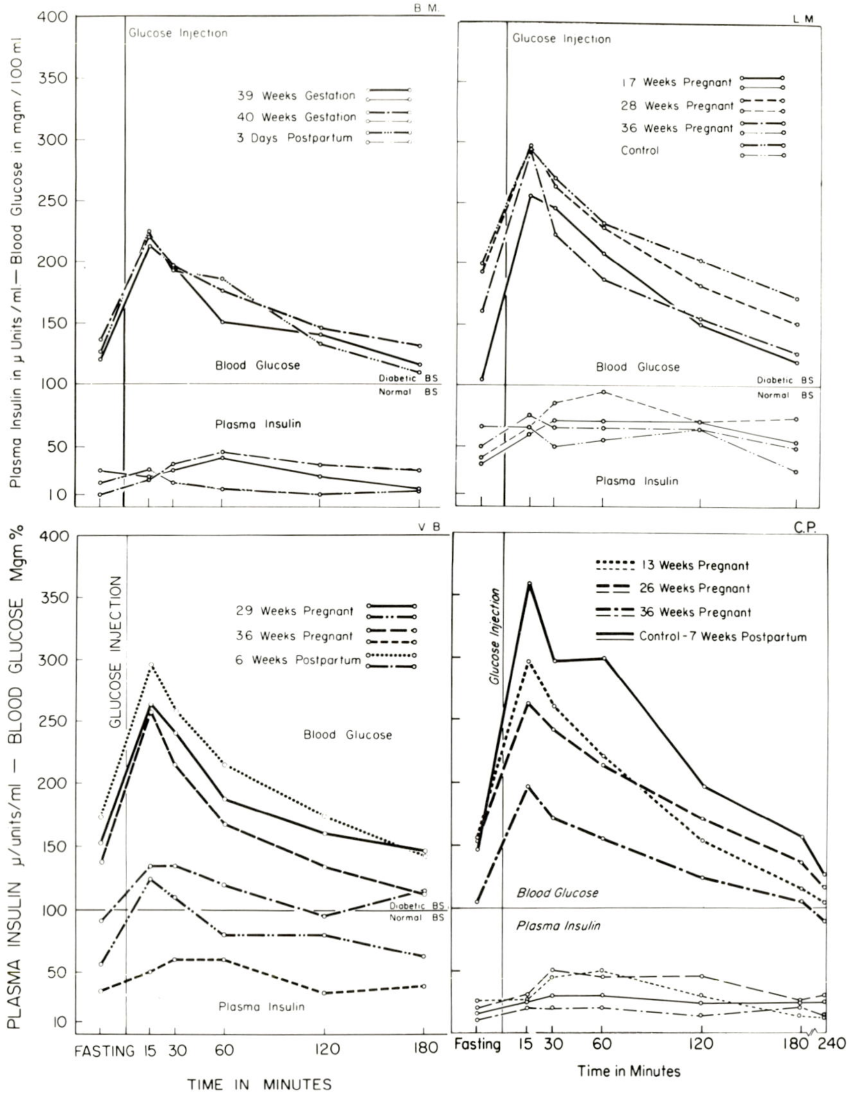

Fig. 9-7. Nine patients with White's class A diabetes mellitus studied serially throughout pregnancy and postpartum. The responses of blood glucose and plasma insulin concentration to an intravenous glucose load are shown.

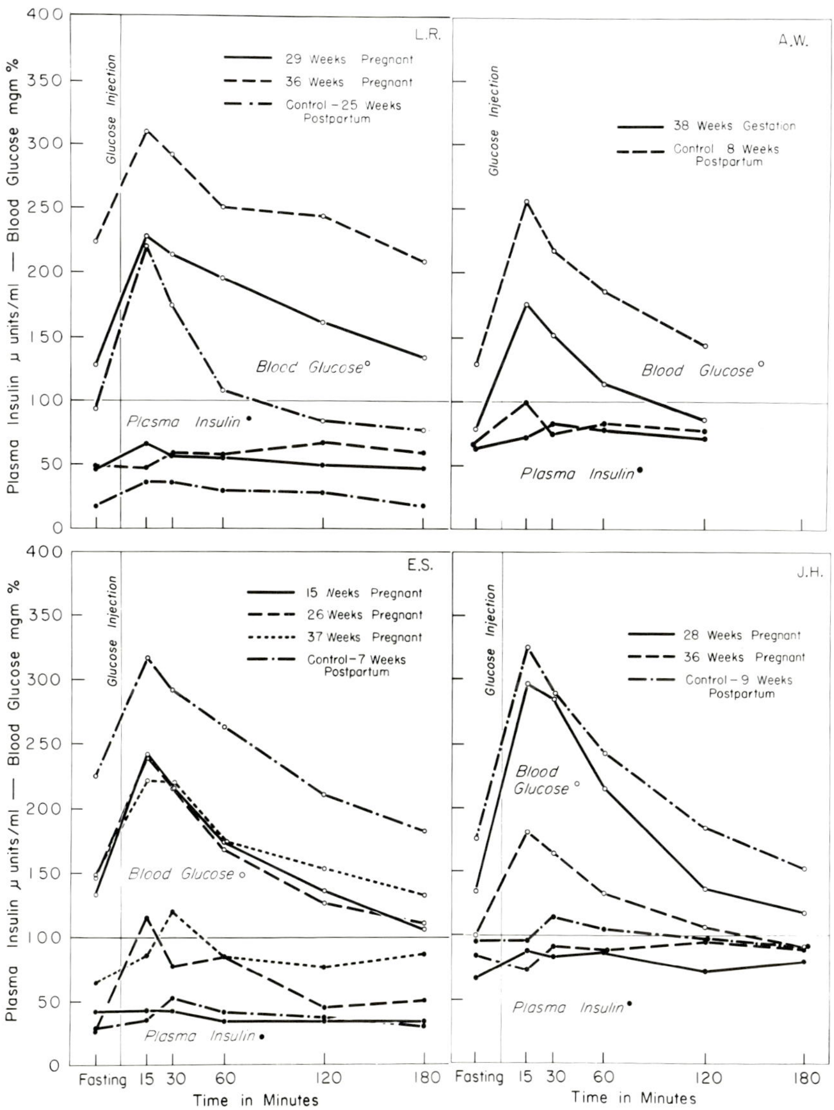

Fig. 9-7. *(continued)*

five subjects (LM,VB,CP,LR,SS). Also of note is the fact that the third trimester insulin values are the lowest of all the test values in three subjects (VB,CP,AW). Second, most of these subjects have a delayed peak in insulin release after the glucose injection as opposed to the normal pregnant and nonpregnant subjects. One may assume that the

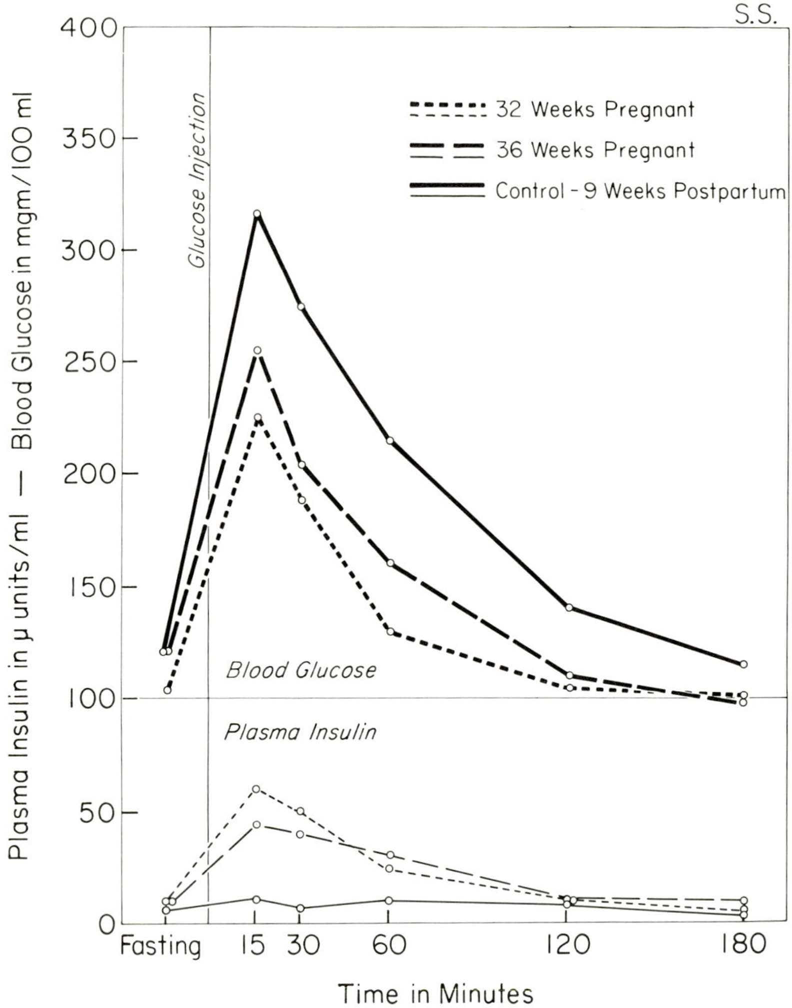

Fig. 9-7. *(continued)*

"diabetogenic" stress of pregnancy is equally active in these patients for they have a functioning placenta, but the pancreatic function is apparently impaired and the beta cells can therefore not release increasing amounts of insulin as pregnancy progresses to term.

A diagrammatic concept of this is shown on Figure 9-8. Here one can see that in the minimally diseased state the pancreatic function may appear normal when the patient is not pregnant or is in early pregnancy.

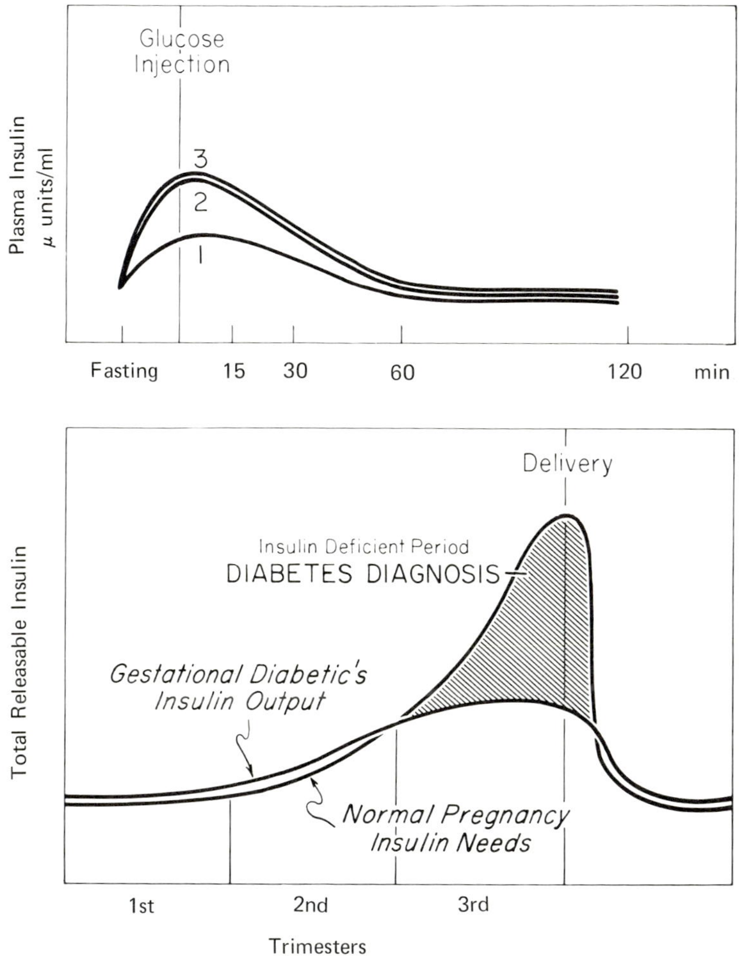

Fig. 9-8. Diagramatic concept of gestational diabetes in pregnancy. The curves 1, 2 and 3 in the upper graph correspond to the first, second and third trimesters.

During these times there is minimum pancreatic stress. By mid or late pregnancy the stress has exceeded the tolerance and overt problems arise. A short period of "relative insulin insufficiency" with resultant abnormally high blood glucose values may be produced. This would represent the "gestational diabetic" syndrome, and the glucose pattern would be expected to revert to normal again in the postpartum period when the pancreatic "stress" is removed. This is indeed what has been found clinically. The term "gestational diabetes" is applied to those patients who develop abnormal glucose tolerance tests only during pregnancy. In a more severely diseased state, as in the overt diabetic, the pancreas is hypofunctioning even before pregnancy begins and this continues throughout pregnancy. The need for excess insulin may become so acute that there is beta cell exhaustion and exogenous insulin is required. In Figure 9-9 are plotted the data of a patient who was frankly diabetic at 32 weeks of gestation, after a normal test in early pregnancy. She then progressed to acidosis at 37 weeks of gestation when exogenous insulin was required to reverse the process. After pregnancy she again had a normal GTT and did not require insulin treatment.

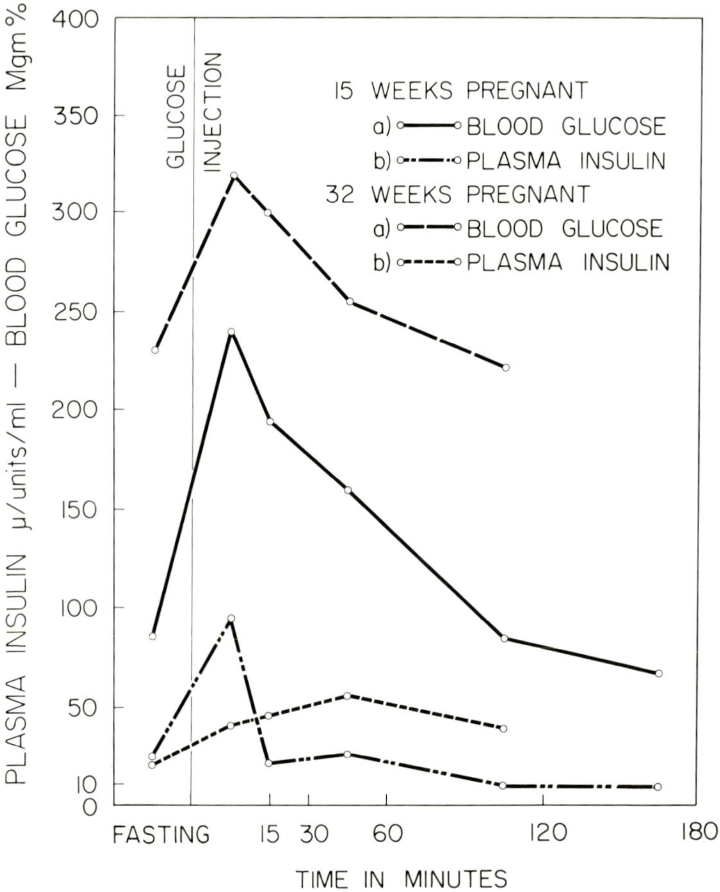

Fig. 9-9. Studies on a subject who had a normal glucose tolerance test in early pregnancy, an abnormal glucose tolerance test in midpregnancy, and a need for exogenous insulin in late pregnancy.

Application

The next question to be raised is how can these data be applied to aid the clinician in his patient management. Several recommendations can be made.

First, pregnancy can be expected to make subclinical diabetes become manifest by virtue of its stress factors. If one has a suspicion that the pregnant patient may have diabetes mellitus because of her family history, or her past history of delivering large infants, or the presence of glucosuria, it would seem that the ideal time to test her would be near term gestation when the pancreas is under its maximum stress. A normal test in early pregnancy may become abnormal as pregnancy progresses.

Secondly, the findings throw some light on the problems of insulin dosage in pregnant juvenile diabetics. It is known that these patients have very little pancreatic beta cell function, and, as a consequence, they are dependent upon an exogenous insulin supply. Since the placental stress factors would be present in these patients, too, one would anticipate that there would be an increasing need for insulin as pregnancy progressed. This has been found to be so in most clinical studies relating total insulin dosage needed during pregnancy. This rising dosage requirement is a good prognostic sign, for it indicates a functioning placenta which is producing insulin antagonism. Conversely, a sudden decrease in the total insulin requirements of a patient may be a signal to the clinician that the placenta is beginning to decrease its production of HPL and may also have become deficient in other respects. This decrease in function may herald fetal disaster.

In Figures 9-2 and 9-3 it can be seen that normally there are only minor changes in glucose tolerance during pregnancy, despite marked plasma insulin changes. Also, in Figure 9-7 it can be seen that the blood glucose patterns of the chemical diabetic retains the abnormal pattern of her nonpregnant state despite the greatly increasing relative deficiency of circulating insulin. If the lack of an adequate amount of circulating insulin is of importance to the outcome of the pregnancy, perhaps because an inadequate amount impairs placental function, one could theorize that the patient should be treated with enough exogenous insulin to make the blood glucose pattern normal. In other words, since the clinical blood glucose pattern in the human acts as an insensitive bioassay for insulin levels, and since clinicians currently use only blood glucose levels in patient management, clinicians cannot be satisfied with anything less than normal blood glucose values. As a test of this concept, the best clinical results in the management of the pregnant diabetic would be expected in those patients who were maintained with nearly normal blood glucose values; this, in fact, has been found to be so. The obstetrician must strive for meticulous glucose control.

FUTURE STUDIES

Our knowledge of insulin metabolism in pregnancy and its relationship to the clinical problems have advanced a great deal in the last decade. We are still only scratching the surface of the intriguing problems of carbohydrate metabolism in pregnancy. Many questions remain to be answered. When does insulin form in the fetal pancreas and what is its role in utero? How does insulin affect the metabolism and function of the placenta? Why do babies die in utero in patients with abnormal carbohydrate metabolism and also in those with only the genetic traits or "prediabetes?" What are the inter-relationships between erythroblastosis fetalis, toxemia, hydramnios, and diabetes mellitus? What tests can best diagnose diabetes in pregnancy? The next decade should offer great research opportunities for those interested in carbohydrate metabolism and pregnancy.

REFERENCES

1. Beck, P., and Daughaday, W. H. Human placental lactogen. Studies of its acute metabolic effects and disposition in normal man. *J. Clin. Invest. 46:*103, 1967.
2. Bleicher, S. J., O'Sullivan, J. B., and Freinkel, N. Carbohydrate Metabolism in pregnancy. V. The interrelations of glucose, insulin and free fatty acids in late pregnancy and postpartum. *New Eng. J. Med. 271:*866, 1964.
3. Burt, R. L. Further observations on reactivity to insulin in normal pregnancy. *Obstet. Gynec. 13:*433, 1959.
4. Buse, M. G., Roberts, W. J., and Buse, J. The role of the human placenta in the transfer and metabolism of insulin. *J. Clin. Invest. 41:*29, 1962.
5. Carrington, E. R., and McWilliams, N. Investigation of serum insulin activity during pregnancy in normal and subclinical diabetic mothers. *Amer. J. Obstet. Gynec. 96:*922, 1966.
6. Freinkel, N., and Goodner, C. J. Carbohydrate metabolism in pregnancy. 1. The metabolism of insulin by human placental tissue. *J. Clin. Invest. 39:*116, 1960.
7. Gestaldi, A., and Crosignani, P. G. Modificazoni, dell'insulinomia in gravidanza dopo carico orale di glucosio. *Ann. Ostet. Ginec. 81:*1171, 1959.
8. Gitlin, D., Kumate, J., and Morales, C. On the transport of insulin across the human placenta. *Pediatrics 35:*65, 1965.
9. Goetz, F. C., Greenberg, B. Z., Ells, J., and Meinert, C. A simple immuno-

assay for insulin: application to human and dog plasma. *J. Clin. Endocr. 23:*1237, 1963.

10. Hellman, B. The islets of Langerhans in the rat during pregnancy and lactation, with special reference to the changes in the cell ratio. *Acta. Obstet. Gynec. Scand. 39:*331, 1960.
11. Kalkhoff, R., Schalch, D. S., Walker, J. L., Beck, P., Kipnis, D. M., and Daughaday, W. H. Diabetogenic factors associated with pregnancy. *Trans. Ass. Amer. Physicians 77:*270, 1964.
12. Josimovich, J. B., and MacLaren, J. A. Presence in the human placenta and term serum of a highly lactogenic substance immunologically related to pituitary growth hormone. *Endocrinology 71:*209, 1962.
13. Leake, N. H., and Burt, R. L. Insulin-like activity in serum during pregnancy. *Diabetes 11:*419, 1962.
14. Martin, J. M. The state of insulin in human plasma. *Diabetes 15:*359, 1966.
15. Nelson, N. Photometric adaptation of Somogyi's method for determination of glucose. *J. Biol. Chem. 153:*375, 1944.
16. Rosenloecher, K. Die Veränderungen des Pankreas in der Schwangerschaft bei Mensch und Tier. *Arch. Gynaek. 151:*567, 1932.
17. Somogyi, M. Determination of blood sugars. *J. Biol. Chem. 160:*69, 1945.
18. Spellacy, W. N., Carlson, K. L., and Birk, S. A. Dynamics of human placental lactogen (HPL) . *Amer. J. Obstet. Gynec. 96:*1164, 1966.
19. Spellacy, W. N., Carlson, K. L., and Birk, S. A. The fetus and the placenta as a source of insulin during pregnancy. *Obstet. Gynec. 29:*74, 1967.
20. Spellacy, W. N., and Goetz, F. C. Plasma insulin in normal late pregnancy. *New Eng. J. Med. 268:*988, 1963.
21. Spellacy, W. N., Goetz, F. C., Greenberg, B. Z., and Ells, J. The human placental gradient for plasma insulin and blood glucose. *Amer. J. Obstet. Gynec. 90:*753, 1964.
22. Spellacy, W. N., Goetz, F. C., Greenberg, B. Z., and Ells, J. Plasma insulin in normal "early" pregnancy. *Obstet. Gynec. 25:*862, 1965.
23. Spellacy, W. N., Goetz, F. C., Greenberg, B. Z., and Ells, J. Plasma insulin in normal "mid" pregnancy. *Amer. J. Obstet. Gynec. 92:*11, 1965.
24. Spellacy, W. N., Goetz, F. C., Greenberg, B. Z., and Schoeller, K. L. Tolbutamide response in normal pregnancy. *J. Clin. Endocr. 25:*1251, 1965.
25. Trayner, I. M., Welborn, T. A., Rubenstein, A. H., and Fraser, T. R. Serum and urine insulin in late pregnancy and in a few pregnant latent diabetics. *J. Endocr. 37:*443, 1967.

Chapter Ten

Thyroid Hormones

Eugene D. Furth and Anthony S. Pagliara

The inter-relationships of thyroid function and human pregnancy are not completely understood because the amount of experimental data is somewhat limited. In addition to clinical data, the present discussion will contain some information derived from animal studies that is helpful in defining concepts. However, there is ample evidence that many aspects of thyroid function vary from species to species,[16] and therefore conclusions derived from animal experiments cannot always be directly applied to man.

This chapter is planned to serve as a brief outline of some of the more important aspects of the inter-relationships of the thyroid and pregnancy. A more detailed account is available in several comprehensive reviews.[15, 18, 28, 34, 51]

NORMAL THYROID PHYSIOLOGY

The normal thyroid gland accumulates dietary iodide at a fairly constant rate, and most of this iodide is incorporated into thyroid hormones or its precursors. The remainder of the ingested iodide is excreted by the kidney. The thyroid hormones are either stored in the gland as colloid or released into the circulation.[10, 46] Figure 10-1 represents an over-all schema of iodine and thyroid hormone metabolism. The two biologically active thyroid hormones secreted by the gland are tetraiodothyronine or thyroxine (T_4) and triiodothyronine (T_3) (Fig. 10-2). Recent evidence suggests that the steric configuration of the thyroid hormone molecule

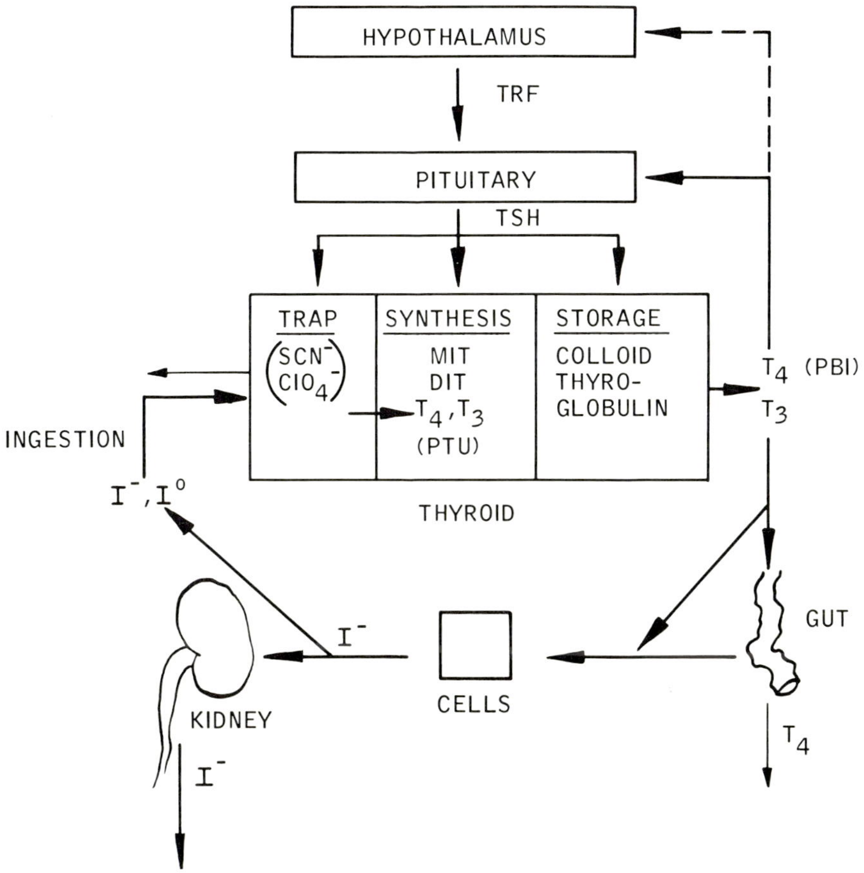

Fig. 10-1. Schema of normal iodine and thyroid hormone metabolism (see text). TRF = thyroid hormone releasing factor, TSH = thyroid stimulating hormone, MIT = monoiodotyrosine, DIT = diiodotyrosine, T_4 = tetraiodothyronine, T_3 = triiodothyronine, PTU = propylthiouracil.

may be more important for biological activity than are the iodine atoms. The steric structure of thyroxine, as interpreted by Jorgensen *et al.*[29] is illustrated in Figure 10-3. If an isopropyl group is substituted on the 3′ position and bromine on the 3 and 5 positions, biological activity is preserved in the absence of iodine, emphasizing the importance of steric configuration for biological activity.

The thyroid hormones are transported in the blood and by way of the extracellular fluid to the cells. Within the cells the hormones may act by mechanisms which involve allosteric modification of existing proteins,

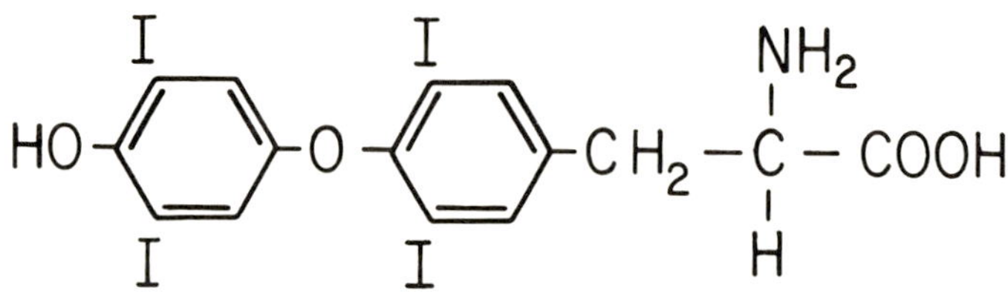

3,5,3',5' TETRAIODOTHYRONINE
(L-THYROXINE)(T_4)

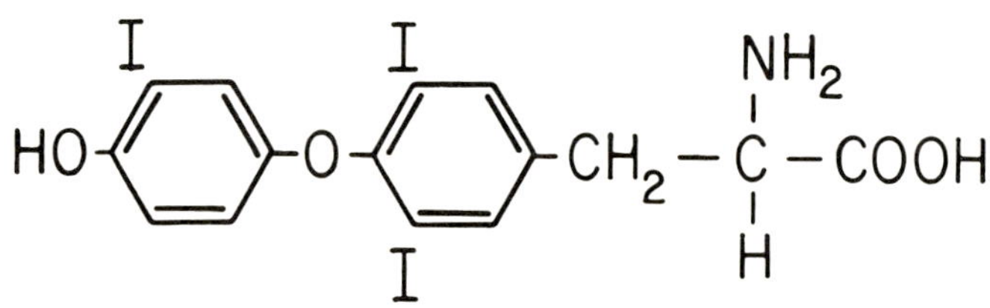

3,5,3'-TRIIODOTHYRONINE(T_3)

Fig. 10-2. Chemical structure of tetraiodothyronine (T_4) and triiodothyronine (T_3).

stimulation of protein synthesis,[50] regulation of oxidative metabolism by mitochondria,[24, 49] and by enhanced production of cyclic AMP through activation of the enzyme adenyl cyclase.[48] The net effects of the hormones are reflected by the metabolic rate of the entire organism and also by some general clinical observations such as pulse rate and body weight. In man, a small fraction of T_4 passes through an enterohepatic pathway, but very little of the hormone is lost in the feces.

The rate of thyroid hormone production is regulated by pituitary thyroid stimulating hormone (TSH), which is in turn regulated by the hypothalamic hormone, thyrotropin releasing factor (TRF)[44] (Fig. 10-1). Details of the inter-relationships among these various hormones in the regulation of thyroid hormone synthesis and release may be found in recent reviews.[5, 44]

Once T_4 and T_3 are metabolized, the hormonal iodide is released

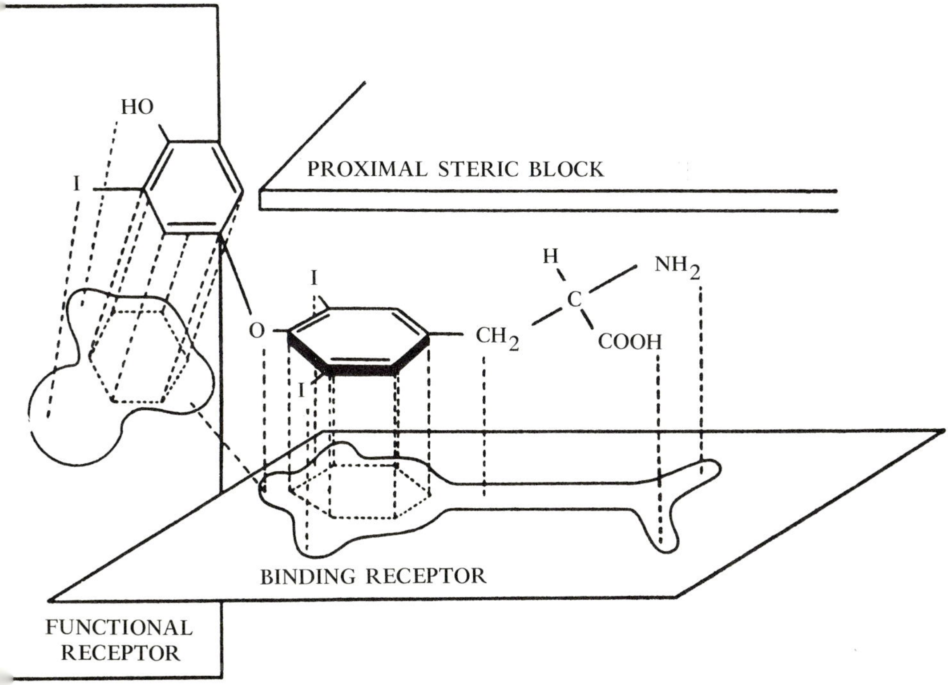

Fig. 10-3. Schematic representation of a hypothetical thyroid hormone receptor interacting with L-triiodothyronine. (From Jorgensen *et al. J. Biol. Chem.* *237*:3832, 1962.)

and enters the body iodide pool where it is available for further hormone synthesis or is excreted in the urine. Quantitative measurements of thyroidal secretion indicate that about 100 μg of T_4 per day and 50 μg of T_3 per day are secreted into the blood.[36] A similar quantity of hormone is metabolized each day, thereby maintaining the hormone concentration constant. Neither net thyroxine metabolism nor hormonal requirements for thyroxine are changed during pregnancy.[11]

Thyroidal iodide trapping may be blocked by thiocyanate (SCN^-) and perchlorate (CLO_4^-) (Fig. 10-1). Organification of iodide and the coupling of monoiodotyrosine (MIT) and diiodotyrosine (DIT) are blocked by propylthiouracil (PTU) and other thioureas (Fig. 10-1).

TESTS OF THYROID FUNCTION

The 24-hour thyroidal radioiodine uptake test reflects thyroidal trapping, organification, storage, and release of iodide. Normal values range between 20 and 50 per cent of an administered tracer dose. It should be noted parenthetically that radioiodine tracer studies are best avoided during pregnancy, although use of the short-lived isotope ^{132}I is considered safe by some.[1]

The blood levels of the circulating thyroid hormones reflect the net result of rates of thyroidal secretion and metabolic degradation rates and are also dependent upon the serum proteins which bind the hormones. T_4 is bound by three circulating serum proteins: pre-albumin, albumin, and an inter-alpha globulin called thyroxine binding globulin (TBG) (Fig. 10-4). An average 4.7 μg of T_4 per 100 ml is bound to protein and 2.76 ng per 100 ml is free in the serum.[47] In contrast to T_4, T_3 is less tightly bound to circulating serum proteins in man. The level of T_3 in the blood is 0.33 μg/100 ml, and of this, 1.51 ng/100 ml is free.[36] The protein-bound iodine (PBI) and the thyroxine by column determinations both measure the iodine contained in the thyroxine which is bound to the circulating serum proteins. In contrast to the PBI and the thyroxine by column tests, the T_3 resin uptake test assesses the interaction of thyroid hormone and serum proteins (Fig. 10-5). Since the resin T_3 test is performed by adding exogenous radioac-

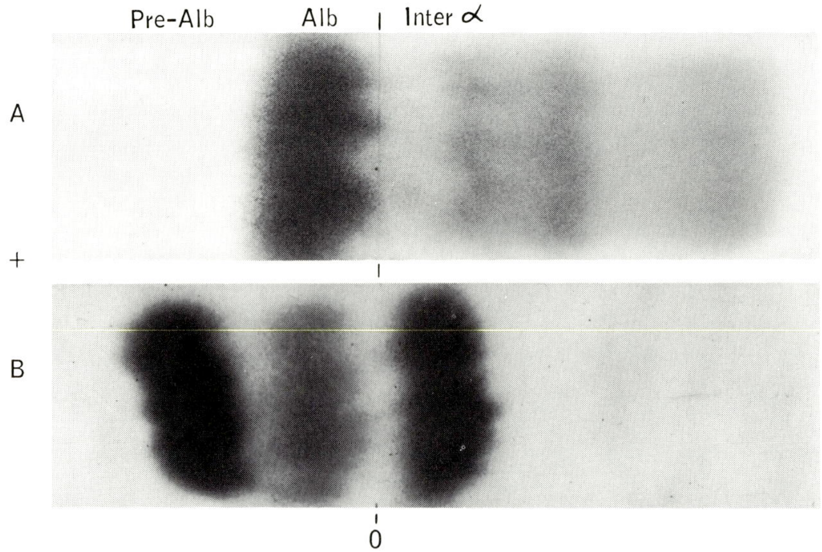

Fig. 10-4. Reverse flow paper electrophoresis of human serum in ammonium carbonate buffer, pH 8.6. *A,* Brom-phenol blue stain of the paper; *B,* radioautograph of the paper before staining. O = origin, + = anode, Alb = albumin, Pre-alb = pre-albumin, inter-α = thyroxine binding globulin.

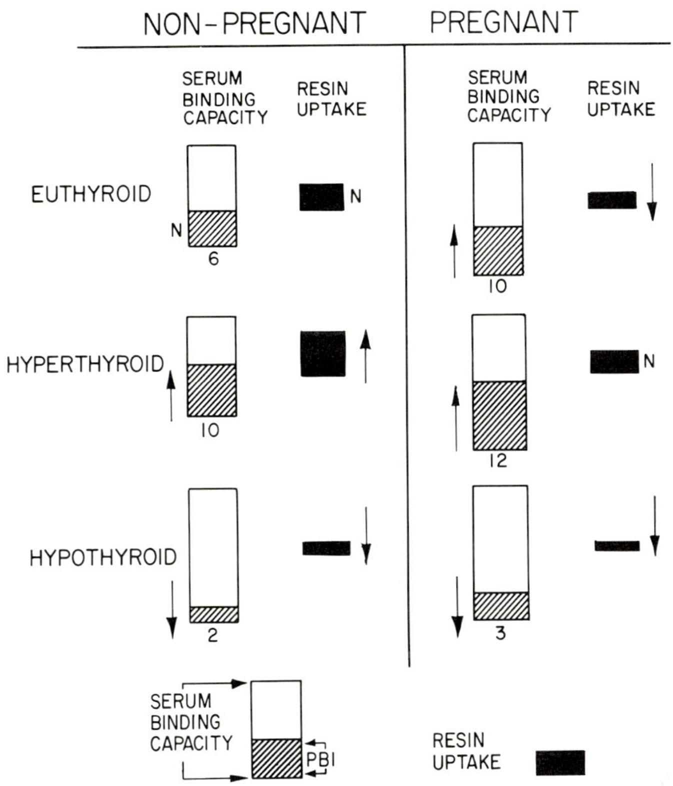

Fig. 10-5. Schematic representation of the PBI, resin uptake, and protein-binding capacity of the serum for thyroxine in pregnant and nonpregnant euthyroid, hyper- and hypothyroid states. N = normal, ↑ = increased, ↓ = decreased. A theoretical PBI value in μg/100 ml is included with each rectangular representation of the binding capacity. Note the increased thyroxine binding capacity in normal pregnancy and in nonpregnant hypothyroidism.

tive T_3 to serum in vitro, this test indirectly measures the binding capacity of the serum proteins for the hormones.

As stated previously, the over-all actions of the thyroid hormones may be determined by measurement of the metabolic rate. Figure 10-6 illustrates the effects of the parenteral injection of equimolar amounts of thyroxine and triiodothyronine. Since T_3 is only minimally bound to serum proteins, its action is more rapid in onset and shorter in duration. In contrast, the action of thyroxine is delayed in onset but longer in total duration. From analysis of such data it is possible to conclude that the total calorigenic activity of the two hormones is very similar.

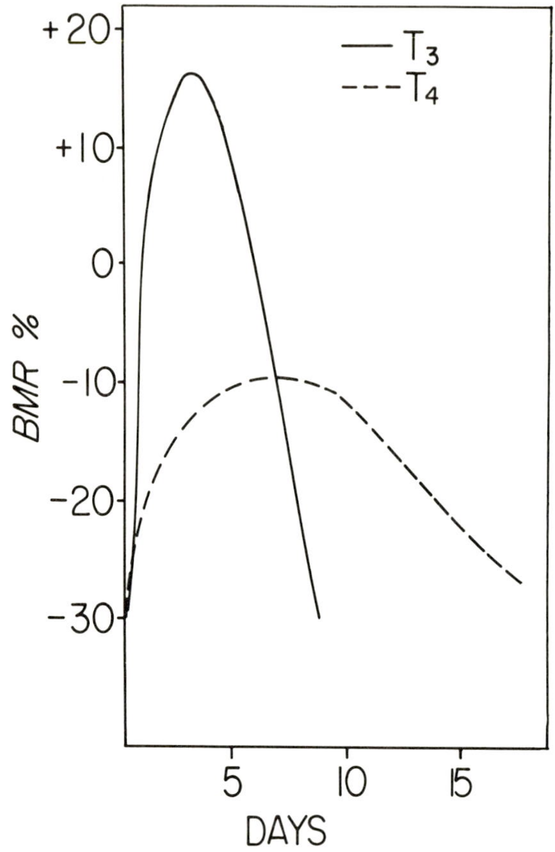

Fig. 10-6. Theoretical effects of a parenteral injection of equimolar amounts of T_4 and T_3 on the BMR of an athyreotic patient. Note the slower onset and longer duration of action of T_4 (dotted line) due to binding to serum proteins. (Modified from Blackburn *et al. J. Clin. Invest. 33*:819, 1954, and Rawson *et al. Trans. Ass. Amer. Physicians 66*:86, 1953.)

An abnormality in the regulation of thyroid hormone secretion due to a defect in the negative feedback mechanism of thyroid hormone upon pituitary TSH release is usually evaluated by the T_3 suppression test. A possible TSH deficiency is usually evaluated by the TSH stimulation test. Both of these involve two consecutive thyroidal radioiodine uptake tests, and they are probably contraindicated in pregnancy. The development of a sensitive radioimmunoassay for plasma TSH may obviate the necessity of the TSH stimulation test. The plasma TSH level in a variety of clinical situations as determined by radioimmunoassay is illustrated in Figure 10-7.

THYROID FUNCTION IN PREGNANCY

One of the most striking changes in thyroid physiology during pregnancy is the rise in the binding capacity of the thyroxine-binding serum proteins. This rise is due to estrogen stimulation and is also seen in the nonpregnant patient receiving exogenous estrogen. The rise in the binding capacity of the protein results in an increase in circulating T_4. Despite this rise in bound T_4, the serum free T_4 remains essentially unchanged.[47] Since the binding capacity of the serum proteins is increased in pregnancy, the resin uptake is decreased. The inter-relation between thyroid hormones and serum-binding proteins in the normal and pregnant women are illustrated in Figure 10-5.

The basal metabolic rate increases in pregnancy, probably as a result of an increase in oxygen-consuming tissue including the fetus and the placenta.[34] There is no evidence to indicate an increase in intracellular metabolism in pregnancy.

The thyroid-pituitary feedback mechanism involving thyroid hormone regulation of TSH secretion appears to be somewhat altered during

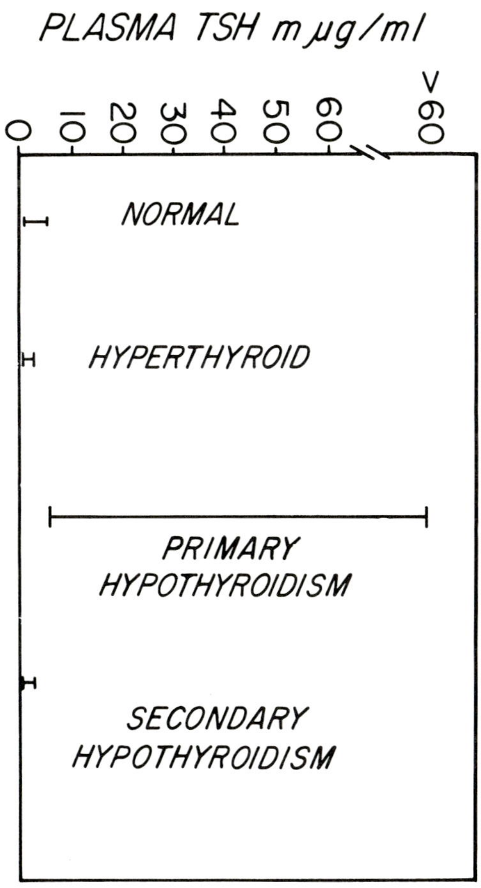

Fig. 10-7. Range of plasma TSH levels in a variety of clinical situations as determined by radioimmunoassay. (Modified from Odell, Wilber, and Utiger. *Recent Progress in Hormone Research.* Academic Press, New York, 1967.)

pregnancy, since administration of exogenous T_3 in large doses does not depress the PBI in the pregnant state to a degree comparable to that seen in similarly treated normal women.[42] The physiological significance of this observation has not been defined.

Human fetal thyroid development begins about the fifteenth week of gestation.[34] The fetal thyroid begins to accumulate iodine and to synthesize colloid, and the fetal pituitary assumes regulation of the fetal thyroid at this time. TSH secretion by the fetal pituitary stimulates the fetal thyroid which in turn regulates fetal pituitary TSH secretion. However, TSH does not cross the placenta during pregnancy (see below), and the fetal and maternal autoregulatory mechanisms for thyroid function operate independently.

Iodine uptake by human fetal thyroid during various stages of development has not been quantitated, but fragmentary radioactive iodine uptake data[14,25] suggest that iodine uptake gradually increases toward term and is then transiently accelerated in the neonatal period.

The thyroxine-binding serum proteins in the fetus are probably synthesized starting about the fifteenth week of gestation.[39] Their binding capacity gradually increases toward term and eventually approaches but does not equal that seen in maternal blood.[13,39] This explains the small difference in cord and maternal PBI and T_4,[13] with the fetal values being slightly lower than maternal values but considerably above the nonpregnant normal adult. As might be expected, the resin T_3 uptakes are usually a bit higher in the fetus than in the mother, supporting the concept that there is a relatively decreased binding capacity in fetal serum.

Transplacental maternal-fetal exchange of thyroid hormones, TSH, iodine, and antithyroid medications constitutes one of the more important aspects of thyroid physiology and pregnancy. Data derived from experiments in animals have indicated that TSH does not cross the placenta.[7,40] In contrast, iodide and even some organic iodine-containing compounds cross the placenta readily.[6,21] The situation with regard to T_4 and T_3 has not been defined precisely, but the bulk of evidence suggests that there is a partial placental barrier to the passage of these hormones in both animals and man.[7,13,19,31,33,39,41] A summary of some of the animal data appears in Table 10-1. In human pregnancy near term large doses of thyroxine administered to the mother do not raise fetal T_4 to maternal levels (Table 10-2).[13] Furthermore, there is also evidence that the transplacental transport of T_3 is retarded since fetal PBI is not suppressed by large maternal doses of T_3 (Table 10-3).[42] Although the data in animals and man suggest a retardation in placental passage of the thyroid hormones, long-term equilibrium studies have not been carried out in man. Based upon experience in a wide variety of clinical situations,

TABLE 10-1
TRANSPLACENTAL TRANSPORT OF SUBSTANCES SIGNIFICANT IN THYROID PHYSIOLOGY

Animal studied	Substances tested	Gestation of animals (days)	Time in pregnancy tested	Characteristics of placental transport	References
	iodide	22	early and	rapid	26, 37
Rat	PTU		late	rapid	26, 37
	T_4			retarded	26, 17
Guinea pig	iodide	68	mid to	rapid	23
	PTU		late	rapid	17, 40
	T_4			retarded	7, 23, 31, 40
	T_3			retarded	7, 31, 41
Rabbit	iodide	32	mid to	rapid	20
	T_4		late	retarded	33, 35
	T_3			retarded	33, 35
Monkey	iodide	168	late	rapid	45
	T_4			retarded	30
	T_3			retarded	45
Man	iodide	278	mid to	rapid	25
	PTU		late	rapid	9
	T_4			retarded	13, 19, 34
	T_3			retarded	19, 34

it seems reasonable to assume that at equilibrium maternal and fetal thyroid hormone levels probably approximate each other. The quantitative aspects of placental T_4 and T_3 transport remain to be precisely delineated.

Propylthiouracil (PTU) readily crosses the placenta in animals and man (Table 10-1).[9] The clinical implications of the rapid transplacental passage of antithyroid drugs will be discussed below.

The long-acting thyroid stimulator (LATS), a 7s-gamma globulin associated with Graves' disease, has been found in the blood of infants with neonatal thyrotoxicosis. This material disappears spontaneously with a half-life characteristic of the serum globulins, suggesting maternal origin[12] and transplacental transport.

A schematic representation of transplacental transport is illustrated in Figure 10-8, and of maternal-fetal thyroid relationships in Figure 10-9.

THYROID DISEASE IN PREGNANCY

The recognition of thyroid disease in pregnancy requires a cognizance of the normal physiological changes of thyroid function as discussed above. In addition, treatment of thyroid disease in pregnancy entails consideration of the effects of thyroid disease and of the antithyroid agents on the fetus.

TABLE 10-2

INDIVIDUAL BUTANOL-EXTRACTABLE IODINE (BEI) AND TRIIODOTHYRONINE ^{131}I UPTAKE VALUES IN 13 PREGNANT WOMEN AND NEWBORN INFANTS AT TERM AFTER MATERNAL THYROXINE LOADING*

Patient No.	Thyroxine dose (μg)	Thyroxine diffusion time (hr)	BEI (μg/100 ml)				Triiodothyronine ^{131}I resin uptake (%)			
			Maternal			Infant	Maternal			Infant
			0	1 hr	Del.		0	1 hr	Del.	
1	500	12.5			5.2	4.2	28	30	25	32
2	1500	33	7.6	23.8	11.3	8.8	26	30	28	36
3	2000	3.5	6.6	24.8	19.0	6.8	23	40	26	28
4	2000	24	6.4	18.3	14.1	5.8	20	35	25	28
5	4000	3.5	5.0		33.2	3.4	24		53	33
6	4000	4	9.0	40.6	39.6	8.4	26	66	50	44
7	4000	7	3.8	23.2	22.4	6.0	27	64	39	29
8	4000	8	7.1	42.2	24.5	7.4	26	49	37	25
9	4000	9	9.2	37.2	36.0	12.6	31	64	52	38
10	8000	3	6.6	60.0	57.4	9.0	22	71	65	33
11	8000	4	5.1	47.0	52.5	12.8	18	68	64	49
12	8000	7	7.4	42.6	42.0	9.9	20	66	56	35
13	8000	52	6.2	77.0	43.0	19.6	22	73	59	56

* From Fisher, Lehman, and Lackey. *J. Clin. Endocr. 24*:393, 1964.

TABLE 10-3

T_4 BY COLUMN AND TBG SERUM LEVELS IN NORMAL PREGNANCY AND AFTER THERAPY WITH T_3

			T_4 by Column (μg/100 ml)				TBG (μg/100 ml)	
Dose of T_3 (μg/day)	Patient	Duration of therapy (wk.)	At 36 wk.	At 38 wk.	Maternal at delivery	Cord at delivery	Maternal	Cord
150	T.S.	3	7.5	4.9	5.2	7.3		
200	E.M.	3	6.7	5.2	4.4	5.2		
	I.J.	3		4.0	4.6	5.1	60.1	27.9
	C.T.	4	6.2	2.9	2.5	3.1		
	B.P.	6		5.4	5.7	5.4		
300	J.P.	10	5.7	1.6	3.7	3.9	32.1	26.2
	B.C.	6	6.9	5.7	4.8	4.0	24.7	40.0
	P.R.	5	6.5	3.2	2.8	3.3	35.6	20.3
	M.W.	4	5.1		1.8	2.6		
	J.C.	4	5.8		0.9	6.5	11.6	25.7
	R.I.	4	6.5	2.6	4.1	7.0	39.1	29.5
	D.C.	3	6.9		2.4	4.1	47.8	25.3
	P.W.	3	7.2	3.2	3.9	6.2		
200†	B.C.*	7		1.8	1.0	4.8	51.7	26.8
200‡	A.S.*	30	4.4	1.0	1.3	3.9	40.5	23.8

* Cretins. From Raiti *et al. New Eng. J. Med.* 277:456, 1967.
† Reduced to 150, 10 days before delivery.
‡ Increased to 300, 10 days before delivery.

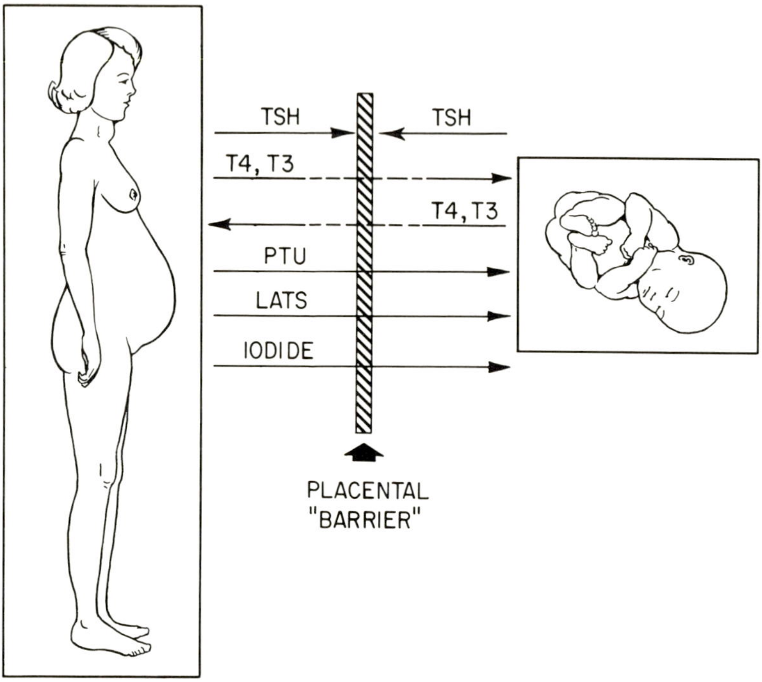

Fig. 10-8. Schematic representation of transplacental transport of pituitary thyrotropin (TSH), thyroxine (T_4), triiodothyronine (T_3), propylthiouracil (PTU), long-acting thyroid stimulator (LATS), and iodide in the human.

Hyperthyroidism

The incidence of hyperthyroidism in pregnancy is low, but untreated thyrotoxicosis in pregnancy is associated with a high incidence of toxemia and fetal wastage.[2] Therapy of hyperthyroidism in pregnancy has been the subject of several extensive reviews,[3, 22, 51] but there is a lack of unanimity as to preferred methods of treatment. Since radioiodine is contraindicated in pregnancy, the therapeutic choices lie between antithyroid drug treatment alone (or combined with thyroid hormone) or followed by surgery. Thiourea drugs readily cross the placenta and are known to be fetal goitrogens. Fetal complications of the antithyroid drugs include simple goiter, with possible airway obstruction, and transient functional hypothyroidism. Furthermore, there is a suggestion that the fetal thyroid may be more "sensitive" to the thiourea drugs than is the maternal thyroid.[7] For these reasons, some authors have suggested that antithyroid drug therapy alone is not ideal, even if the mother is maintained in a "slightly hyperthyroid" state.

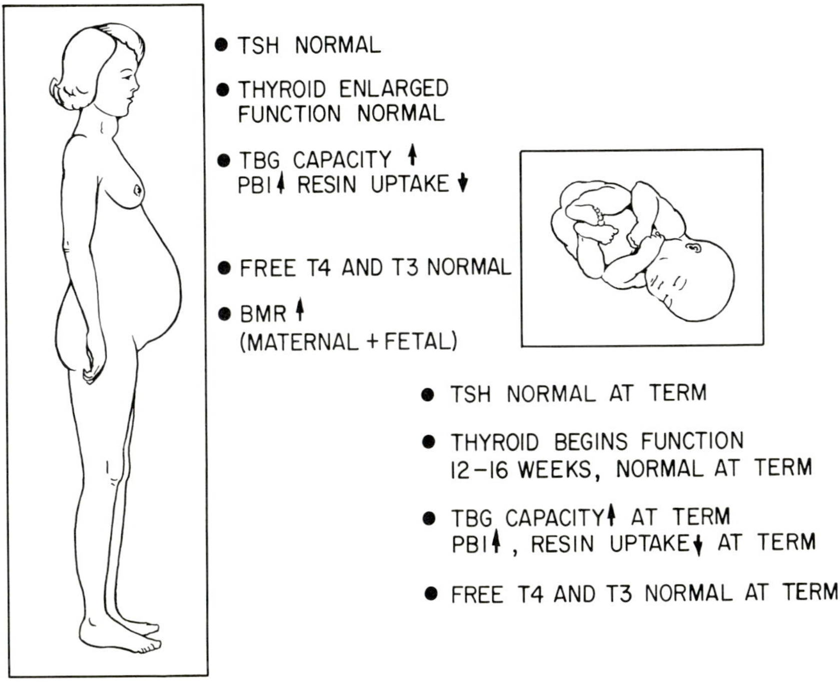

Fig. 10-9. Summary of the changes of maternal and fetal thyroid physiology.

To circumvent the fetal effects of the thioureas, exogenous thyroid hormone administration combined with blocking doses of antithyroid drugs has received support.[22,51] This combination therapy assumes that adequate exogenous thyroid administered to the mother will reach the fetus, suppress fetal TSH, and prevent fetal goiter. In addition, the thyroid hormone will prevent fetal hypothyroidism. The excess thyroid hormone production by the maternal thyroid is blocked with the thiourea. As indicated in the preceding sections, the extent of maternal to fetal placental transport of thyroid hormones is not clearly defined, and there is a possibility that the combination of antithyroid drug-thyroid hormone therapy may be better in theory than in practice. Unfortunately, a lack of controlled prospective studies using thiourea agents alone or in combination with thyroid hormones makes objective evaluation of the various therapeutic programs difficult.

There are advocates of subtotal thyroidectomy in the second trimester of pregnancy, followed by postoperative thyroid hormone therapy to the mother.[2,21] Although a time-tested form of therapy, such surgery is not without maternal and fetal hazard. Advocates of definitive radioiodine therapy for thyrotoxicosis to all adults prefer the administration of antithyroid drugs with or without exogenous hormone during pregnancy which permits the use of radioiodine as definitive therapy post partum. Both antithyroid drugs and iodide are secreted in the milk, and mothers receiving such therapy should not nurse.

In the last analysis, all methods of therapy cited above are probably quite effective if certain principles are considered. First and foremost, the antithyroid drugs should be used in the smallest effective dose consistent with reasonable control of maternal hyperthyroidism. Frequent clinical observations and tests of thyroid function should be performed in order to maintain the mother in a "slightly hyperthyroid" condition. The protein-bound iodine and T_4 by column should be in the high normal range for pregnancy, a range that is clearly abnormally high for a euthyroid person (Fig. 10-5).[8] The resin T_3 test, normally low in pregnancy, should be maintained in the normal range for a euthyroid patient. When thyroid medications are administered together with antithyroid drugs, the combination of T_4 and T_3 as proposed by Wool and Selenkow may be advantageous, since this combination results in a protein-bound iodine value consistent with the patient's metabolic status.[52] If subtotal thyroidectomy is elected, it should be performed in the second trimester, and following surgery the patient should be maintained in a "high normal" metabolic state. Since iodide crosses the placenta readily and is a fetal goitrogen, it should be used cautiously and for a limited time only in the preoperative management of the patient.

Hypothyroidism

Hypothyroidism in pregnancy should be promptly and vigorously treated to maintain the clinical and laboratory status of the patient in the high normal range. Once again, there is a lack of unanimity of opinion regarding the drug of choice, namely, thyroxine or triiodothyronine. Advocates of thyroxine claim that it permits use of the protein-bound iodine or thyroxine by column as an index of adequate replacement. Advocates of triiodothyronine point out that the hormone is not bound by the serum proteins and may cross the placenta more readily. Since we have presented evidence above that both hormones may cross the placenta slowly, we again would be inclined to advocate the mixture of thyroxine and triiodothyronine which permits a reasonably accurate assessment of replacement therapy by use of the PBI.

Other Thyroid Disease

Cancer of the thyroid detected in pregnancy should be handled as it would be in the nonpregnant state, namely by appropriate surgical intervention. Needless to say, large tracer doses of radioiodine and radioiodine therapy should be withheld until the pregnancy terminates.

Neonatal hyperthyroidism, associated with transplacental transfer of long-acting thyroid stimulator (LATS), has been mentioned in the preceding section and has been reviewed recently.[12] Brief and vigorous treatment of the infant is satisfactory since the process is self-limiting.

Since many aspects of the relationship between maternal and fetal thyroid physiology, remain unexplained, thyroid function in pregnancy should prove to be a fertile area for future investigation.

REFERENCES

1. Aboul-Khair, S. A., Crooks, J., Turnbull, A. C., and Hytten, F. E. The physiological changes in thyroid function during pregnancy. *Clin. Sci. 27:*195, 1964.
2. Becker, W. F., and Sudduth, P. G. Hyperthyroidism and pregnancy. *Ann. Surg. 149:*867, 1959.
3. Bell, G. O., and Hall, J. Hyperthyroidism and pregnancy. *Med. Clin. N. Amer. 44:*363, 1960.
4. Blackburn, C. M., McConahey, W. M., Keating, F. R., and Albert, A. Calorigenic effects of single intravenous doses of L-triiodothyronine and L-thyroxine in myxedematous persons. *J. Clin. Invest. 33:*819, 1954.
5. Bowers, C. Y., Schally, A. V., Reynolds, G. A., and Hawley, W. D. Interactions of L-thyroxine or L-triiodothyronine and thyrotropin-releasing factor on the release and synthesis of thyrotropin from the anterior pituitary gland of mice. *Endocrinology 81:*741, 1967.
6. Burrow, G. N. Neonatal goiter after maternal propylthiouracil therapy. *J. Clin. Endocr. 25:*403, 1965.
7. D'Angelo, S. A. Pituitary-thyroid interrelations in maternal, fetal and neonatal guinea pigs. *Endocrinology 81:*132, 1967.
8. Danowski, T. S. *Clinical Endocrinology,* Vol. 2, Williams & Williams, Baltimore, 1962, p. 94.
9. Davis, L. J., and Forbes, W. Thiouracil in pregnancy—effect on fetal thyroid. *Lancet 2:*740, 1945.
10. DeGroot, L. J. Current views on the formation of thyroid hormones. *New Eng. J. Med. 272:*243, 297, 355, 1965.
11. Dowling, J. T., Appleton, W. G., and Nicoloff, J. T. Thyroxine turnover during human pregnancy. *J. Clin. Endocr. 27:*1749, 1967.
12. Elsas, L. J., Whittemore, R., and Burrow, G. N. Maternal and neonatal Graves' disease. *J.A.M.A. 200:*250, 1967.
13. Fisher, D. A., Lehman, H., and Lackey, C. Placental transport of thyroxine. *J. Clin. Endocr. 24:*393, 1964.
14. Fisher, D. A., Oddie, T. H., and Burroughs, J. C. Thyroidal radioiodine uptake rate measurement in infants. *Amer. J. Dis. Child. 103:*738, 1962.

15. Freedberg, I. M., Hamolsky, M. W., and Freedberg, A. S. The thyroid gland in pregnancy. *New Eng. J. Med. 256:*505, 1957.
16. Furth, E. D., Becker, D. V., Nunez, F. A., and Reid, C. F. Thyroxine metabolism in the dog. *Endocrinology 82:*976, 1968.
17. Geloso, J. P., and Bernard, G. Effets de l'ablation de la thyroide maternelle ou foetale sur le taux des hormones circulantes chez le foetus de rat. *Acta Endocr.* (Kobenhavn) *56:*561, 1967.
18. Greenman, G. W., Gabrielson, M. O., Howard-Flanders, J., and Wessell, M. A. Thyroid dysfunction in pregnancy. *New Eng. J. Med. 267:*426, 1962.
19. Grumbach, M. M., and Werner, S. C. Transfer of thyroid hormone across the human placenta at term. *J. Clin. Endocr. 16:*1392, 1956.
20. Hall, P. F., and Myant, N. B. Passage of exogenous thyroxine and of iodide between mother and foetus in pregnant rabbits. *J. Physiol. 133:*181, 1956.
21. Hawe, P. The management of thyrotoxicosis during pregnancy. *Brit. J. Surg. 52:*731, 1965.
22. Herbst, A. L., and Selenkow, H. A. Combined antithyroid-thyroid therapy of hyperthyroidism in pregnancy. *Obstet. Gynec. 21:*543, 1963.
23. Hirvonen, L., and Lybech, H. On the permeability of guinea pig placenta for thyroxine. *Acta. Physiol. Scan. 36:*17, 1956.
24. Hoch, F. L. Thyrotoxicosis as a disease of mitochondria. *New Eng. J. Med. 266:*446, 498, 1962.
25. Hodges, R. E., Evans, T. C., Bradbury, J. T., and Keettel, W. C. The accumulation of radioactive iodine by human fetal thyroids. *J. Clin. Endocr. 15:*661, 1955.
26. Hoskins, L. C., Van Arsdel, P. P., Jr., and Williams, R. H. Placental transmission and mammary gland secretion of thyroxine in the rat. *Amer. J. Physiol. 193:*509, 1958.
27. Hung, W. Elevation of protein-bound iodine in an 8-year-old due to transplacental passage of an organic dye. *Pediatrics 37:*677, 1966.
28. Ingbar, S. H., and Woeber, K. A. "The Thyroid Gland." In *The Textbook of Endocrinology,* R. H. Williams (Ed.), Saunders, Philadelphia, 1968.
29. Jorgensen, E. C., Lehman, P. A., Greenberg, C., and Zenker, N. Thyroxine analogues. VII. Antigoitrogenic, calorigenic, and hypocholesterolemic activities of some aliphatic, alicyclic, and aromatic ethers of 3, 5 diiodotyrosine in the rat. *J. Biol. Chem. 237:*3832, 1962.
30. Kock, H. C., Reichert, W., Stolte, L., VanKessel, H., and Seelen, J. Placental thyroxine transfer and foetal thyroxine utilization. *Acta Physiol. Pharmacol. Neerl. 13:*363, 1965.
31. London, W. T., Money, W. L., and Rawson, R. W. Placental transport of ^{131}I labelled thyroxine and triiodothyronine in the guinea pig. *Endocrinology 73:*205, 1963.
32. Myant, N. B. The passage of thyroxine and triiodothyronine from mother to foetus in pregnant rabbits, with a note on the concentration of protein-bound iodine in foetal serum. *J. Physiol. 142:*329, 1958.

33. MYANT, N. B. Passage of thyroxine and triiodothyronine from mother to foetus in pregnant women. *Clin. Sci. 17*:75, 1958.
34. MYANT, N. B. "The Thyroid and Reproduction in Mammals." In *The Thyroid Gland,* R. Pitt-Rivers and W. R. Trotter (Eds.), Butterworth, London, 1964.
35. MYANT, N. B., and OSORIO, C. The passage of thyroxine-binding substances between mother and foetus in pregnant rabbits. *J. Physiol. 151*:66, 1960.
36. NAUMAN, J. A., NAUMAN, A., and WERNER, S. C. Total and free triiodothyronine in human serum. *J. Clin. Invest. 46*:1346, 1967.
37. NIKITOVITCH, M., and KNOBIL, E. Placental transfer of thyrotropic hormone in the rat. *J. Clin. Endocr. 15*:837, 1955.
38. ODELL, W., WILBER, J. F., and UTIGER, R. D. "Studies of Thyrotropin Physiology by Means of Radioimmunoassay." In *Recent Progress in Hormone Research,* Vol. 23, G. Pincus (Ed.), Academic Press, New York, 1967, p. 47.
39. OSORIO, C., and MYANT, N. B. The binding of thyroxine by human foetal serum. *Clin. Sci. 23*:277, 1962.
40. PETERSON, R. R., and YOUNG, W. C. The problem of placental permeability for thyrotropin, propylthiouracil and thyroxine in the guinea pig. *Endocrinology 50*:218, 1952.
41. POSTEL, S. Placental transfer of perchlorate and triiodothyronine in the guinea pig. *Endocrinology 60*:53, 1957.
42. RAITI, S., HOLZMAN, G. B., SCOTT, R. L., and BLIZZARD, R. M. Evidence for the placental transfer of triiodothyronine in human beings. *New Eng. J. Med. 277*:456, 1967.
43. RAWSON, R. W., RALL, J. E., PEARSON, O. H., ROBBINS, J., POPPELL, H. F., and WEST, C. D. L-triiodothyronine versus L-thyroxine. A comparison of their metabolic effects in human myxedema. *Trans. Ass. Amer. Physicians 66*:86, 1953.
44. REICHLIN, C. "Control of Thyrotropic Hormone Secretion." In *Neuroendocrinology,* L. Martini and W. F. Ganong (Eds.), Academic Press, New York, 1966.
45. SCHULTZ, M. A., FORSANDER, J. B., CHEZ, R. A., and HUTCHINSON, D. L. The bi-directional placental transfer of I-131 3:5:3′ triiodothyronine in the rhesus monkey. *Pediatrics 35*:743, 1965.
46. STANBURY, J. B. "Familial Goiter." In *The Metabolic Bases of Inherited Disease,* J. B. Stanbury, J. B. Wyngaarden, and D. S. Fredrickson (Eds.), McGraw-Hill, New York, 1966.
47. STERLING, K., and BRENNER, M. A. Free thyroxine in human serum: simplified measurement with the aid of magnesium precipitation. *J. Clin. Invest. 45*:153, 1966.
48. SUTHERLAND, E. W., and ROBISON, G. A. The metabolic effects of catecholamines. A. The role of cyclic-3′,5′ AMP in responses to catecholamines and other hormones. *Pharmacol. Rev. 18*:145, 1966.

49. Tapley, D. F. Mode and site of action of thyroxine. *Mayo Clin. Proc. 39:*626, 1964.
50. Tata, J. R. "Thyroid Hormone Action." In *Actions of Hormone on Molecular Processes,* G. Litwack and D. Kritchevsky (Eds.), Wiley, New York, 1964.
51. Werner, S. C. (moderator). Hyperthyroidism in the pregnant woman and the neonate. *J. Clin. Endocr. 27:*1637, 1967.
52. Wool, M. S., and Selenkow, H. A. Physiologic combinations of synthetic thyroid hormones in myxedema. *Clin. Pharm. Ther. 6:*710, 1965.

Chapter Eleven

Neurohypophyseal Hormones

Roberto Caldeyro-Barcia, Stig Melander, and Juan A. Coch

The posterior lobe of the pituitary gland, the neurohypophysis, is an endocrine gland with many features which make it distinctly different from most of the other endocrine organs. It is the source of two highly potent hormones, oxytocin and vasopressin, both polypeptides of closely related chemical structure, and both able to act on the same target organs, namely the kidneys, mammary glands, uterus, and fallopian tubes. These organs show marked differences in their relative sensitivity to the two hormones. The kidney responds to very small amounts of vasopressin, but it is also sensitive to the dose of oxytocin currently employed for induction of labor. During lactation, the mammary gland responds to both hormones, but is 80–100 times more sensitive to oxytocin than to vasopressin. In the nonpregnant woman, the uterus and Fallopian tubes respond better to vasopressin than to oxytocin. During pregnancy, the uterine response to oxytocin markedly increases, while the response to vasopressin does not change significantly.

Oxytocin is essential for lactation in the human and in all other mammals studied, and it is probably essential for parturition as well. Vasopressin has derived its name from its vasoconstrictor effect; this effect is minimal with the concentrations found in blood in the human and other mammals, where the prime target organ is the kidney. Vasopressin regulates the water balance and maintains the osmotic pressure of the plasma by control of the reabsorption of water in the renal tubules—

hence the name antidiuretic hormone (ADH). Notwithstanding the fact that ADH more adequately describes the main role in man, the original name vasopressin will be used predominantly in this chapter.

Both neurohypophyseal hormones are released by nervous stimuli, originating from peripheral receptors, usually located in or in close functional relation to the target organs.

The purpose of this chapter is to give the pertinent facts about the structure and the release of the two neurohypophyseal hormones. The effect of oxytocin on the uterus under various circumstances will then be described and the evidence for its playing a physiological role in the mechanism of parturition in the human will be examined. This will be followed by a brief review of the enzymes which degrade oxytocin and of the assays available for oxytocin determination in biological fluids. For exhaustive reviews and more complete lists of references the reader is referred to the chapter on "Neurohypophysial Hormones and Similar Polypeptides" in the recently published *Handbook of Experimental Pharmacology*.[7]

STRUCTURE OF OXYTOCIN AND VASOPRESSIN

The structure of oxytocin was elucidated independently and at about the same time by du Vigneaud, Ressler, and Tripett[145] and by Tuppy.[135] Du Vigneaud deduced the sequence of the amino acids in oxytocin on the basis of the amino acid composition of the different peptides obtained after mild hydrolysis and from the results given by Edman's degradation of some of these fragments. Postulating that all the amino acids were most probably bound together by α-amide linkages, and that the three moles of ammonia amidified the three carboxyl groups not taking part in peptide linkages, du Vigneaud proposed the following structure for oxytocin:

$$\text{Cys-Tyr-Ile-Gln-Asn-Cys-Pro-Leu-Gly-NH}_2$$

(with a bracket linking the two Cys residues)

Working with oxidized oxytocin and applying slightly different techniques, Tuppy[135] arrived simultaneously and independently at the same structure, which, some months later, was confirmed by the brilliant total synthesis by du Vigneaud *et al.*[144]

The method used to elucidate the structure of vasopressin[108] was very similar to that used for oxytocin. Vasopressin from cattle was oxidized with performic acid and yielded the same amino acids as the intact material except that two equivalents of cysteic acid were found in place of cystine. The following structure was therefore proposed for vasopressin:

Cys-Tyr-Phe-Gln-Asn-Cys-Pro-Arg-Gly-NH_2

Total hydrolysis of highly purified vasopressin from hog's yielded phenylalanine, tyrosine, glutamic acid, aspartic acid, proline, glycine, lysine, and cystine in approximately equimolar ratio, as well as three equivalents of ammonia. Thus, the amino acid contents of vasopressin from cattle and from hogs were identical, except for the basic amino acids arginine and lysine. The following structure for lysine-vasopressin was therefore proposed, merely on the grounds of analogy:[143]

Cys-Tyr-Phe-Gln-Asn-Cys-Pro-Lys-Gly-NH_2

This provisional structure was fully confirmed by total synthesis which was achieved by du Vigneaud's team in 1954.

NEUROSECRETION

Oxytocin and vasopressin are produced in the perikarya of the neurons of the supraoptic and paraventricular nuclei of the hypothalamus. The process is known as neurosecretion.[5]

The neurons secreting polypeptide hormone (oxytocin, vasopressin, releasing factors, etc.) are described as peptidergic neurons,[6] using a similar terminology as that employed for adrenergic and cholinergic nerves. Each neurosecretory cell synthesizes, stores, and secretes only one of the hormones.[8]

Much evidence indicates that the paraventricular nucleus contains mainly oxytocinergic neurons, while the supraoptic nucleus contains vasopressinergic ones.[13, 104, 150]

Oxytocin and vasopressin are stored within microvesicles probably made up of a protein, the neurophysin, which acts as an inert carrier for the polypeptide hormones. Several microvesicles join forming the "elementary granules" (with a diameter of 800–3000 Å). These microvesicles are separated from the neuroplasm by an enveloping membrane and enclose an electron-dense substance. The "elementary granules" are distributed in the neuroplasm of the axons of the neurosecretory cells. They are transported from the hypothalamus into the posterior lobe of the pituitary by means of the "axonal flow" via the unmyelinated axons of the neurosecretory cells of the supraoptic and paraventricular nuclei (for references cf. Bargmann[5]). The size of the granules increases as they move towards the ends of the axons, suggesting progressive synthesis of material.[150] The experimental section of the hypothalamic-hypophyseal pathway causes accumulation of the neurosecretory granules in the proximal stumps of the interrupted nerve fibers. In the posterior lobe the axons end near capillary vessels where the neurosecretion will be released into the bloodstream. This is the main final pathway for neurosecretion. Small amounts of neurosecretory material have been found in the interstices of the ependymal cells and within the third ventricle. Controversial reports have been published about the detection of neurohypophyseal hormones in the cerebrospinal fluid.

The release of oxytocin and vasopressin can be produced by several physiological and nonphysiological stimuli. After the action of any of such stimuli there is a diminution of the number of granules of neurosecretion in the axon of the posterior lobe, whereas the proportion of empty vesicles is increased.

The release of the neurohypophyseal hormones occurs when the neurosecretory neurons are stimulated. These cells conduct nerve impulses,[13] and when these impulses reach the end of the neurosecretory axons at the posterior lobe, acetylcholine is liberated from the synaptic vesicles which are present at that site. It has been postulated that acetylcholine increases the permeability to oxytocin and vasopressin of the membrane which envelops the elementary granules.[110] The hormones leave the granules (which become empty vesicles) and enter the surrounding axoplasm. Acetylcholine probably also increases the permeability of the plasmalemma of the axonal endings. Before entering the bloodstream the hormones must go through the basement membrane and the capillary endothelium. The latter is provided with so-called pores ("fenestrated endothelium"). The pores are closed by a diaphragm.[5]

FACTORS INFLUENCING THE SECRETION AND RELEASE OF OXYTOCIN AND VASOPRESSIN

The most important stimuli known to cause the release of one or both neurohypophyseal hormones are: (1) increased osmotic pressure of the plasma; (2) suckling of the teat; (3) stimulation of the female genitalia; (4) stimulation of the male genitalia; (5) hemorrhage; (6) administration of various pharmacological agents; (7) emotion and nociceptive stimuli; (8) birth *per vias naturalis* (stimulus for the fetus).

The following agents are known to inhibit the release of one or both neurohypophyseal hormones: (1) ethanol, which inhibits the release of both hormones; (2) overhydration, which inhibits antidiuretic hormone but not oxytocin release; (3) chlorpromazine and related substances; (4) epinephrine in low doses; (5) adrenergic blocking agents inhibit vasopressin release.

Before discussing in detail the three most important stimuli (hypertonic solutions, suckling, and stimulation of the female genitalia) a short review of the other factors which are capable of releasing neurohypophyseal hormones is presented.

Emotion and pain are able to cause release of vasopressin in dogs and in man (for references cf. Ginzburg[75]). Hemorrhage, with a fall in arterial pressure, causes a remarkable release of vasopressin with little or no release of oxytocin. These effects are mediated by the vagus nerve which normally carries afferent stimuli from the right atrium which inhibit vasopressin release.[75] Ether, chloroform, cyclopropane, halothane, and barbiturates are capable of increasing vasopressin release. Similar antidiuretic effect has been observed after injection of morphine or pethidine.[75] Morphine and pethidine increase the contractions of the pregnant human uterus.[18] It is not yet known whether the oxytocic effect is mediated by the release of neurohypophyseal hormones or by other mechanisms. In women, the injection of acetylcholine stimulates the secretion of vasopressin and oxytocin. The physiological stimuli of hypertonicity and suckling (see below) do not seem to be mediated by the cholinergic mechanism since they are not inhibited by atropine.[71] Nicotine elicits the release of vasopressin, but not that of oxytocin. Whereas the injection of small amounts (15 μg) of adrenaline prevents the release of vasopressin and oxytocin, higher doses of catecholamines may cause the release of neurohypophyseal hormones.[75]

Increased Osmotic Pressure of the Plasma

Increased osmotic pressure of the plasma causes the release of the antidiuretic hormone (ADH or vasopressin) in all species studied. In the dog, sustained intracarotid infusion of hypertonic NaCl solution at a rate that increased the osmotic pressure of the blood by only 1.8 per cent, produced an antidiuretic effect[142] that could be matched in every aspect by the intravenous infusion of 0.07 mU/minute of posterior pituitary extract. "Osmoreceptors" specifically adapted to respond to changes in osmotic pressure in the "milieu interieur"[142] are probably located within the supraoptic nuclei or in their proximity.[13, 91]

In the resting subject in water balance, the osmotic pressure of the blood seems to be sufficient to allow some secretion of ADH (less than 0.1 mU/min). Overhydration decreases plasma osmotic pressure and inhibits the secretion of ADH with a resulting increase in urinary volume ("water diuresis"). During dehydration the increased osmotic pressure of plasma stimulates secretion of ADH which has an important role in water conservation.[75]

The intracarotid injection of hypertonic NaCl solution causes the release of ADH and oxytocin in the goat, rabbit, and conscious bitch.[2] In the latter, the amount of oxytocin released is 10 to 20 times greater than that of ADH. In pregnant and puerperal women during water diuresis, the intravenous injection of hypertonic (3%) NaCl solution (600 ml containing 18 gm of NaCl injected in 20 minutes) produced clear signs of ADH release, namely, a fall in the free water clearance and a rise in urinary osmolality. However, no signs of release of oxytocin were detected in the records of intrauterine and intramammary pressures,[28, 30, 70] suggesting that in man oxytocin and ADH are released independently. The independence of oxytocin and vasopressin release has already been postulated by Theobald[132] and by Dicker.[43]

Suckling of the Nipple

A very efficient stimulus to cause reflex release of oxytocin (and in some species also vasopressin) is the mechanical stimulation of the nipples, preferably by suckling. The released oxytocin will stimulate the myoepithelium of the mammary gland (milk ejection) and the myometrium.

Milk ejection can be quantitatively studied by recording the intramammary pressure by means of one or several polyethylene tubes introduced into the mammary ducts and connected to pressure transducers.[124]

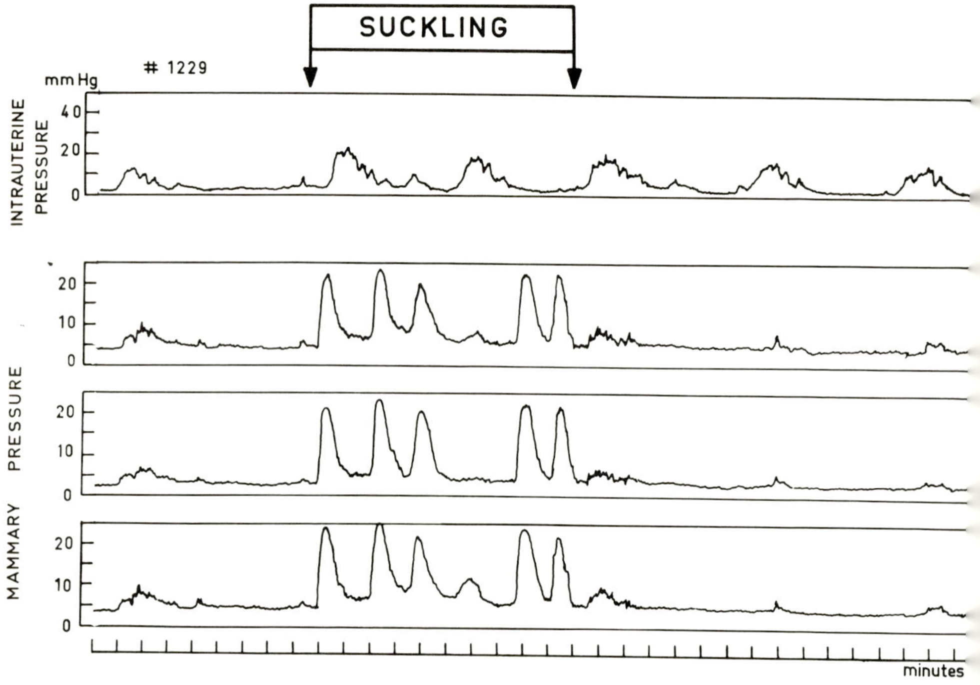

Fig. 11-1. Records obtained in a woman on the third postpartum day. (From Sica-Blanco, Sala, and Caldeyro-Barcia. Unpublished data, 1960.)

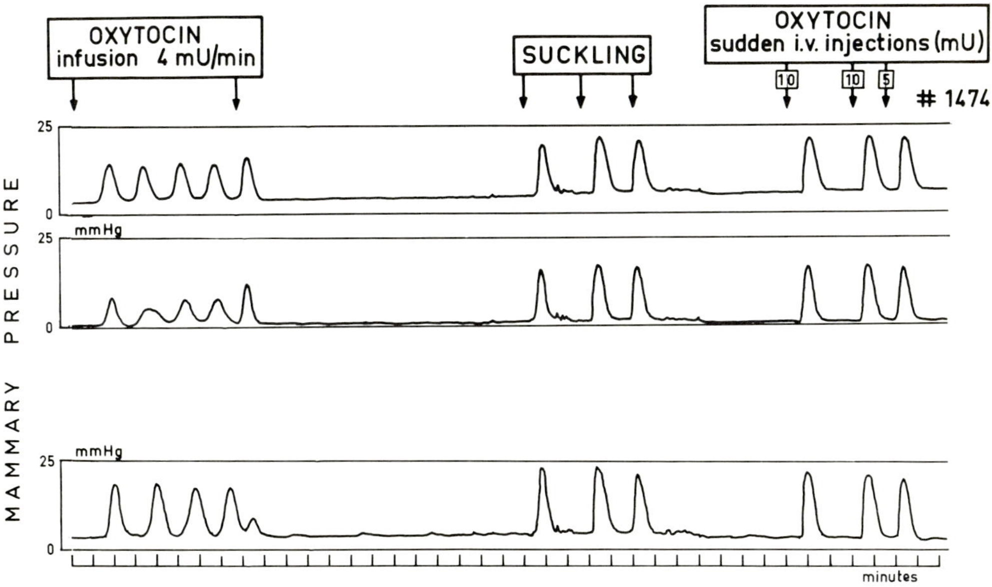

Fig. 11-2. Records obtained in a woman 4 days after delivery. Effects of suckling are better reproduced by sudden injections of oxytocin than by continuous intravenous infusion. (From Sica-Blanco, Sala, González-Panizza, and Caldeyro-Barcia. *III Congr. Uruguayo Ginecotocología 2*:283, 1960.)

Reflex milk ejection has been studied by recording intramammary pressure in one breast and placing a baby to suck on the contralateral breast.[16, 22, 124] Usually the first contraction of the mammary myoepithelium is recorded within 60 seconds of the onset of suckling (Fig. 11-1). Rhythmic mammary contractions continue to be produced for as long as suckling continues[16, 124] and cease very shortly after termination of the stimulus (Fig. 11-1). The amplitude of mammary pressure rises ranges between 5 and 25 mm Hg and the frequency ranges between 4 and 10 contractions per 10 minutes.[124, 126]

Figure 11-2 shows that in puerperal women the mammary response to suckling can be reproduced best by a series of rapid intravenous injections of oxytocin in doses of 1 to 10 milliunits given with an adequate rhythm.[28, 126] The milk ejection effect of a continuous intravenous infusion of oxytocin is less similar to the response to suckling than that obtained with repeated, rapid intravenous injections. This suggests that oxytocin release during suckling in women occurs in repeated spurts of variable amounts. It has been calculated that in lactating women oxytocin secretion during suckling averages 4 to 8 mU/minute and that each spurt releases 1 to 10 mU.[16] Some authors estimated a higher secretion.[28,126,146] The quantity of oxytocin released probably depends on the intensity and frequency of the stimuli.[146]

In puerperal women, several authors graphically recorded uterine contractions and clearly demonstrated the stimulation of the myometrium caused by suckling.[84,89,102,124,126,147] This stimulation could be matched by 100–250 mU oxytocin injected intravenously.[147] The quantitative analysis of the response of the pregnant uterus to suckling was made by recording intrauterine (amniotic) pressure. In 8 out of 10 women, uterine activity increased more than 80 Montevideo Units when the baby suckled for 20 minutes.[30] In 15 pregnant women at term, suckling by a newborn baby caused a marked increase of the intensity and frequency of uterine contractions which developed labor-like characteristics (Fig. 11-3).[4] When suckling was discontinued uterine activity diminished to the initial level. Suckling of the nipple was successful in inducing labor in 10 of the 15 women studied. In pregnant women, the augmentation of uterine activity

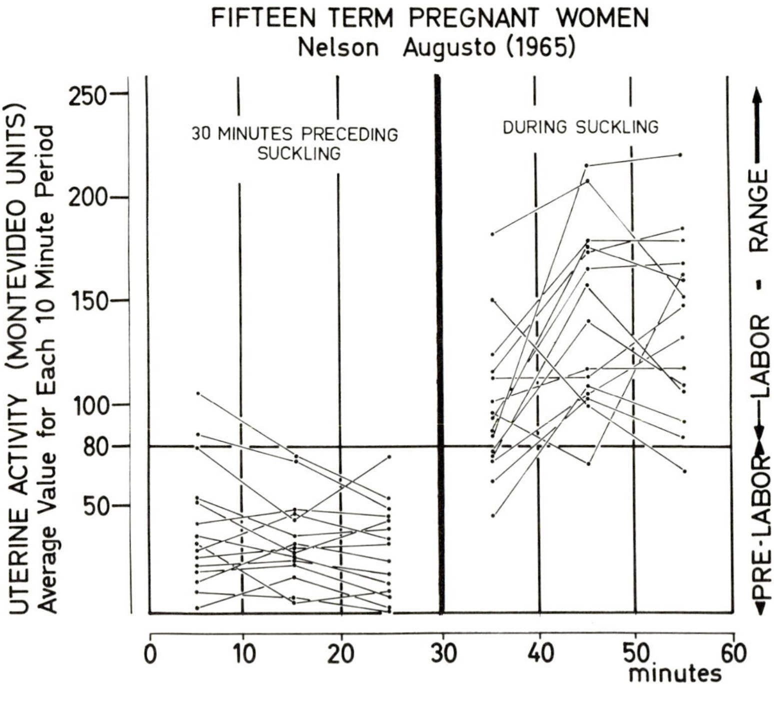

Fig. 11-3. Effects of suckling on uterine activity of 15 pregnant women at term. (From Augusto. *Tese de Doutoramento.* Faculdade de Medicina, Ribeirao Preto, Brasil, 1965, p. 73.)

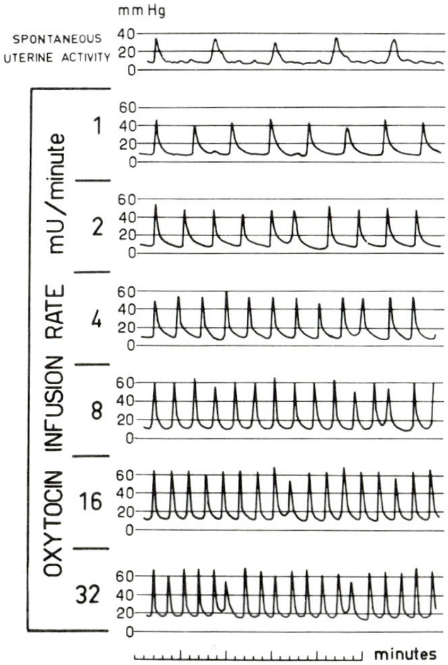

	TONUS	CONTRACTIONS		UTERINE ACTIVITY
		INTENSITY	FREQUENCY contractions	
	mm Hg	mm Hg	per 10 min.	Montev. Units
Spontaneous	8	27	1.5	40
1	8	35	2.4	85
2	9	40	3.	120
4	9	45	3.8	174
8	10	50	4.8	233
16	12	53	5.1	270
32	16	51	6.	306

Fig. 11-4. *Left,* seven parts of a continuous record of amiotic pressure obtained in a pregnant woman near term. Each part corresponds to a different rate of infusion of oxytocin. *Right,* average values (for each record) of the tonus, intensity, and frequency of the contractions, and of the uterine activity. Spontaneous activity is too low for promoting the progress of labor. Intravenous infusion of synthetic oxytocin (Syntocinon) at the rates of 2, 4, and 8 mU/min, respectively, increases uterine activity to values like those recorded in early first stage, advanced first stage, and second stage of normal labor. Infusion of 32 mU/min produces uterine trachysystolia and hypertonus. (From Caldeyro-Barcia. *Modern Trends in Gynaecology and Obstetrics,* Librairie Beauchemin Limité, Montreal, 1959, 1:65.)

caused by suckling[22,109] is similar to that produced by the continuous intravenous infusion of 4–8 mU of oxytocin per minute[109] (Fig. 11-4). The progressive development of uterine activity after the onset of suckling, as well as its gradual disappearance after termination of the stimulus (Fig. 11-1), are very similar to the changes seen at the beginning and after the end of an oxytocin infusion[125] (Fig. 11-5).

In the puerperal unanesthetized rabbit, suckling causes an increase of uterine contractions,[67] attributed to the release of oxytocin. The amount released depends on the strength of the stimulus, and this depends on the number of young suckling simultaneously and on their physical maturity.

In pregnant and parturient women, stimulation of the nipple was performed for 20 minutes by rubbing cotton soaked in oil circularly over the nipple. A consistent stimulation of uterine contractions (which were recorded with an external tocograph) occurred in all the 22 patients studied. Labor was induced by this method in 4 patients.[95] The instrumental dilation of the mammary ducts induced milk ejection and increased uterine activity similar to that caused by suckling.[28,30,70]

Conditioned reflexes can produce milk ejection which may occur in cows at milking time before suckling starts. In women, milk ejection has been reported in response to conditioned stimuli associated with nursing or a spontaneous surge of maternal feeling. The recording of intramammary pressure shows that mammary response of the mother on seeing the baby or hearing it cry is similar to that caused by suckling.[126]

In puerperal women it was found that during suckling a substance appears in the blood of the internal jugular vein[33] with the chromatographic, electrophoretic and pharmacological properties of oxytocin.[14] The concentration of this substance in the jugular plasma during suckling is equivalent to 12–25 μU/ml of synthetic oxytocin (Table 11-1). These values are higher than in blood withdrawn from women at times when

TABLE 11-1
VALUES FOR THE OXYTOCIN-LIKE ACTIVITY IN THE JUGULAR BLOOD OF PUERPERAL WOMEN DURING SUCKLING

	Experiment Number	Number of Patients	Extraction Method*	Assay Method†	Oxytocin-Like Activity (μU/ml plasma)
Pooled Samples	1	3	E	ME	19
	2	4	E	ME	15
	3	2	C	IM	12
	4	8	E	IM	6
Individual Samples	10	1	C	IM	18
	11	1	C	IM	23
	20	1	E	IM	25
	21	1	E	IM	11
Control Samples	20	1	E	IM	<10†
	25	1	E	IM	<10
	31	1	E	IM	<14
	36	1	E	IM	<12
	37	1	E	IM	< 6

(From Coch, Fielitz, Brovetto, Cabot, Coda, and Fraga. *J. Endocr. 40*:137, 1968.)
* E = electrophoresis, C = chromatography.
† ME = milk ejection, IM = isolated strip of rat mammary gland.
‡ <10 indicates that no activity could be detected when threshold of the method was 10μU/ml plasma.

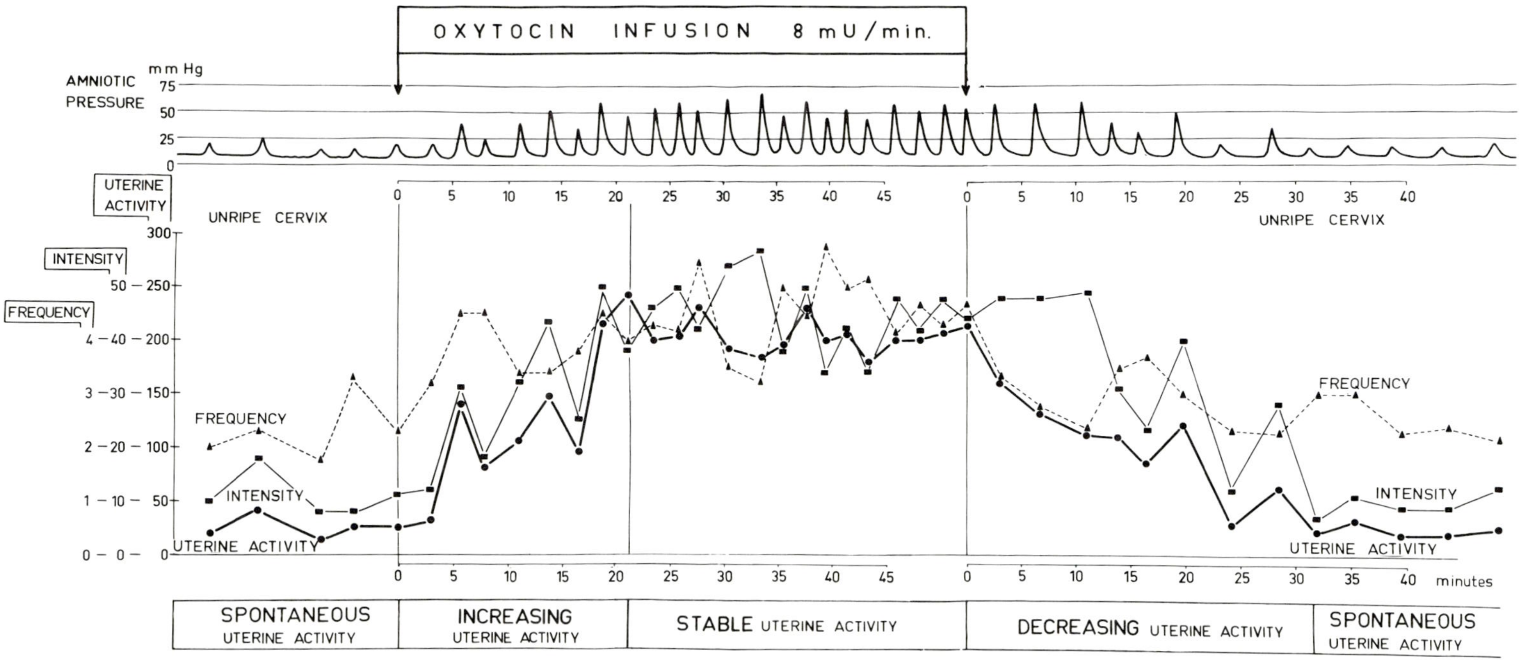

Fig. 11-5. Uterine contractility, before, during and after the infusion of oxytocin at the rate of 8 mU/min in a full term, pregnant woman not in labor. Tracing of amniotic pressure is shown at the top. Below the tracing, the values for the frequency, intensity, and uterine activity corresponding to each uterine contraction are plotted at the time of the respective contraction. (Note that there are three scales on the left of the graph for the three parameters measured.) The infusion lasted 22 minutes before the full effects of the dose were seen. When the infusion was discontinued, 32 minutes elapsed before the uterine activity fell to pre-infusion level.

they were not nursing their babies.[33] The concentration of oxytocin in jugular blood withdrawn from women during suckling is in good agreement with that calculated from the rate of infusion of oxytocin necessary to elicit a milk ejection response similar to that produced during suckling.[33] These values found in nursing women also agree with the concentration of oxytocin reported in ewes, [54] and in sows and cows[59] during suckling or milking.

Suckling is an almost specific stimulus for the release of oxytocin. However, it may also release a small amount of vasopressin. The ratio of vasopressin/oxytocin released is 1/30 in the dog[107] and 1/100 in the rabbit. In these two species, as well as the cow,[105] the small amount of vasopressin released during suckling may be able to reduce the urine flow, provided that sufficient water has been given to establish water diuresis. In lactating women conflicting evidence has been reported: Kalliala and Karvonen found antidiuresis,[93] Theobald reported that this effect was not always present and that there may be a pronounced time lag between the start of suckling and the onset of antidiuresis.[132] Other authors did not find any antidiuresis during suckling in women, and state that there is an independent release of oxytocin and antidiuretic hormone, each elicited by specific stimuli.[26,30,70]

In women, milk ejection can be inhibited by factors such as cold, emotion, and pain which may interfere with the release of oxytocin by means of a discharge of epinephrine. Ethanol is able to block the increased uterine activity in postpartum women and rabbits during suckling.[66,68] The degree of inhibition of the oxytocin release is dependent on the alcohol concentration in the blood.[68] When the concentration was 70 mg/100 ml in lactating women, the uterine response to suckling during one nursing period was less than half of that observed under normal conditions.[146] Ethanol also inhibits the milk ejection response and the increased uterine activity in pregnant and parturient as well as puerperal women.[27] For the last purpose, alcohol must reach concentrations of 200–400 mg/100 ml of blood, which are higher than those needed to block the release of vasopressin. The effect of alcohol seems to be central, preventing the release of oxytocin, since the responses of the mammary gland and the myometrium to injected oxytocin are not changed by alcohol.

In a postpartum woman with diabetes insipidus, suckling of the nipple by the baby caused a clear mammary response (Fig. 11-6), although it was weaker and of shorter duration than in normal women (Figs. 11-1 and 11-2).[12] In blood withdrawn from the jugular vein at the time of the mammary contraction, the concentration of oxytocin was estimated to be 8 μU per ml of plasma,[47] i.e., much lower than the concentration found in normal women,[32] using the same method of extraction and bioassay. After the patient was given 40 ml of Scotch whisky orally, suckling elicited no further contractions of the mammary gland (Fig. 11-6), whereas milk ejection response was still produced by the intravenous administration of oxytocin (10 mU given in doses of 1 mU every 30 seconds). The milk yield was low and breast feeding had to be supplemented with bottle feeding. The results illustrated in Figure 11-6 suggest that this patient partially retained the ability to synthesize and release oxytocin, despite the fact that she was unable to release vasopressin. This patient had three normal spontaneous labors several years after the onset of the diabetes insipidus (Fig. 11-7). Her third child was born seven days before the study illustrated in Figure 11-6. In another patient with diabetes insipidus, the baby's suckling during prelabor resulted in a clear mammary response.[28]

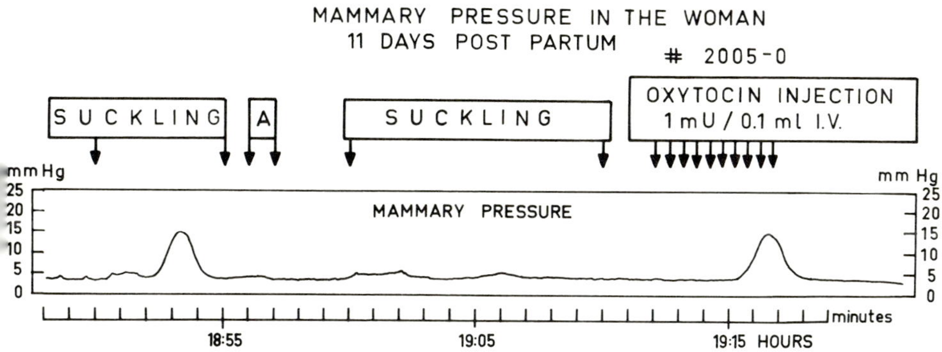

Fig. 11-6. Record obtained in a woman with diabetes insipidus, eleven days after delivery. A = ingestion per mouth of 40 ml of Scotch whisky which blocked the mammary response to suckling. Ethanol did not inhibit the response to injected oxytocin. (From Branda, Fielitz, and Roca. Annual Meeting of the Royal College of Physicians and Surgeons. Canada, Jan. 1970.)

Artificial Stimulation of the Female Genitalia

It is well known that in several species the contractile activity of the uterus increases following stretching or other mechanical stimulation of the uterine cervix, vagina, or vulva (for references cf. Fitzpatrick[55]). Thus, vaginal and cervical distension in lactating cows and ewes causes milk ejection and antidiuresis, corresponding to the effects of 20–50 mU of oxytocin and 2 mU of vasopressin.[40, 41, 106] In puerperal rabbits and cats, Ferguson found that the contractions of one uterine horn increased as a response to distension of the other horn or of the cervix or vagina.[46, 83] Dilatation of the cervix in term rabbits also was found to increase uterine

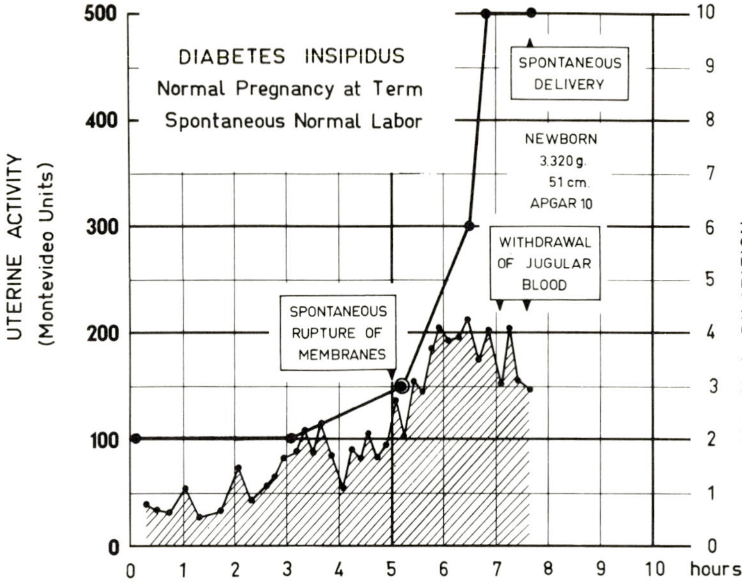

Fig. 11-7. *B,* Normal uterine activity (shaded area) and progress of cervical dilatation during spontaneous labor at term pregnancy in a patient with diabetes insipidus. (From Fielitz, Cabot, Brovetto, and Coch. *IV Congr. Uruguayo Ginecotocología II*:614, 1964.)

activity, and this effect was abolished by transection of the spinal cord.[42] Ferguson ascribed the effect, which has since been called the Ferguson reflex, to a release of oxytocin. Neither Cross[37] nor Fuchs, Olsen, and Petersen[65] were able to confirm this; they explained the increased uterine activity after vaginal dilatation as a sympathetic reflex.

In pregnant women near term, the stretching of the uterine cervix by means of a balloon produced an immediate and significant increase of uterine contractility with improved coordination of the contractions;[50] labor was initiated in almost all cases. However, milk ejection (studied by recording intramammary pressure) occurred only in two of the nine women, and even in these two women, the amount of oxytocin released (estimated from the milk ejection response) was insufficient to account for the increased uterine contractility caused by cervical distension. In a similar study conducted in nine puerperal women, cervical dilatation failed to cause milk ejection in eight patients. In the remaining woman, cervical dilatation produced six mammary contractions similar to those produced in the same woman by injection of 0.25–0.75 mU of oxytocin.

The mechanism by which artificial stretching of the cervix increases the activity of the pregnant human uterus is not yet known. The uterine response is blocked by spinal anesthesia, suggesting that a reflex is involved.[123] The efferent limb of such reflex may be mediated by the sympathetic innervation of the uterus, as suggested for the rabbit, or by the release of norepinephrine from the adrenal medulla.[123] It is known that the intravenous infusion of norepinephrine in doses of 5–10 μg/minute enhances the activity of the pregnant human uterus and that the stimulation pattern is very similar to that occurring during artificial distension of the uterine cerivx.[123] These authors found an increased blood level of catecholamines when the uterine cervix was stretched.

The participation of a reflex release of acetylcholine is discarded[123] because atropine does not interfere with uterine stimulation caused by cervical dilatation but it does block the direct effect of acetylcholine.[120] Furthermore, the uterine stimulation caused by acetylcholine (continuous intravenous infusion of 10 μg/minute) is much slower and less marked than that produced by cervical dilatation.

Coitus

The view that neurohypophyseal hormones are released in the female during mating has received support from the response seen in three different target organs, namely the uterus, mammary gland, and kidney.[55]

Increased uterine activity has been observed associated with mating in several species, and this has been attributed to the release of oxytocin. However, the more specific observation of a milk ejection reflex has been reported at coitus in man, horse, and cattle. Furthermore, antidiuresis occurs in females after coitus in both the rat and man. Similar antidiuretic effects have been recorded in males at coitus.

Using very reliable and specific methods, Walmsley was able to detect increased concentration of oxytocin (800 μU/ml) in jugular blood in only one of the four mares studied during mating.[147] It has been suggested by Harris that the release of neurohypophyseal hormones in the female at mating, by inducing contractions of the uterus and the fallopian tubes, may accelerate the transport of spermatozoa towards the ova.[82] Despite the considerable work performed in this field, Harris' suggestion has not yet received satisfactory confirmation.[55]

Labor and Delivery

The view that oxytocin (and vasopressin) may be released from the neurohypophysis during labor and delivery is based on two sets of facts: (1) the lower uterine segment, cervix, and vagina are considerably stretched during parturition; (2) there is a remarkable similarity between the pattern of uterine contractions recorded during normal spontaneous labor and the contractions artificially elicited by the intravenous injection of synthetic oxytocin. This similarity has been demonstrated in women[20] and in rabbits.[60, 61]

The study of the release of oxytocin and vasopressin during labor has been approached by recording the activity of oxytocin-responsive organs and by measuring the oxytocin concentration in blood.

Mammary Activity

Mavis Gunther observed during labor in a woman who was still lactating from a previous pregnancy that milk was expelled from the breast coincidentally with labor pains, and that this milk-ejecting effect was duplicated by the injection of pituitrin after delivery.[80] In pregnant women, the mammary myoepithelium is usually quiescent, unless oxytocin (or vasopressin) is injected or the nipples are stimulated by suckling or artificial mechanical stimulation. The appearance of "spontaneous" contractions of the mammary myoepithelium (i.e., in the absence of the above mentioned agents) is a good argument in favor of the release of endogenous oxytocin and/or vasopressin which are about the only endogenous factors which in physiological concentrations are known to stimulate the mammary contraction.

In our Service of Obstetrical Physiology in Montevideo, such activity of the mammary myoepithelium has been recorded in several women during labor, although it is not present in all cases.[15, 22, 124, 126] Figure 11-8*A* shows a record obtained during normal spontaneous labor after rupture of the membranes (cervical dilatation between 7 and 8 cm). Uterine contractions are normal and intramammary pressure shows intermittent rises which are not synchronous with those recorded in the amniotic pressure tracing. There is no coincidence between each individual contraction of the myometrium and those of the mammary myoepithelium. This fact disagrees with the description made by Gunther by simple visual inspection of milk ejection in a parturient woman.[80]

Figure 11-8*B* corresponds to the same labor 45 minutes later. Full cervical dilatation is attained. At hour 12:40 the second stage of labor begins, and in 7 more minutes, the fetus is delivered. Uterine contractions are stronger and more frequent in Figure 11-8*B* than in Figure 11-8*A;* a similar augmentation has occurred in the contractions of the mammary myoepithelium.

In a pregnant woman at term but not in labor, the mammary myoepithelium is usually quiescent, and uterine contractions, although present, are much weaker and less frequent than those illustrated in Figure 11-8. By intravenous administration of oxytocin it is possible to evoke mammary and myometrial activity similar to that illustrated in this figure. The best duplication is obtained with a series of successive injections made at irregular intervals, ranging from 2 to 5 minutes, the individual doses varying from 1 to 4 mU. The average dose per minute would be 2–4 mU/minute for Figure 11-8*A* and 4–8 mU/minute for Figure 11-8*B*.

On the other hand, the continuous intravenous injection in such doses per minute would produce mammary (Fig. 11-2) and uterine (Fig. 11-5) contractions having a much more regular rhythm and with less variability in amplitude than in the example illustrated in Figure 11-8. Since in spontaneous labor there is usually some irregularity in the rhythm and amplitude of uterine and mammary contractions (Fig. 11-8), it is assumed that the release of oxytocin by the neurohypophysis is also made in a series of spurts rather than in a perfectly continuous and even secretion.

Cobo did not detect contractions of the mammary gland in 10 out of 13 normal subjects, whom he recorded during normal spontaneous labor.[26] Mammary activity was present in only 3 subjects and it appeared only sporadically during labor. Cobo suggested that the release of oxytocin, which caused mammary contractions such as those illustrated in Figure 11-8, was elicited by the artificial stimulation of the receptors in the nipple. This stimulation was caused by the catheter inserted into the mammary duct in order to record intramammary pressure. He concluded that the release of oxytocin occurring during normal labor in women

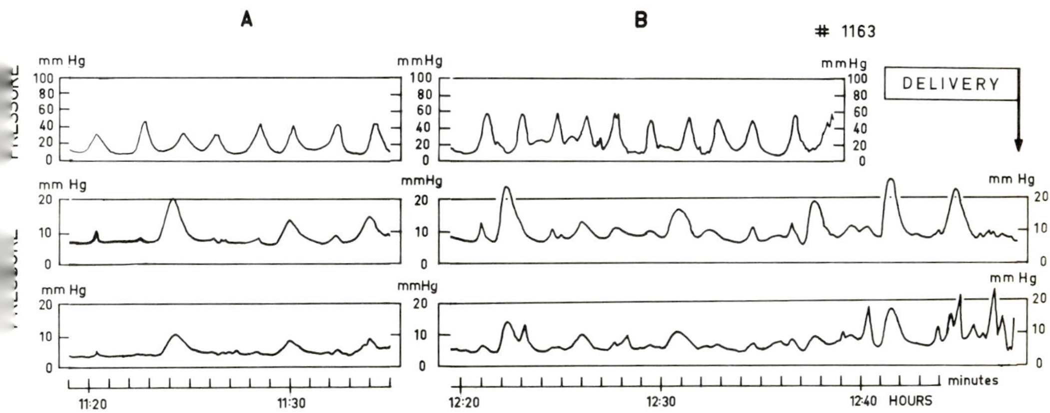

Fig. 11-8. *A,* Spontaneous mammary contractions recorded in a woman during the first stage of normal spontaneous labor. Cervical dilatation is 7 cm at 11:20. Membranes had ruptured at 9:30. *B,* Greater activity of the mammary gland and of the uterus at the end of the first stage (12:30) and during the second stage of labor (12:40 onwards). (From Sica-Blanco, Sala, and Caldeyro-Barcia. Unpublished data, 1960.)

was too small to account for the induction of uterine contractions and that other factors must be responsible.

In the parturient rabbit, Cross recorded milk ejection immediately preceding the delivery of the litter.[38] The milk ejection effect was somewhat greater than that produced by the intravenous injection of 50 mU of exogenous oxytocin. The release of the oxytocin-like factor occurred apparently as a single spurt.

The findings of Cross are in keeping with those of Anna-Riitta Fuchs,[60] also obtained in the parturient rabbit. In her remarkable studies intrauterine pressure was recorded continuously throughout the last 48 hours of pregnancy and also throughout labor in unanesthetized, unrestrained rabbits. Uterine activity was low until a few minutes before parturition. Then, quite suddenly, uterine contractions of considerable intensity and frequency occurred and caused the delivery of the whole litter within a few minutes. Uterine contractions continued for more than one hour after the last pup was delivered. A similar activation of the postpartum uterus was produced by a single intravenous injection of 200–300 mU of oxytocin.

Ethanol

The effect of ethanol on parturition was also studied by Anna-Riitta Fuchs in the rabbit.[61,63] The onset of labor was predicted by an oxytocin sensitivity test. With concentrations of ethanol of 250–350 mg/100 ml blood, the onset of labor was inhibited and typical uterine contractions were absent. Delivery was postponed for about 30 hours. Since uterine response to exogenous oxytocin was not impaired by ethanol, the interference with parturition is attributed to central inhibition of the sudden release of oxytocin, which seems to be indispensable for normal labor in the rabbit.

The information obtained in rabbits regarding the effect of ethanol was applied to the treatment of threatened premature labor in women by Fuchs *et al.*[70] Alcohol was given to 68 patients in threatened premature labor, including 52 with intact and 16 with ruptured membranes. The alcohol was given intravenously as a 9.5% solution in dextrose/water. A loading dose was given during the first one or two hours, followed by a maintenance dose of one-tenth of the loading dose per hour. Of the 52 patients with intact membranes, delivery was postponed for three days or more in 35; 30 of them carried their pregnancy to 37 weeks or more. In 10 patients labor was arrested initially but recurred and was allowed to progress, and in 7 patients labor could not be arrested. In all 16 patients with ruptured membranes the treatment with alcohol failed to postpone delivery significantly. However, an inhibitory effect on the uterine contractions was observed in all 68 cases, as well as in 10 cases of labor at term and in 3 cases of threatened premature labor in connection with a Shirodkar procedure. It is concluded that alcohol can inhibit the uterine activity during labor and that this presumably is due to an inhibition of the release of oxytocin from the neurohypophysis. These results have been confirmed by other investigators.[96]

During labor in term pregnant women, Cobo was able to inhibit uterine contractions when a concentration of 200–400 mg of ethanol per 100 ml of blood was reached.[27] After the intravenous infusion of alcohol was discontinued, the uterus rapidly recovered its initial activity at a time when the milk ejection response to suckling was still inhibited. Cobo concluded that other factors, independent of the neurohypophysis, were responsible for this recovery in activity of the parturient uterus.

Overhydration

In overhydrated women during spontaneous labor Cobo *et al.* observed a marked increase in urinary osmolality;[29] this effect became more pronounced during the second stage of labor and disappeared after delivery. Labor antidiuresis was attributed to increased release of antidiuretic hormone, mostly elicited by pain and emotional stress. Spinal anesthesia with tetracain to a level of D-8 relieved labor pains and markedly reduced antidiuresis.

In mid-first stage of labor, the administration of ethanol in doses which greatly diminished both uterine activity and reflex milk ejection response to suckling, produced only a mild inhibition of antidiuresis.[27] Overloading with water inhibited antidiuresis in early labor but not in more advanced stages when the high rate of vasopressin release is apparently unimpaired by overhydration.[27] The increased release of vasopressin, which is supposed to occur in women during parturition,[31] has not been confirmed by Hoppenstein *et al*[88] who did not find any change in the concentration in maternal blood throughout labor and delivery (see below.

Determination of Oxytocin Levels

If oxytocin is released during labor, it should be theoretically possible to detect the hormone in blood, but the unequivocal identification of oxytocin in blood and the accurate measurement of its concentration is a difficult and yet unsolved problem. One source of trouble is the very low concentration of the hormone which in peripheral blood of parturient women has been estimated to be 5–20 μU/ml or less.[20,52,78,94,133] These estimations are based on the dose which would have to be injected intravenously every minute to pregnant women at term in order to produce mammary and uterine activity similar to that recorded during normal spontaneous labor. To partially overcome this problem of low concentrations, determinations can be made on blood withdrawn from the jugular vein which drains the head and therefore should have a greater concentration of oxytocin than peripheral blood. To identify and measure such low concentrations of oxytocin requires procedures of chemical extraction and bioassay or radioimmunoassay of very high specificity and sensitivity. Much progress has been made in this field during the past decade (see later).

Jugular blood of ewes, cows, mares, goats, and rabbits has been examined for oxytocin during parturition.[53, 54, 55, 57, 58, 63] In the majority of these investigations, all oxytocin-like activity was extracted by gel filtration and sheet paper chromatography, using synthetic oxytocin as control. The activity found by these authors was assayed by procedures based on the milk ejection response of the rabbit or guinea pig,[53, 54, 134] which is much more specific than the uterine response. Furthermore, the extraction procedure and method of bioassay eliminate from consideration many substances which could otherwise be considered as having oxytocin-like activity.[55]

With these improved techniques, the British workers were able to find oxytocin-like activity in the jugular blood of ewes, cows, and goats. In all species the maximum activity was detected in the expulsive stage of labor (several hundreds of μU/ml), while much lower activity was detected in earlier stages of labor. After parturition there was a rapid decline in activity to prepartum values within 5 or 10 minutes. Similar results were found in the unextracted blood plasma of cows[138] and rabbits.[63]

Table 11-2 summarizes the results obtained in ruminants by several groups of investigators, together with those found in women by the Montevideo group,[31] who employed similar extraction procedures and bioassay methods. Blood of pregnant women has a high content of oxytocinase, and special techniques had to be employed to prevent inactivation of oxytocin as the blood was withdrawn and processed. Two samples of blood were obtained simultaneously from the internal jugular vein and a peripheral vein. Maximum values for oxytocin-like activity (350–900 μU/ml) were found in jugular blood during the second stage of labor (Fig. 11-9). These values were six to nine times higher than those of the corresponding samples of peripheral blood taken simultaneously. This difference is in keeping with the view that the active substance originates from a source in the head of the woman and moreover that it has a short life in circulation. It should be pointed out that the half-life of exogenous oxytocin in pregnant women has been estimated to range

TABLE 11-2

OXYTOCIN-LIKE ACTIVITY DETECTED IN JUGULAR BLOOD OR PLASMA IN RELATION TO PARTURITION. ACTIVITY EXPRESSED AS μU/ml OXYTOCIN AND GIVEN AS THE RANGE OF OBSERVATIONS REPORTED FOR EACH GROUP*

	Stage of Parturition				
		Intrapartum			
Species	Prepartum	Early	Late	Postpartum	Author
Cows	0–100	0–150	350–1,000	0–400	Fitzpatrick and Walmsley, 1965[57]
Ewes	0–10	10–65	100–3,000	0–10	Fitzpatrick, 1961[53]
Mares	0–250	0–140	250–800	0–300	Fitzpatrick and Walmsley, 1965[57]
Goats	0–20	0–90	90–300	0–80	Folley and Knaggs, 1966[59]
Women		50–400	350–900	50–350	Coch *et al.*, 1965[32]
Cows		0–0.001	1–3,000	0.005–0.1	Van Dongen and Hays, 1966[139]

* From Fitzpatrick, *The Pituitary Gland,* Harris and Donovan (Eds.), Butterworths, London, 1966, p. 453.

between 1.2 and 4.0 minutes.[78,116] In early labor and also after delivery, the oxytocin-like activity of jugular blood was much lower than during the expulsive period. The values found in women are of the same order as those reported in all animal species studied (Table 11-1). The oxytocin-like factor extracted from the jugular blood of parturient women was rapidly inactivated by incubation at 38° C with plasma from a pregnant woman. This fact is in agreement with the view that the substance responsible is oxytocin or a mixture of oxytocin and vasopressin. A personal communication from Dr. T. Chard at St. Bartholomew's Hospital in London indicates that a very sensitive and specific radioimmunoassay for oxytocin has been developed by his group. It was notable that no oxytocin was detected by this assay in maternal plasma at any stage of pregnancy or labor (sensitivity limit 0.7 μU/ml). By contrast, a high proportion of cord plasmas did contain oxytocin, higher quantities being present in the arterial than in the venous blood.

Endogenous Oxytocin and Vasopressin

The role of endogenous oxytocin in labor will be considered briefly, although it is also discussed in Chapter Thirteen. In this discussion the expulsive period should be considered apart from the first stage of labor.

It has been estimated that during the infusion of 8 mU/minute of oxytocin to pregnant women at term, the concentration in peripheral blood should be 20 μU/ml.[78,94] The Montevideo group has estimated that during a normal first stage of labor the secretion rate of oxytocin should average between 2 and 8 mU/minute.[20,126] The corresponding concentration in peripheral blood should be between 5 and 20 μU/ml. Theobald

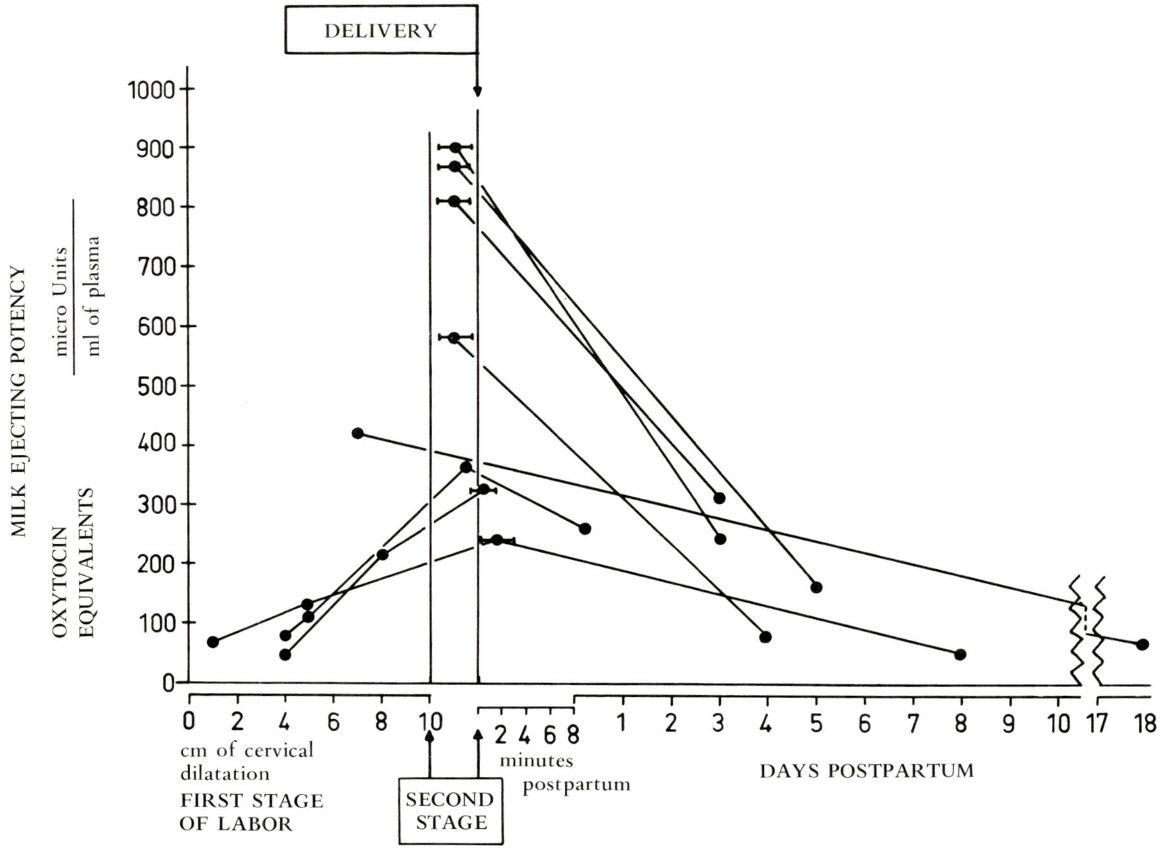

Fig. 11-9. Concentration of oxytocin-like substance in jugular blood of women during labor, delivery and puerperium. (From Coch, Brovetto, Cabot, Fielitz, and Caldeyro-Bracia. *Amer. J. Obstet. Gynec.* *91*:10, 1965.)

estimated a lower secretion rate, namely 0.5 to 1 mU/minute.[133] The corresponding concentrations in peripheral blood should be 1 to 2 μU/ml. Such low levels of oxytocin in blood would not be detectable with the currently available methods.

Just prior to and during the delivery of the fetal head, surprisingly high concentrations of an oxytocin-like substance have been found in the jugular blood of women, goats, cows, ewes, and mares. These findings suggest a massive release of oxytocin in the form of one or several spurts, which would be in keeping with the observations in the rabbit just prior to the delivery of the litter.[38,60]

In the woman, as well as in large animals with a single fetus, such a massive release of oxytocin could subserve several possible roles.

1. Acceleration of the expulsion of the fetus which is already in the birth canal, thus preventing prolongation of asphyxia which could be produced by the compression of the umbilical cord and by the partial separation of the placenta.
2. Stimulation of the retraction of the uterus as the fetus is expelled. Uterine retraction, in turn, fulfills several functions: (a) contributes to fetal propulsion, (b) separates the placenta, (c) contributes to hemostasis at the site of placental detachment by distorting and compressing the maternal vessels which irrigate the intervillous space, and (d) prevents uterine inversion which is facilitated by lack of uterine atony.

The mechanism eliciting the massive discharge of oxytocin is unknown. The distension of the vagina and perineum, which is maximal during expulsion of the fetus, may play a role. Another alternative is that the great release of oxytocin is a nonspecific and biologically purposeless response to pain or stress.[55]

In this connection it is interesting to point out that in peripheral fetal blood obtained from the umbilical vessels at the moment of vaginal birth, a surprisingly high concentration of vasopressin (35 μU/ml) was found by Hoppenstein, Miltenberger, and Moran.[88] In contrast, two babies delivered by cesarean section had a mean concentration in cord blood of only 0.38 μU/ml. In the maternal peripheral blood, the mean values were 2.2 μU/ml during labor and 1.5 μU/ml during cesarean section. During the course of labor and vaginal delivery the concentration of vasopressin in the maternal blood remained essentially unchanged, despite the magnitude of the stimuli present (pain and stress). The concentration of vasopressin in the blood of the newborn baby rapidly declined after normal delivery. During the second through the 22nd postpartum hours, the level averaged 0.46 μU/ml. If these findings are confirmed, it may be concluded that during vaginal birth a remarkably high release of vasopressin occurs in the human fetus. The mechanism and role of such release deserve much attention. The Montevideo group was unable to detect oxytocin in fetal blood obtained at birth from the umbilical cord of one case recently studied; the sensitivity of the method was 5 μU oxytocin per ml of plasma.[34]

Hypothalamo-neurohypophyseal System

There is little doubt that stimulation of the hypothalamo-neurohypophyseal system can initiate parturition. Whether destruction of the system prevents labor and delivery is more ambiguous.[55]

Electrical stimulation of the pituitary stalk in postparturient rabbits and cats resulted in increased uterine activity, strikingly similar to the responses to intravenous oxytocin (200–500 mU).[83] Spinal transection in the thoracic region, vagotomy, or section of splanchnic nerves, did not affect the uterine responses.[46] Electrolytic lesions in the pituitary stalk or the destruction of the pituitary body did abolish response to subsequent stimulation. Electrical stimulation of the supraoptic and paraventricular nuclei[38] and of the supraoptic-hypothalamic tract,[82] but not other areas of the hypothalamus, evokes uterine and mammary contractions in the rabbit similar to those seen after injection of oxytocin. Electrical stimulation of the neural stalk in an anesthetized rabbit initiated the birth of the litter in a normal manner.[38]

Electrolytic lesions in the anterior hypothalamus produce interruption of the hypothalamo-neurohypophyseal tracts and result in degenerative changes in the neurohypophysis distal to the lesion. Antidiuretic and oxytocic substances disappear from the gland, and this is accompanied by the onset of permanent diabetes insipidus.[51] In sevens cats subjected to this treatment in pregnancy, all showed dystocia of extreme severity. Four animals died in labor either totally unable to deliver young or delivering only part of the litter. Of the surviving three animals, two lost their litters and only one successfully delivered and reared her litter (even though she exhibited diabetes insipidus). In all seven cases labor was prolonged. Similar results were obtained in guinea pigs.[42]

Lesions in the paraventricular region of the cat may cause severe dystocia and prolongation of labor without concurrent diabetes insipidus.[104] These results support the view that the paraventricular nucleus is the main site of oxytocin production and also that this hormone plays a role in parturition.

Section of the pituitary stalk in women causes severe diabetes insipidus but is not incompatible with normal labor.[55] This should not be regarded as conclusive evidence against the participation of oxytocin in labor since in rats, after section of the stalk, the median eminence appears to retain functional innervation and to undergo reorganization, and may well produce some oxytocin. On the other hand, it is possible that oxytocin may be advantageous for normal parturition but not absolutely essential.[55]

Two women with diabetes insipidus have been described who were unable to accomplish parturition without the help of administration of exogenous oxytocin.[55] On the other hand, several cases of women with diabetes insipidus, in whom labor was unimpaired, have been reported.[55] One patient with diabetes insipidus was thoroughly studied at the Service of Obstetrical Physiology in Montevideo during three consecutive pregnancies. The disease started when the patient was 16 years old. When she was without treatment, the urinary volume was 18–25 liters/day. With nasal administration of antidiuretic hormone the diuresis was maintained at 3–5 liters/day. Pregnancies occurred at the ages of 24, 26, and 29 years. On all three occasions labor started spontaneously at term and proceeded normally. Figure 11-7 shows the plotting of uterine activity and cervical dilatation against time. The quantitative analysis of these records[47] showed that the values for uterine contractility were very close to the average obtained in normal labor in healthy women. However, the oxytocin-like activity measured in the blood of the internal jugular vein failed to show the marked rise which was usually found by the same authors in healthy women during the expulsive period of normal labor.[32] In the puerperal period, suckling caused reflex milk ejection in the contralateral breast (Figure 11-6) but the response was definitely weaker than in healthy lactating women (Figs. 11-1 and 11-2). A possible interpretation of these findings is that this patient was unable to produce vasopressin but that she was able to release some oxytocin, although in smaller amounts than healthy women.

EFFECTS OF EXOGENOUS OXYTOCIN

Fallopian Tube

The contractions of the human Fallopian tube in vivo have been recorded in the nonpregnant woman by means of indwelling catheters placed in the tubal lumen after abdominal surgery.[97] The intravenous injection of 1000 mU of oxytocin increased tubal activity. A similar dose of ADH depressed tubal activity, whereas continuous infusion at the rate of 5 mU/minute had a stimulant effect.[36]

The contractions of the salpinx in a tubal pregnancy at term have been recorded by means of a catheter introduced into the amniotic sac through puncture of the abdominal wall and connected with a pressure transducer.[19] The spontaneous contractions were very small (average intensity 7 mm Hg) and had a very low frequency (1.3 contractions per 10 minutes) (Fig. 11-10). The intravenous infusion of oxytocin at rates of 1,2, and 4 mU/minute caused a marked rise in the frequency (3 contractions every 10 minutes for an infusion rate of 4 mU/minute) but very little augmentation of the intensity which increased only to 10 mm Hg. Higher doses of oxytocin (32, 64, and 128 mU/minute) caused an even further increase in frequency, but no change in the intensity, of the tubal contractions. The base line tonus was 10 mm Hg and did not change during the infusion of oxytocin, even with very high doses.

Nonpregnant Human Uterus

In the nonpregnant woman no significant effects of uterine activity were obtained in vivo with infusion rates up to 128 mU/minute.[22] Very high doses (1000 mU by rapid intravenous injection) were needed to give

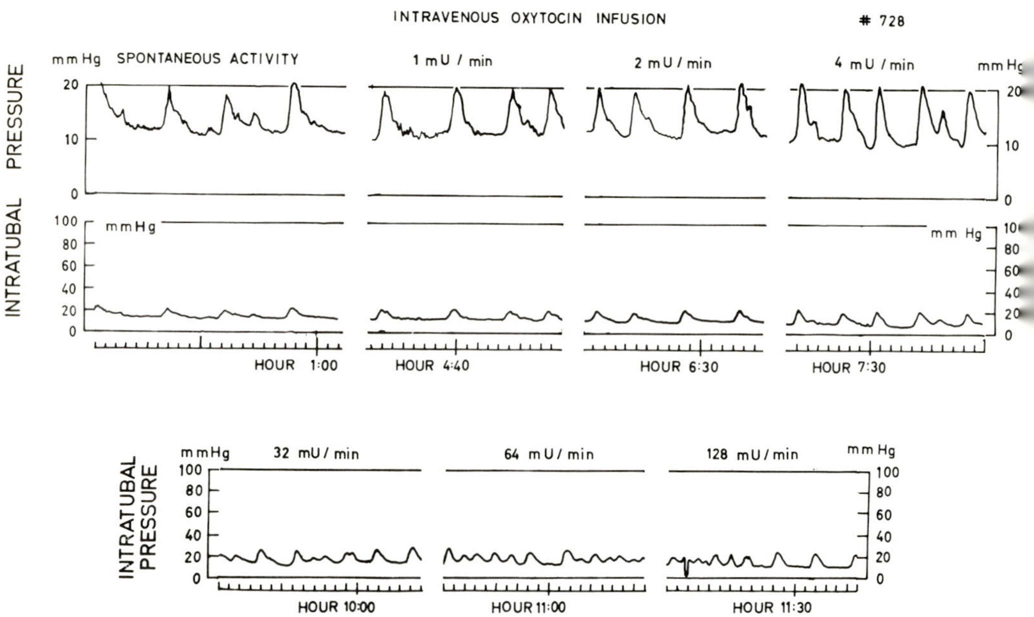

Fig. 11-10. Record of the spontaneous contraction of the pregnant fallopian tube in a woman at term pregnancy compared to the contraction during infusion of oxytocin at various rates. (From Caldeyro-Barcia, Alvarez, Pose, Poseiro, Méndez-Bauer, and Sica-Blanco. Unpublished data, 1958.)

a distinct response at the most favorable stage of the cycle, i.e., around menstruation.[35,64] The response to 1000 mU of oxytocin was absent in the late proliferative phase and the early secretory phase. During menstruation, vasopressin had a stimulant effect more potent than oxytocin. The vasopressin effect diminished progressively throughout the proliferative phase and at midcycle shifted successively from no effect to a depressive effect on the uterine tonus. At the beginning of the secretory phase this negative response reverted to positive.[35] Administration of ethanol during menstruation inhibited the contractions of the nonpregnant uterus but did not prevent its response to exogenous oxytocin or vasopressin.[64] The infusion of vasopressin at the rate of 4 mU/minute restored the initial contractility in spite of continued alcohol administration. Expansion of the plasma volume by infusion of iso-oncotic solutions also inhibited uterine activity during menstruation, supporting the hypothesis that vasopressin is the cause of the uterine activity in the nonpregnant woman, at least during menstruation (A.-R. Fuchs and E. M. Coutinho, personal communication).

Term Pregnant Human Uterus

In women, during the last 8 weeks of pregnancy, pure synthetic oxytocin given by continuous intravenous infusion at "physiological" doses (1 to 8 mU/minute) causes a marked increase in the intensity and frequency of uterine contractions without significantly raising the uterine tonus (Fig. 11-4). Visual inspection of amniotic fluid pressure and intramyometrial pressure tracings reveals only a small difference between the contractions produced by oxytocin and those of normal spontaneous labor. However, oxytocin accelerates and coordinates the spread of the contractile wave through the uterus,[20,23] and a fine quantitative analysis of the shape of the contractions shows differences between the two groups. Furthermore, during oxytocin infusion there is less variability in the intensity of the contractions and also in the intervals between them. The amount of uterine "work" required for dilating the cervix in labor induced with an oxytocin infusion is greater than that required in normal spontaneously-beginning labor.[130] This difference is attributed to the greater resistance in induced labor of a cervix not yet ready for labor.

By increasing the infusion rate of oxytocin it is possible to produce, at will, all the types of uterine contractility which occur spontaneously in normal labor (Fig. 11-4). Uterine activity (i.e., the product of the intensity of the contractions multiplied by their frequency) increases as an exponential function of the rate of oxytocin infusion.[23] In women in late pregnancy, but not in labor, infusion rates of 8–16 mU/minute are usually adequate to raise uterine contractility to maximum values recorded during normal labor: intensity of the contractions, 50 mm Hg; frequency, 5 contractions per 10 minutes; tonus, 12 mm Hg.

In pregnant women near or at term, oxytocin given at infusion rates higher than 8–16 mU/minute causes abnormally frequent contractions (more than 5 per 10 minutes—tachysystolia), and abnormally high tonus (more than 12 mm Hg—hypertonicity) (Fig. 11-4). The intensity of the contractions diminishes as tachysystolia and hypertonicity develop. Very high infusion rates (8000 mU/minute) cause an immediate and very pronounced rise in tonus, which may reach 50–60 mm Hg, devoid of rhythmic contractions.[109] This "contracture" persists for the duration of the macroinfusion.

After the start of an infusion at "physiological" rates, the intensity and frequency of uterine contractions rise progressively, and it takes from 15–60 minutes before they become stabilized (Fig. 11-5). Uterine activity decreases gradually after cessation of the infusion, and it takes 30–40 minutes before the effects of the infusion have disappeared. If descending uterine activity is plotted against time, an exponential curve is obtained. During the last four weeks of pregnancy the average T-50% of such curves is 15 minutes. At earlier stages of pregnancy T-50% values range from 3 to 13 minutes.[125]

MECHANISM OF ACTION OF OXYTOCIN ON THE UTERUS

Oxytocin acts on the membrane of the myometrial cell and not on the contractile myoplasm.[39] Jung postulates that oxytocin increases membrane permeability to potassium, thus lowering the membrane potential and the excitability threshold.[92] According to Marshall and Csapo, if the membrane has the normal resting polarization, the stimulatory effect of oxytocin is associated with a depolarization towards the "critical" level; but if the membrane has been previously depolarized below the "critical" level for excitation, oxytocin repolarizes the membrane towards this "critical" level.[98] It has been suggested that oxytocin may act by mobilizing Ca^{++} and possibly other ions to act as inward current carriers during the upstroke of the action potential.[98] Increasing Na^{+} and Ca^{++} concentrations enhance the oxytocin effects, whereas Na^{+}-free and Ca^{++}-free solutions abolish the oxytocin effects.

In the superfused rat uterus, oxytocin in physiological concentrations (0.002 mU/ml) markedly enhanced the tension developed by isometric contractions caused by threshold electrical stimulation.[48] Similar results had been obtained in the rabbit uterus using much higher concentrations of oxytocin (0.1 mU/ml).[39] It is probable that oxytocin acts by lowering the excitability threshold of the myometrial fibers which would enable a larger number of units to respond to the threshold stimulus. In the "calcium-deficient uterus" the enhancing effect of oxytocin on the isometric response of the uterus to electrical stimulation is a function of the concentration of oxytocin;[39] it has been suggested that this method could be used to assay for the hormone.[149]

These observations suggest that in vivo, under the influence of physiological doses of oxytocin, a greater number of uterine fibers would respond to any threshold stimulus originating spontaneously in some "pacemaker" of the intact uterus. Csapo has found that physiological concentrations of oxytocin increase the frequency of the action potentials and the total duration of the electrical discharge which causes each uterine contraction.[39] All the above described mechanisms may explain the augmentation of the intensity of the contractions which is produced in vivo by physiological doses of oxytocin.[22] The lowering of the excitability threshold in the pacemaker fibers can explain the increased frequency of the contractions.

An overdose of oxytocin depresses the resting membrane potential beyond physiological limits. This abnormal depolarization of the cell membrane makes the production of action potentials impossible, which in turn prevents the production of the rhythmic contractions which are caused by trains of action potentials.[39] According to Jung, the uterine tonus depends on a contractile mechanism different from that of the rhythmic contractions;[92] uterine tonus rises in linear relationship to the lowering of the resting membrane potential caused by an overdose of oxytocin. This mechanism explains the production of uterine contracture (a rise in the tonus and suppression of rhythmic contractions) which is caused by an overdose of oxytocin. In contracture there is a depolarization of the cell membrane and an absence of normal trains of action potentials.

Some octapeptides (such as carbamylated and acetylated analogues of oxytocin) are able to prevent the uterostimulating effects of oxytocin. It has also been suggested that they act by competing with oxytocin at hypothetical receptors located in the membrane of the myometrial fiber.[103] A similar antagonistic effect to oxytocin has been found in the rat with the octapeptide penicillamine-oxytocin,[24] but the effect was absent in the rabbit (Fuchs and Lopes, to be published).

CHANGES OCCURRING THROUGHOUT PREGNANCY IN THE UTERINE RESPONSE TO OXYTOCIN

Pregnancy increases the uterine response to oxytocin. Our earliest studies were carried out at the 12th week (Fig. 11-11). At this stage spon-

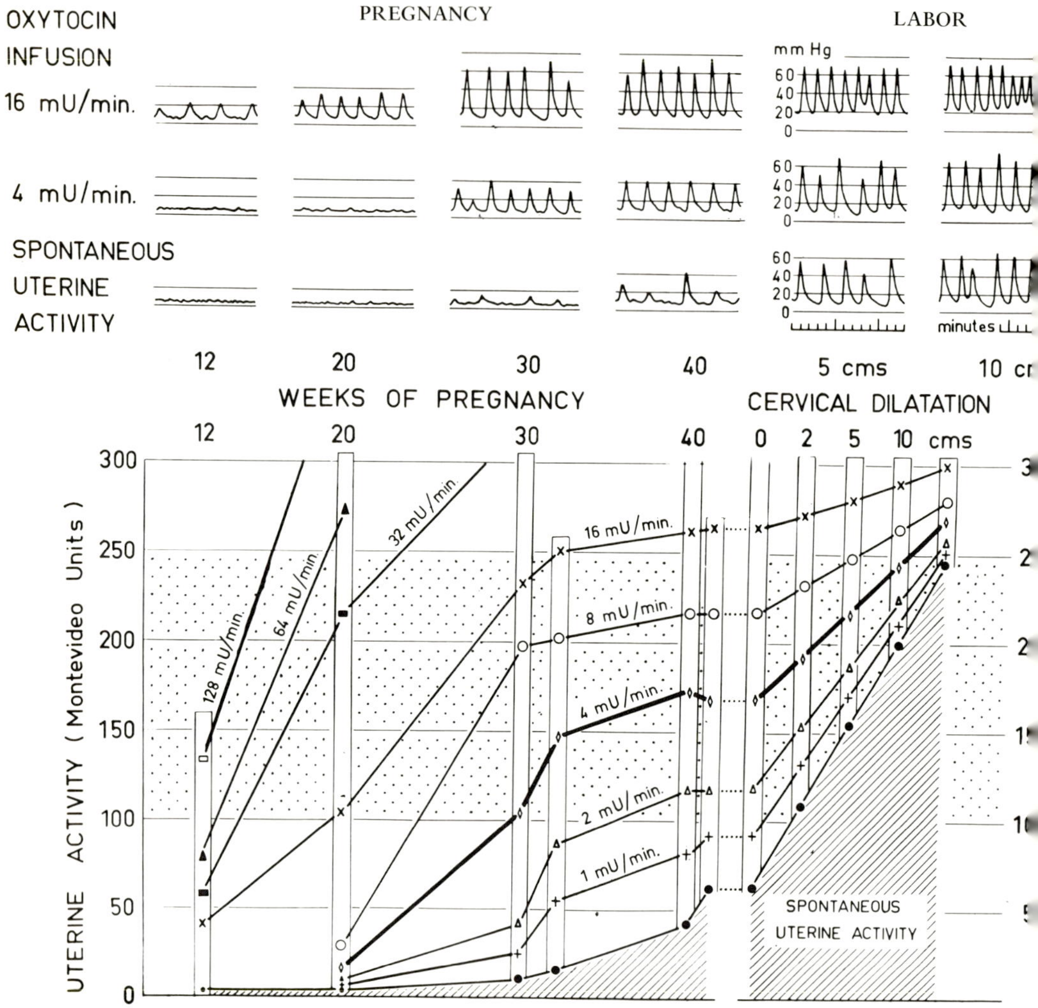

Fig. 11-11. Upper part of figure shows typical segments of original records of uterine contractions. In each vertical column the segments belong to the same record and illustrate the spontaneous uterine activity, the effect of an oxytocin infusion of 4 mU/minute, and of an infusion of 16 mU/minute at a given gestational age or during labor. In lower part of figure, the mean values of uterine activity are plotted against duration of pregnancy and against cervical dilatation during labor. Dotted area indicates normal range of uterine activity during labor. (From Caldeyro-Barcia and Sereno. *Oxytocin*. Caldeyro-Barcia and Heller (Eds.), Pergamon Press, Oxford, 1961, p. 177.)

taneous uterine activity is very low and an infusion of oxytocin at rates up to 8 mU/minute had almost no effect.[20,21] Infusion of 16–32 mU/minute produced a noticeable increase in uterine activity, indicating that even at this early stage of pregnancy the uterine response to oxytocin is already much higher than before pregnancy. Infusion of 128 mU/minute stimulated the uterus to an extent which demonstrated that the myometrium was already able to contract strongly. Figure 11-11 shows that the response of the uterus to oxytocin increases progressively as pregnancy advances. Between the 12th and 20th weeks there was a marked increase of the uterine response to very high rates of infusion (32, 64, and 128 mU/minute) and a much smaller increase to high rates (8 and 16 mU/minute). There was no visible change in the uterine response to low rates of infusion (1, 2, and 4 mU/minute) which produced no significant effect. Even at the 20th week these low rates failed to have significant effects on the uterus.[20,21] At midpregnancy, at least 16 mU/minute were required to produce uterine contractions which would cause amniotic pressure changes similar to those recorded in the term pregnant uterus during the first stage of spontaneous labor.

Because of the differences in uterine volume and radius of curvature at midpregnancy and at term, equal rises in amniotic pressure do not mean that the contractions are equally strong. For the same rise in amniotic pressure, the force and tension developed by the uterine contraction are much greater at term than at midpregnancy. Between the 20th and 30th weeks the response to high rates of infusion (8 and 16 mU/minute) increased markedly, whereas there was very little rise in the response to low rates (1, 2, and 4 mU/minute). After the 30th week, the increase in the uterine response to oxytocin was more marked for low rates of infusion (1, 2, and 4 mU/minute) than for high rates (8 and 16 mU/minute). The maximum response to high doses of oxytocin is reached between the 34th and 36th weeks, and no further changes occur during the last weeks of pregnancy[15,20,21] (Fig. 11-11). The response to low doses (0.5–1 mU/minute) continues to increase until the onset of labor.[133]

Up to the 30th week, spontaneous uterine activity remains low, showing no significant changes. After the 30th week, it begins to increase gradually and progressively. This increase becomes faster as labor is approached.[21] Figure 11-11 also shows that similar increments of activity (over spontaneous activity) are produced during the 32nd to the 40th weeks by any given rate at which oxytocin is infused. If the rise occurring in spontaneous activity between the 32nd and the 40th weeks is overlooked, it may be erroneously concluded that the response to oxytocin is slightly higher at the 40th than at the 32nd week. During labor, spontaneous uterine activity usually increases markedly as cervical dilatation progresses (Fig. 11-11). Hence, if the same rate of infusion of oxytocin is maintained throughout labor, the resultant uterine activity usually increases as labor advances. However, the increments of activity caused by oxytocin actually diminish as the spontaneous activity increases and approaches the maximum activity of which the uterus is capable,[15] leaving little margin for further augmentation.

The divergent results obtained by other workers[129, 133] may be explained by differences in the methods employed for measuring the uterine response to oxytocin.[21] For example, Theobald maintains that uterine sensitivity to oxytocin increases greatly and often immediately before the onset of labor.[133] The reason for this apparent discrepancy lies in the fact that Theobald was referring to the uterine response to what he considers physiological amounts of oxytocin (0.5–1 mU/minute), whereas Caldeyro-Barcia and Sereno[21] were describing the effects of large doses (4, 8, and 16 mU/minute) (Caldeyro-Barcia and Theobald, to be published). According to Smyth, uterine excitability, as measured by the oxytocin sensitivity test, increases 10 times during the last week of pregnancy, since a single intravenous injection of 10 mU is sufficient to produce one contraction on the day before labor, whereas 10 injections of 10 mU each at intervals of one minute are required one week earlier.[129] This author found a consistent relationship between uterine reactivity to oxytocin and the interval required for the onset of labor, whether spontaneous or after the rupture of membranes. Several authors have confirmed Smyth's results.[129]

However, Göltner, using the same "oxytocin sensitivity test," found that during the last weeks of pregnancy the response of the uterus to small doses of oxytocin shows large individual variations and concludes that the results of such tests do not permit a reliable prediction of the date of onset of labor.[77]

Uterine Response to Oxytocin in Complicated Pregnancies

No differences were found among primigravidas, multiparas, and grand multiparas. Uterine response to oxytocin was found to be normal in diabetes mellitus, in Rh-negative patients with erythroblastotic fetuses, and in toxemic patients, as long as the fetuses remained alive.

Figure 11-12 shows the response obtained in 19 patients with intrauterine fetal death, in whom the fetus had been dead for more than one week, in some cases up to 4 weeks. On the right side are plotted eight dose-response curves which are not significantly different from those obtained in the control group of uncomplicated pregnancies between the

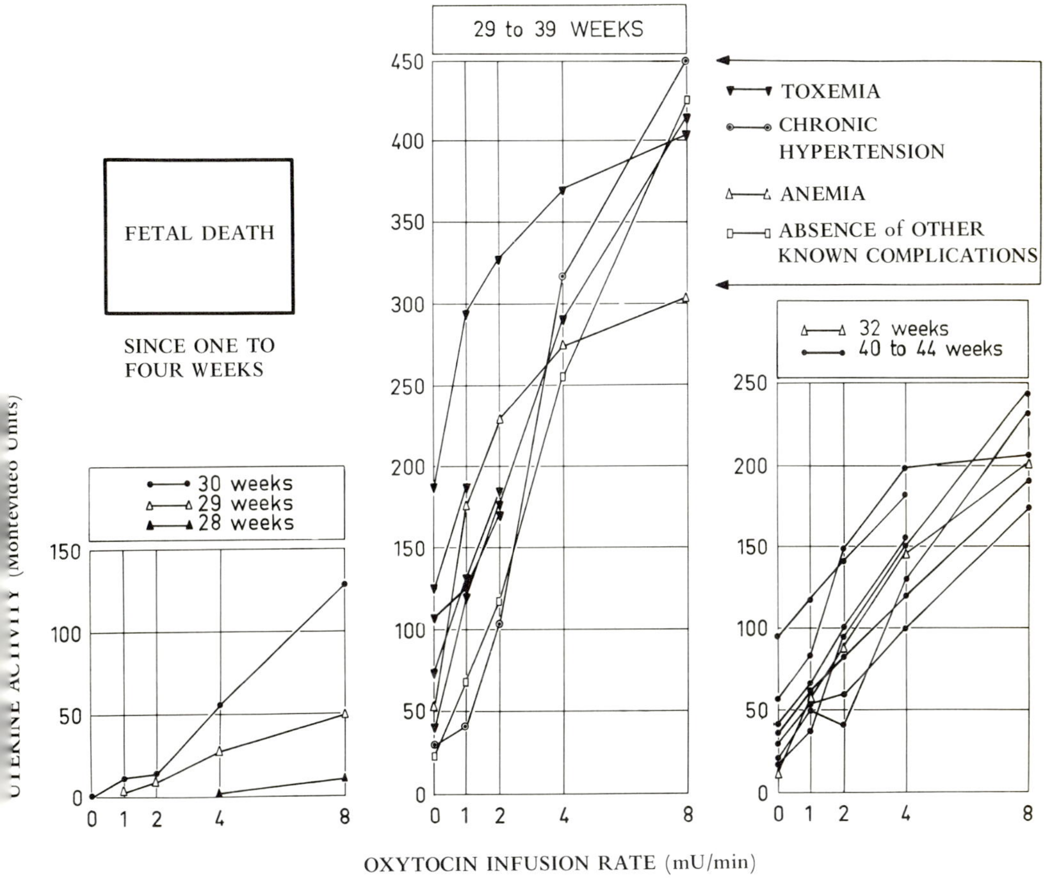

Fig. 11-12. Dose response curve to oxytocin infusion in patients with intrauterine fetal death for seven days or longer. (Modified from Noriega-Guerra, Sereno, Cobo, Gómez-Rogers, Fernández, González-Panizza, and Poseiro. *Arch. Ginec. Obstet.* (*Uruguay*) *18*:3, 1960.)

36th and 40th weeks. The gestational ages of these eight patients ranged from 40 to 44 weeks in seven cases and was 32 weeks in one case. In the middle are plotted eight dose-response curves which were much higher and steeper than those of the control group of uncomplicated term pregnancies. The gestational age of this group, showing an abnormally high response to oxytocin, ranged from 29 to 39 weeks. The reasons for the high response are unknown. The three curves plotted on the left side of Figure 11-12 correspond to very low responses and were obtained at 28, 29, and 30 weeks of pregnancy. The two lower curves were obtained in the same patient at the 28th and 29th weeks. This patient was the only one in this series in whom induction of labor with oxytocin infusion failed. In all other 18 patients with intrauterine fetal deaths, labor was successfully induced by this method.

Caldeyro-Barcia describes two types of spontaneous uterine activity in abruptio placentae.[15] In type I there is moderate hypertonus (10–20 mm Hg) with superimposed uterine contractions of medium intensity (15–20 mm Hg). In type II the tonus is very high, greater than 30 mm Hg, and uterine contractions have a high frequency (one per minute) and low intensity (10 mm Hg). According to Cobo *et al.,* in type I oxytocin infusion increases the intensity and frequency of uterine contractions very much like in uncomplicated pregnancies.[31] In type II oxytocin has no effect on uterine contractions or tonus.

In Figure 11-13 15 patients with polyhydramnios have been divided into two groups according to their response to oxytocin. In group 1 the response is not different from that obtained in uncomplicated pregnancies. In group 2 the uterus does not respond to oxytocin infusion.

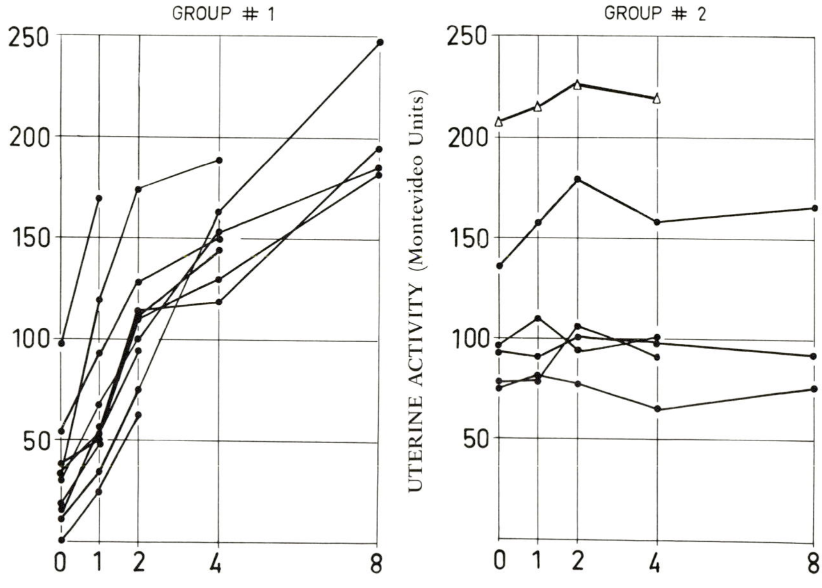

Fig. 11-13. Dose response curve to oxytocin in 15 patients with polyhydramnios. *Group 1,* response to oxytocin is same as in uncomplicated pregnancies. *Group 2,* uterus does not respond to oxytocin. Lack of response can be corrected by withdrawal of excess amniotic fluid. (Drawn from data in Noriega-Guerra, Sereno, Cobo, Gómez-Rogers, Fernández, González-Panizza, and Poseiro. *Arch. Ginec. Obstet.* (*Uruguay*) *18:3,* 1960.)

The spontaneous uterine activity (oxytocin infusion rate equal to zero) of group 2 is much higher than that of group 1. In group 2 the uterine tonus is higher than normal and the uterus behaves as if it were overdistended. In this group the withdrawal of the excess of amniotic fluid corrects the overdistension; the uterine tonus decreases, the contractions become stronger, and labor is usually induced by this procedure. In group 1 uterine contractions and tonus have normal values for the gestational age, and labor is usually successfully induced by oxytocin infusion because of the normal response.

COMPARISON OF OXYTOCIN, VASOPRESSIN, AND DEAMINO-OXYTOCIN

In early pregnancy, arginine-vasopressin and oxytocin are equiactive on the human uterus.[102] As pregnancy advances, the response to oxytocin is greatly augmented in a selective manner, since no significant changes occur in the response to vasopressin. In late pregnancy the effects on uterine contractions of infusions of 64 mU of vasopressin per minute are quantitatively equivalent to those of 2 mU of oxytocin per minute. The contractions elicited by vasopressin are uncoordinated and have an irregular rhythm, whereas those produced by oxytocin are regular and well coordinated. The uterine tonus is increased by 64 mU/minute of vasopressin, whereas it is not affected by 2 mU/minute of oxytocin.[25]

Deamino-oxytocin is a synthetic analogue of oxytocin in which the N terminal amino group has been removed. It stimulates the contraction of the pregnant human uterus in a manner very similar to oxytocin, but deamino-oxytocin is 2.6 times more potent per unit weight than oxytocin when they are given as intravenous infusions.

Response of Mammary Myoepithelium

The intravenous infusion of oxytocin at doses of 4–8 mU/minute in lactating women produced rhythmical contractions of the mammary gland with an intensity of 10–20 mm Hg and a frequency of 3–5 contractions per 10 minutes (Fig. 11-2).[124,126] In addition to the rhythmical contractions, a rise in the tonus was produced in the human mammary gland when the rate of the infusion was higher than 16 mU/minutes. Similar effects, lasting 20–40 minutes, were caused by intramuscular injections of high doses (1,000 mU) of oxytocin. In almost every aspect the effects of oxytocin infusion on the mammary gland are strikingly similar to those on the pregnant human uterus. The only clear difference lies in the fact that when the infusion is discontinued, the contractions of the mammary gland stop almost immediately (Fig. 11-2), whereas it takes about one-half hour for the disappearance of the uterine effects (Fig. 11-5).

In nonpregnant women, no response to oxytocin has been obtained, even with high doses (1,000 mU in a rapid intravenous injection).[117] During pregnancy, weak milk-ejecting responses are obtained. In the first weeks, the threshold dose is about 100 mU[117] and then drops markedly to about 1 mU between the 18th and 20 weeks. Little change occurs in the threshold dose during the second half of pregnancy. In the first days of lactation, the threshold dose decreases even further to about 0.5 mU on the fifth postpartum day.[119] After weaning, the threshold increases progressively and in 30 days reaches 100 mU.[126]

The threshold dose for arginine-vasopressin is higher than 100 mU at the beginning of pregnancy and decreases at the 18th to 20th week to about 50–60 mU.[118] No changes occur in the second half of pregnancy. The changes in the slope of the dose-response curve for arginine-vasopressin, its values, and the induced pressure are similar to those of oxytocin.[117] In order to induce a similar mammary response, the dose of vasopressin should be 50 times higher than that of oxytocin during pregnancy,[117] and 100 times higher during lactation.[118] The specificity of the response of the human mammary myoepithelium to oxytocin increases during lactation. This specificity is greater than in other species, where the relationship is only 10 to 1.[45] Arginine-vasopressin and synthetic lysine-8 vasopressin have the same milk-ejecting potency on the human myoepithelium.[118] Deamino-oxytocin was found to be 1.5 times as potent as oxytocin when measured in women at the third postpartum day.[1] Deamino-oxytocin is the only polypeptide known to be more active on the human mammary myoepithelium than natural oxytocin.

OXYTOCINASE

In human beings, enzymatic activity capable of inactivating oxytocin has been found in plasma (or serum) of pregnant women, extracts of placenta, decidua, pregnant and nonpregnant myometrium, liver, kidney, and erythrocytes. The enzyme, oxytocinase, has been found in plasma of pregnant Rhesus monkeys and in many animal tissue extracts such as placenta, decidua, pregnant and nonpregnant myometrium, pancreas, ovary, liver, kidney, erythrocytes, hypothalamus, and mammary gland. No, or only traces, of oxytocinase activity have been found in plasma of men, nonpregnant women, human fetal plasma, liquor amnii, and pregnancy or nonpregnancy plasma of rats, guinea pigs, rabbits, pigs, cats, dogs, sheep, cows, and horses (for references cf. Tuppy[136]).

Activity in Plasma of Pregnant Women

Fekete discovered the oxytocinase activity of plasma of pregnant women.[45] The enzyme responsible for this activity has been called oxytocinase or cystine aminopeptidase because of its ability to attack N-terminal half-cystine bonds. In this chapter, the designation plasma oxytocinase will be used to indicate the enzyme specific for human pregnancy plasma.

It has long been suggested that plasma oxytocinase originates from the placenta. Ryden compared the oxytocinase activity in homogenates of various tissues of pregnant and nonpregnant women with that of plasma.[114] The placenta was the only organ that contained an oxytocinase activity with properties resembling those of plasma oxytocinase (pH optimum, stability, progress curve). Other arguments are: (1) the absence of plasma oxytocinase in nonpregnant women, (2) its absence in fetal blood, (3) the decline of plasma activity starting immediately after expulsion of the placenta in normal deliveries, (4) the high activity values in multiple pregnancies.[100]

Almost all studies of plasma oxytocinase activity in pregnancy are based on determinations of the rate of cleavage of oxytocin or L-cystine di-β-naphthylamide.[137] There is general agreement that plasma oxytocinase activity starts to rise around the fourth month of pregnancy and that there is a curvilinear increase during pregnancy with the highest activity values at term. No decline has been noticed just before or at the start of spontaneous labor. No correlation has been found between the stage of labor and the plasma oxytocinase activity. Transient fluctuations or decreases of enzyme activity sometimes occur during normal pregnancy and labor.

Many studies have tried to correlate the plasma oxytocinase activity with various disorders of pregnancy and parturition, but generally without success. Determinations of the activity have been found to be of no clinical help in threatened or incomplete abortions, hydatiform mole, premature labor, intrauterine fetal death, prolonged pregnancy, or toxemia.[100] A report that plasma oxytocinase activity is decreased in preeclampsia needs confirmation.[90]

The physiological significance of the increased plasma oxytocinase activity during pregnancy is not known. The assumption that oxytocinase serves to regulate the oxytocin level is logical. However, effective mechanisms exist for the clearance of oxytocin from the circulation in the absence of oxytocinase activity. Men, sheep, rats, and rabbits have the same half-lives (1–3 minutes) for circulating oxytocin after exogenous administration.[74] The assumption that plasma oxytocinase prevents premature labor or that a decrease of activity precedes the beginning of labor, receives no support from the available data.

It has been suggested that plasma oxytocinase acts at its site of production and protects the placental vessels from the constrictory action of vasopressin.[114] It is interesting to note that the oxytocinase level of intervillous blood was about 3 times higher than that of cubital blood of pregnant women.

Tissue Oxytocinase

Extracts or homogenates of many mammalian organs inactivate oxytocin and vasopressin (lysine- and arginine-vasopressin), including liver, kidney, uterus, placenta, hypothalamus, and mammary gland of rats, rabbits, dogs, and human beings (see Tuppy[136]).

The inactivation of oxytocin in liver extracts and uterine homogenates involves a two-step reaction.[3,113] The first step is a reductive rupture of the disulfide linkage of the molecule which thus loses its ring structure. The rupture is catalyzed by a thiol oxidoreductase (disulfide transhydrogenase) system. The first step is followed by an aminopeptidase attack on the dihydro-oxytocin, step by step liberating the first three amino acids of reduced oxytocin. The aminopeptidase seems to be able to attack only reduced oxytocin, not the intact molecule. Conversely, plasma oxytocinase attacks intact oxytocin. The tissue aminopeptidase is probably identical with kidney leucine-aminopeptidase.[113]

Particular interest has been shown in the oxytocinase activity of uterine homogenates. Some authors reported that the nonpregnant rat myometrium possessed a low oxytocinase activity.[44,122] During pregnancy the activity increased four- to eightfold until term. At the time of delivery a sudden decline was noticed. These findings were not confirmed by Ryden who could not demonstrate any significant difference between the oxytocinase activity of the pregnant and nonpregnant rat myometrium.[114] Melander was unable to demonstrate any difference in activity between human pregnant and nonpregnant uteri.[100]

The human placenta exhibits a special feature, since it is the only placenta investigated that shows two oxytocinase activities, one with the same properties as plasma oxytocinase, the other with properties like those of tissue oxytocinase.[114]

It seems likely that enzymatic degradation by tissue oxytocinase plays an important role in the metabolism of oxytocin and vasopressin. In intact animals, both peptide hormones are rapidly removed from the circulation by the kidneys, liver, and mammary glands.[74] Some data are available on renal excretion of oxytocin in human beings. González-Panizza,

Sica Blanco, and Méndez-Bauer reported that in a nonpregnant woman after macroinfusion, approximately 20 per cent of the injected oxytocin was recovered in the urine.[78] In pregnant women less than 1 per cent was recovered in the urine. Although these results have been obtained with unphysiologically high doses, it seems as if there is a diminished urinary excretion of oxytocin during pregnancy.

Studies with a sulfur-free analogue of oxytocin, in which both sulfur atoms of oxytocin have been replaced by methylene groups, have yielded interesting results.[112] This analogue should be resistant to the attack of a thiol oxidoreductase and the subsequent attack by the aminopeptidase. Nevertheless, the time-course of its antidiuretic action is not increased in comparison with that of vasopressin. Other inactivating systems than tissue oxytocinase might thus be operating in the regulation of the neurohypophysial hormones.

The presence of enzyme systems capable of degrading oxytocin and vasopressin in the hypothalamus of dogs and rabbits is interesting.[85,87] Significantly higher enzyme activity was reported six hours after parturition and in lactation than in late pregnancy.

ASSAY OF OXYTOCIN

The International Standard is a dry powder which is prepared from the fresh posterior lobes of pituitary glands by acetone extraction. The International Unit of pituitary (posterior lobe) extract is, by definition, the amount of oxytocin and vasopressin contained in 0.5 mg of the International Standard in use.

Bioassay Procedures

The oxytocin activity of a posterior pituitary peptide must be compared with the oxytocin component of the standard in a test organ sensitive to oxytocin. Some of the test organs most frequently employed for standardizing the oxytocic activity of peptide solutions are described below.

In the avian blood pressure test, the arterial blood pressure of a young anesthetized rooster is recorded. The intravenous injection of oxytocin causes a fall in the blood pressure. This is the only officially recognized method in the USA for the standardization of oxytocin.[131]

The in vitro rat uterus assay is a very simple procedure for determinations of oxytocin.[86] However, there are many sources of error. The results may be influenced by components of the unknown solutions which may stimulate or inhibit an oxytocic response. Organ or blood extracts may contain 5-hydroxytryptamine, acetylcholine, substance P, plasmakinine, bradykinin, angiotensin, unidentified oxytocic peptides, calcium or potassium ions, all of which can induce the rat uterus to contract. It follows, therefore, that a uterine contraction in vitro by no means indicates the presence of oxytocin.[131] If the method is confined in application to the standardization of synthetic oxytocin or hypophyseal extracts, the above-mentioned source of error can be largely ignored. The determination of the oxytocin activity of blood and tissue extracts requires more specific methods.[56]

The ionic composition and the temperature of the organ bath may alter the uterine response qualitatively as well as quantitatively. Other difficulties are the spontaneous uterine contractions and the low uterine sensitivity to oxytocin.

In the in situ rat uterus, assay, intrauterine pressure is recorded.[10] This is a sensitive and highly specific bioassay for oxytocin. A dose of 100 μU/ml of the peptide can usually be detected, and even more important, oxytocin is the only substance which causes contraction of the uterus without producing any change in arterial blood pressure.

In the milk ejection assay in situ, the intramammary pressure is recorded and oxytocin is injected intravenously. The usual threshold dose is 2–3 mU in the lactating rabbit,[45] and 0.5–1 mU in the lactating guinea pig.[134] Most substances which are troublesome sources of interference in the chicken blood pressure and isolated rat uterus assays are without effect on the milk-ejection response to oxytocin. A further increase in sensitivity by a factor of 10–20 is achieved by administering the hormone solutions by close arterial injection into the blood supply of the mammary gland.[17,54,134] In the lactating rat, the threshold is 10 μU.[10] However, with the intra-arterial injection technique the specificity of the intravenous milk-ejection method is forfeited. Acetylcholine, 5-hydroxytryptamine, and, in the guinea pig but not in the rabbit, histamine, can evoke a milk-ejection response when injected intra-arterially.

The in vitro method using mammary strips from lactating rabbits[101] and rats [128] shows good discrimination in a dose range of 0.5–10 mU/ml and a linear relationship between oxytocin concentration and response. The strips show no spontaneous activity, but unfortunately many other substances besides oxytocin cause contractions of the rabbit and rat mammary strips. The isolated strip of the mouse mammary gland is very sensitive to oxytocin (usual threshold dose 5–25 μU/ml), and the specificity is higher than that of the corresponding rabbit and rat preparations. The mouse mammary strip at present appears to be the most suitable preparation for oxytocin bioassay because of its sensitivity, precision, and specificity.[49]

A very sensitive method for detection of oxytocin is based upon observation of pieces of lactating rat mammary gland through a dissecting microscope.[139] The time interval between exposure to solutions containing oxytocin and the expulsion of milk from the tissue bears a linear relationship to the oxytocin concentration over a range of 0.1 μU–10 mU/ml. This is by far the most sensitive test for detection of oxytocin in biological fluids, but because of its very low precision, the method is unsuitable for bioassay procedures.[140]

The extraction procedures are crucial for the quantitative assay of oxytocin in biological fluids. This is due to the very low concentrations of the neurohypophysial polypeptides or, conversely, to the remarkably high potency of these molecules, and to their instability in biological fluids. Many workers, including Bisset, Hilton, and Poisner,[11] Coch *et al.*,[33] Roberts and Share,[111] and Ryden and Sjöholm,[115] have described extraction procedures or modifications of previous methods, all with the purpose of separating oxytocin from all other substances that might interfere in the bioassay while maintaining a high and reasonably constant recovery rate. A detailed discussion of these procedures is beyond the scope of this review; the problems have not been completely solved in spite of recent progress, but it is possible that the development of more specific and sensitive radioimmunoassays may obviate further attempts to improve the extraction procedures.

Radioimmunoassays

The development of radioimmunoassay methods for oxytocin have received considerable attention during the last two years. The main prerequisites for a radioimmunoassay are: (1) a specific antibody, (2) a labeled antigen of sufficiently high specific activity, and (3) a method for separation and estimation of free or antibody-bound labeled antigen. Specific antibodies to oxytocin have been produced in rabbits with unconjugated oxytocin.[72,76,81] The antibody-titer and the affinity were, however, rather low. Coupling of oxytocin as hapten to larger molecules, in order to get a larger complex and increase antigenicity, has been made by chemically coupling to rabbit serum albumin and by ionic binding to a special carboxymethyldextran.

Radioiodination of oxytocin with ^{131}I has been reported[73] with specific activities of 40 μC/μg.[76] Several different methods have been used for the separation of free and antibody-bound labeled antigen.[79,148] The solid-phase separation seems to offer the best possibilities. Two varieties of this method exist: (1) coupling the antibodies chemically to insoluble Sephadex-isothiocyanate particles,[148] and (2) using antibody-coated tubes.[79] Separation is easily achieved by centrifugation or washing out of free antigen. Radioimmunoassay methods have been capable of detecting

25 μU of oxytocin per milliliter.[76] This sensitivity is not yet high enough to quantitate physiological concentrations of oxytocin in peripheral plasma. Antiserum with greater affinity should improve the sensitivity.

REFERENCES

1. Althabe, O., Jr., Arnt, I. C., Branda, L. A., and Caldeyro-Barcia, R. Comparison of the milk-ejecting potencies of oxytocin and deamino-oxytocin in lactating women. *J. Endocr. 36:*7, 1966.
2. Andersson, B. Some observations on the neuro-humoral regulation of milk-ejection. *Acta Physiol. Scand. 23:*1, 1951.
3. Audrain, L., and Clauser, H. Mécanisme de l'inactivation de l'oxytocine par le tissue utérin. *Biochim. Biophys. Acta 38:*494, 1960.
4. Augusto, N. Indução do parto pela mamada. Tese de Doutoramento, Faculdade de Medicine, Ribeirao Preto, Est. S. P., Brasil, 1965, p. 73.
5. Bargmann, W. "Neurohypophysis. Structure and Function." In *Neurohypophysial Hormones and Similar Polypeptides,* B. Berde (Ed.), Springer, Heidelberg, 1968, p. 1.
6. Bargmann, W., Linder, E., and Andres, K. H. Über Synapsen an endokrinen Epithelzellen und die Definition sekretorischer Neurone. Untersuchungen am Zwischenlappen der Katzenhypophyse. *Z. Zellforsch. 77:*282, 1967.
7. Berde, B. (Ed.) "Neurohypophysial Hormones and Similar Polypeptides." *Handbook of Experimental Pharmacology,* XXIII, Springer, Heidelberg, 1968.
8. Bindler, E., Labella, Fr. S., and Sanwal, M. Isolated nerve endings (neurosecretosomes) from the posterior pituitary. Partial separation of vasopressin and oxytocin and the isolation of microvesicles. *Cell Biol. 34:*185, 1967.
9. Bisset, G. W., Clark, B., Haldar, J., Harris, M. C., Lewis, C. P., and Rocha e Silva, M. The assay of milk-ejecting activity in the lactating rat. *Brit. J. Pharmacol. 31:*537, 1967.
10. Bisset, G. W., Haldar, J., and Lewin, J. E. "Action of Oxytocin and Other Biologically Active Peptides on the Rat Uterus." In *Memoirs of the Society for Endocrinology,* No. 14, V. R. Pickles and R. Fitzpatrick (Eds.), Cambridge University Press, Cambridge, 1966, p. 185.
11. Bisset, G. W., Hilton, S. M., and Poisner, A. M. Hypothalamic pathways for independent release of vasopressin and oxytocin. *Proc. Roy. Soc.* (*Biol.*) *166:*422, 1967.
12. Branda, L. A., Fielitz, C., and Roca, R. Oxytocin release in diabetes insipidus. Ann. Meet. Royal Coll. Phys. Surg. Canada, Jan. 1970.
13. Brooks, C. M. C., Ishikawa, T., Koizumi, K., and Lu, H. H. Activity of neurons in the paraventricular nucleus of the hypothalamus and its control. *J. Physiol.* (London) *182:*217, 1966.
14. Brovetto, J., Olhaberry, J., Gioia de Coch, M. N., Coda, H., Fielitz, C.,

Cabot, H. M., Fraga, A., and Coch, J. A. Separation of oxytocin from the substances that interfere with its biological assay on the isolated rat mammary gland. *J. Endocr. 38:*355, 1967.

15. Caldeyro-Barcia, R. "Uterine Contractility in Obstetrics." In *Modern Trends in Gynaecology and Obstetrics,* Vol. 1, Librairie Beauchemin Limitée, Montreal, 1959, p. 65.
16. Caldeyro-Barcia, R. Oxytocin in pregnancy and labour. *Acta Endocr.* (*Suppl.*) *50:*41, 1960.
17. Caldeyro-Barcia, R. "Factors Controlling the Actions of the Pregnant Human Uterus." In *Physiology of Prematurity, Transact. 5th Conf.,* M. Kowlessar (Ed.), Josiah Macy, Jr. Foundation, Princeton, N.J., 1961, p. 11.
18. Caldeyro-Barcia, R., Alvarez, H., and Poseiro, J. J. Action of morphine on the contractility of the human uterus. *Arch. Int. Pharmacodyn. 101:*171, 1955.
19. Caldeyro-Barcia, R., Alvarez, H., Poseiro, J. J., Pose, S. V., and Méndez-Bauer, C. Contractions of the term pregnant Fallopian tube. Spontaneous activity and response to oxytocin and ergonovine. Unpublished data, 1958.
20. Caldeyro-Barcia, R., and Poseiro, J. J. Oxytocin and contractility of the pregnant human uterus. *Ann. N.Y. Acad. Sci. 75:*813, 1959.
21. Caldeyro-Barcia, R., and Sereno, J. A. "The Response of the Human Uterus to Oxytocin Throughout Pregnancy." In *Oxytocin,* R. Caldeyro-Barcia and H. Heller (Eds.), Pergamon Press, Oxford, 1961, p. 177.
22. Caldeyro-Barcia, R., Sica-Blanco, Y., Alvarez, H., Pose, S. V., Poseiro, J. J., Méndez-Bauer, C., Fielitz, C., González-Panizza, V. H., Cabot, H. M., Branda, L., Escarcena, L., Coch, J. A., and Brovetto, J. "Oxytocin in Labor and in Milk Ejection." In *Perspectives in Biology,* C. F. Cori, V. G. Foglia, L. F. Leloir, and S. Ochoa (Eds.), Elsevier, Amsterdam, 1962, p. 62.
23. Caldeyro-Barcia, R., Sica-Blanco, Y., Poseiro, J. J., González-Panizza, V., Méndez-Bauer, C., Fielitz, C., Alvarez, H., Pose, S. V., and Hendricks, C. H. A quantitative study on the action of synthetic oxytocin on the pregnant human uterus. *J. Pharmacol. Exp. Ther. 121:*18, 1957.
24. Chan, W. Y., Fear, R., and du Vigneaud, V. Some pharmacologic studies on 1-L-penicillamine-oxytocin and 1-deaminopenicillamine-oxytocin: two potent oxytocin inhibitors. *Endocrinology 81:*1267, 1967.
25. Cibils, L. A., Poseiro, J. J., and Noriega Guerra, L. Comparison of the effects on the pregnant human uterus of highly-purified natural oxytocin, pitocin, synthetic oxytocin (Syntocinon), valyl^3-oxytocin and arginine vasopressin. In *Oxytocin,* R. Caldeyro-Barcia and H. Heller (Eds.), Pergamon Press, Oxford, 1961, p. 266.
26. Cobo, E. Uterine and milk-ejection activities during human labor. *J. Appl. Physiol. 24:*317, 1968.
27. Cobo, E. Inhibición de la neurohipófisis humana, usando alcohol y sobrecarga de agua. *Proc. 3rd Meeting Latin-American Assoc. Human Reprod.* (ALIRH), Salvador, Bahia, Brasil, 1968, p. 82.

28. Cobo, E., Bernal, M.M.de, Gaitán, E., and Quintero, C. Neurohypophyseal hormone release in the human. II. Experimental study during lactation. *Amer. J. Obstet. Gynec. 97:*519, 1967.

29. Cobo, E., de Bernal, M. M., Quintero, C. A., and Cuadrado, E. Neurohypophyseal hormone release in the human. III. Experimental study during labor. *Amer. J. Obstet. Gynec. 101:*479, 1968.

30. Cobo, E., Gaitán, E., Mizrachi, M., and Strada, G. Neurohypophyseal hormone release in the human. I. Experimental study during pregnancy. *Amer. J. Obstet. Gynec. 91:*905, 1965.

31. Cobo, E., Quintero, C. A., Strada, G., and Zambrana, M. A. Uterine behavior in abruptio placentae. *Amer. J. Obstet. Gynec. 93:*1151, 1965.

32. Coch, J. A., Brovetto, J., Cabot, H. M., Fielitz, C. A., and Caldeyro-Barcia, R. Oxytocin equivalent activity in the plasma of women in labor and puerperium. *Amer. J. Obstet. Gynec. 91:*10, 1965.

33. Coch, J. A., Fielitz, C., Brovetto, J., Cabot, H. M., Coda, H., and Fraga, A. Estimation of an oxytocin-like substance in highly purified extracts from the blood of puerperal women during suckling. *J. Endocr. 40:*137, 1968.

34. Coch, J. A., Melander, S., Garófalo, E., Gioia de Coch, M. N., Roca, R., Mattei, A., and Caldeyro-Barcia, R. Concentration of oxytocin in human fetal blood at birth. In preparation, 1969.

35. Coutinho, E. M., and Lopes, A. C. V. Response of the nonpregnant uterus to vasopressin as an index of ovarian function. *Amer. J. Obstet. Gynec. 102:*479, 1968.

36. Coutinho, E. M., and Maia, H. Atividade espontanea e resposta da trompa de Fallopia humana *in vivo* aos hormonios neuro-hipofisarios. In *Proc. 3rd Meeting-American Assoc. Res. Human Reprod.* (ALIRH), Salvador, Bahia, Brasil, 1968, p. 79.

37. Cross, B. A. The motility and reactivity of the oestrogenized rabbit uterus *in vivo;* with comparative observations on milk ejection. *J. Endocr. 16:*237, 1958.

38. Cross, B. A. On the mechanism of labour in the rabbit. *J. Endocr. 16:*262, 1958.

39. Csapo, A. "The Effects of Oxytocic Substances on the Excitability of the Uterus." In *Oxytocin,* R. Caldeyro-Barcia and H. Heller (Eds.), Pergamon Press, Oxford, 1961, p. 100.

40. Debackere, M., and Peeters, G. The influence of vaginal distension on milk ejection and diuresis in the lactating cow. *Arch. Int. Pharmacodyn. 123:*462, 1960.

41. Debackere, M., Peeters, G., and Tuyttens, N. Reflex release of an oxytocic hormone by stimulation of genital organs in male and female sheep studied by a cross-circulation technique. *J. Endocr. 22:*321, 1961.

42. Dey, F. L., Fisher, C., and Ranson, S. W. Disturbances in pregnancy and labor in guinea pigs with hypothalamic lesions. *Amer. J. Obstet. Gynec. 42:*459, 1941.

43. Dicker, S. E. Possible independence of oxytocin and vasopressin secretion in the human being. *J. Physiol.* (London) *147:*25P, 1959.
44. Dicker, S. E., and Whyley, G. A. The role of oxytocinase during pregnancy in man and animals. *Acta Endocr. 34,* Suppl. *51:*145, 1960.
45. Fekete, K. Beiträge zur Physiologie der Gravidität. *Endokrinologie 7:*364, 1930.
46. Ferguson, J. K. W. A study of the motility of the intact uterus at term. *Surg. Gynec. Obstet. 73:*359, 1941.
47. Fielitz, C. A., Cabot, H. M., Brovetto, J., and Coch, J. A. Embarazo, parto y lactancia en una mujer con diabetes insípida. *IV Congr. Uruguayo de Ginecotocología 2:*614, 1964.
48. Fielitz, C., González Panizza, V. H., and Caldeyro-Barcia, R. Effect of low concentration of oxytocin on the uterine response to electrical stimulation. *Acta Physiol. Lat. Amer. 10:*201, 1960.
49. Fielitz, C., Roca, R., Mattei, A., Garófalo, E., Gioia de Coch, M. N., and Coch, J. A. "The Use of the Strips of Lactating Mouse Mammary Gland on the Bioassay of Oxytocin." *Proc. 3rd Meeting Latin-American Assoc. Res. Human Reprod.* (ALIRH), Salvador, Bahia, Brasil, 1968, p. 86.
50. Fisch, L., Sala, N. L., and Schwarcz, R. L. Effect of cervical dilatation upon uterine contractility in pregnant women and its relation to oxytocin secretion. *Amer. J. Obstet. Gynec. 90:*108, 1964.
51. Fisher, C., Magoun, H. W., and Ranson, S. W. Dystocia in diabetes insipidus. The relation of pituitary oxytocin to parturition. *Amer. J. Obstet. Gynec. 36:*1, 1938.
52. Fitzpatrick, R. J. "On Oxytocin and Uterine Function." In *The Neurohypophysis,* H. Heller (Ed.), Butterworth, London, 1957, p. 203.
53. Fitzpatrick, R. J. "The Estimation of Small Amounts of Oxytocin in Blood." In *Oxytocin,* R. Caldeyro-Barcia and H. Heller (Eds.), Pergamon Press, Oxford, 1961, p. 360.
54. Fitzpatrick, R. J. Blood concentration of oxytocin in labour. *J. Endocr. 22:*xix, 1961.
55. Fitzpatrick, R. J. "The Posterior Pituitary Gland and the Female Reproductive Tract." In *The Pituitary Gland,* G. W. Harris and B. T. Donovan (Eds.), Butterworth, London, 1966, p. 453.
56. Fitzpatrick, R. J., and Bentley, P. J. "The Assay of Neurohypophysial Hormones in Blood and Other Body Fluids." In *Neurohypophysial Hormones and Similar Polypeptides,* B. Berde (Ed.), Springer, Heidelberg, 1968, p. 190.
57. Fitzpatrick, R. J., and Walmsley, C. F. "The Release of Oxytocin During Parturition." In *Advances in Oxytocin Research,* J. H. M. Pinkerton (Ed.), Pergamon Press, Oxford, 1965, p. 51.
58. Folley, S. J., and Knaggs, G. S. Levels of oxytocin in the jugular vein blood of goats during parturition. *J. Endocr. 33:*301, 1965.
59. Folley, S. J., and Knaggs, G. S. Milk-ejection activity (oxytocin) in

the external jugular vein blood of the cow, goat and sow, in relation to the stimulus of milking or suckling. *J. Endocr. 34:*197, 1966.

60. FUCHS, A.-R. Oxytocin and the onset of labour in rabbits. *J. Endocr. 30:*217, 1964.
61. FUCHS, A.-R. The role of oxytocin in the initiation of labour. *Excerpta Med. Int. Congr. Sr. 83*:753, 1965.
62. FUCHS, A.-R. The inhibitory effect of ethanol on the release of oxytocin during parturition in the rabbit. *J. Endocr. 35:*125, 1966.
63. FUCHS, A.-R. The physiological role of oxytocin in the regulation of myometrial activity in the rabbit. *Mem. Soc. Endocr. 14:*229, 1966.
64. FUCHS, A.-R., COUTINHO, E. M., XAVIER, R., BATES, P. E., and FUCHS, F. Effect of ethanol on the activity of the nonpregnant human uterus and its reactivity to neurohypophyseal hormones. *Amer. J. Obstet. Gynec. 101:*997, 1968.
65. FUCHS, A.-R., OLSEN, P., and PETERSEN, K. Effect of distension of uterus and vagina on uterine motility and oxytocin release in puerperal rabbits. *Acta Endocr.* (Kobenhavn) *50:*239, 1965.
66. FUCHS, A.-R., and WAGNER, G. Effect of alcohol on release of oxytocin. *Nature* (London) *198:*92, 1963.
67. FUCHS, A.-R., and WAGNER, G. Quantitative aspects of release of oxytocin by suckling in unanesthetized rabbits. *Acta Endocr.* (Kobenhavn) *44:*581, 1963.
68. FUCHS, A.-R., and WAGNER, G. The effect of ethyl alcohol on the release of oxytocin in rabbits. *Acta Endocr.* (Kobenhavn) *44:*593, 1963.
69. FUCHS, F., FUCHS, A.-R., POBLETE, V. F., and RISK, A. Effect of alcohol on threatened premature labor. *Amer. J. Obstet. Gynec. 99:*627, 1967.
70. GAITÁN, E., COBO, E., and MIZRACHI, M. Evidence for the differential secretion of oxytocin and vasopressin in man. *J. Clin. Invest. 43:*2310, 1964.
71. GAITÁN, E., JUBIZ, W., and PAZ, A. Studies of the mechanisms which regulate the secretion of oxytocin and vasopressin in human beings. *Excerpta Med. Int. Congr. Sr. 99:*E108, 1965.
72. GILLILAND, P. F., and PROUT, T. E. Production and detection of antibodies to oxytocin. *Metabolism 14:*918, 1965.
73. GILLILAND, P. E., and PROUT, T. E. Radioiodination of oxytocin. *Metabolism 14:*912, 1965.
74. GINSBURG, M. "Fate and Transport of Neurohypophysial Hormones." In *Proc. 2nd Internat. Pharmacology Meeting,* J. Rudinger (Ed.), Pergamon Press, London, 1964, p. 87.
75. GINSBURG, M. "Production, Release, Transportation and Elimination of the Neurohypophysial Hormones." In *Neurohypophysial Hormones and Similar Polypeptides,* B. Berde (Ed.), Springer, Heidelberg, 1968, p. 286.
76. GLICK, M., WHEELER, M., KAGAN, A., and KUMARESAN, P. "Radioimmunoassay of Oxytocin." In *Pharmacology of Hormonal Polypeptides and Proteins,* Plenum, New York, 1968, p. 93.

77. GÖLTNER, E. Erkennung des bevorstehenden Geburtsbeginnes mittels "Oxytocin-sensitivity Test." *Zbl. Gynaek. 81:*113, 1959.

78. GONZÁLEZ PANIZZA, V. H., SICA BLANCO, Y., and MÉNDEZ-BAUER, C. "The Fate of Injected Oxytocin in the Pregnant Woman Near Term." In *Oxytocin,* R. Caldeyro-Barcia and H. Heller (Eds.), Pergamon Press, Oxford, 1961, p. 347.

79. GOODFRIEND, T. L., BALL, D. L., and FARLEY, D. B. Radioimmunoassay of angiotensin. *J. Lab. Clin. Med. 72:*648, 1968.

80. GUNTHER, M. The posterior pituitary and labour. *Brit. Med. J. I:*567, 1948.

81. GUDSON, J. P. An antibody to oxytocin. *Amer. J. Obstet. Gynec. 98:*526, 1967.

82. HARRIS, G. W. The innervation and actions of the neurohypophysis; an investigation using the method of remote-control stimulation. *Phil. Trans Roy. Soc. B232:*385, 1947.

83. HATERIUS, H. O., and FERGUSON, J. K. W. Evidence for the hormonal nature of the oxytocic principle of the hypophysis. *Amer. J. Physiol. 124:*314, 1938.

84. HENDRICKS, C. H., ESKES, T. K. A. B., and SAAMELI, K. Uterine contractility at delivery and in the puerperium. *Amer. J. Obstet. Gynec. 83:*890, 1962.

85. HOLTON, P. A. A modification of the method of Dale and Laidlaw for standardization of posterior pituitary extracts. *Brit. J. Pharmacol. 3:*328, 1948.

86. HOPPENSTEIN, J. M., MILTENBERGER, F. W., and MORAN, W. H., Jr. The increase in blood levels of vasopressin in infants during birth and surgical procedures. *Surg. Gynec. Obstet. 127:*966, 1968.

87. HOOPER, K. C. The catabolism of bradykinin, oxytocin, substance P and vasopressin by homogenate of dog hypothalamus. *Biochem. J. 81:*44P, 1961.

88. HOOPER, K. C. The metabolism of oxytocin during lactation in the rabbit. *Biochem. J. 100:*893, 1966.

89. HUBER, R., and NOLD, B. Ueber die Rolle des Wehenhormons bei der Laktation. *Z. Geburtsh. Gynaek. 145:*325, 1956.

90. ICHALIOTIS, S. D., and LAMBRINOPOULOS, TH. C. Preeclampsia associated with decrease in serum oxytocinase. *Obstet. Gynec. 24:*659, 1964.

91. JEWELL, P. A., and VERNEY, E. B. An experimental attempt to determine the site of the neurohypophysial and osmoreceptors in the dog. *Phil. Trans. Roy. Soc. B240:*197, 1957.

92. JUNG, H. "The Effect of Oxytocin on the Mechanism of Uterine Excitation." In *Oxytocin,* R. Caldeyro-Barcia and H. Heller (Eds.), Pergamon, Oxford, 1961, p. 87.

93. KALLIALA, H., and KARVONEN, M. Antidiuresis during suckling in women. *Ann. Med. Exp. Biol. Fenn. 29:*233, 1951.

94. LAUSON, H. D. "Vasopressin and Oxytocin in the Plasma of Man and Other Mammals." In *Hormones in Human Plasma,* H. N. Antoniades (Ed.), Little, Brown, Boston, 1960, p. 225.

95. Leinzinger, E., and Rainer, A. Tokometrische Untersuchungen Über die Wehen bereitschaft mit Hilfe der Mamillenfriktion in Kombination mit Partergin Sandoz. *Geburtsh. Frauenheilk. 14:*257, 1954.
96. Luukkainen, T., Väistö, L., and Järvinen, P. A. The effect of oral intake of ethyl alcohol on the activity of the pregnant human uterus. *Acta Obstet. Gynec. Scand. 46:*486, 1967.
97. Maia, H., and Coutinho, E. M. A new technique for recording human tubal activity in vivo. *Amer. J. Obstet. Gynec. 102:*1043, 1968.
98. Marshall, J. M., and Csapo, A. I. Hormonal and ionic influences on the membrane activity of uterine smooth muscle cells. *Endocrinology 68:*1026, 1961.
99. de Mattos, C. E. R., and Coutinho, E. M. "O reflexo de Ferguson em coelhas grávidas." *Proc. 3rd Meeting Latin-American Assoc. Res. Human Reprod.* (ALIRH), Salvador, Bahia, Brasil, 1968, p. 81.
100. Melander, S. E. J. Plasma oxytocinase activity. *Acta Endocr.* (Kobenhavn) 49, *Suppl. 96:*1, 1965.
101. Méndez-Bauer, C., Cabot, H. M., and Caldeyro-Barcia, R. A new test for the biological assay of oxytocin. *Science 132:*299, 1960.
102. Moir, J. C. The effect of posterior lobe pituitary gland fractions on the intact human uterus. *J. Obstet. Gynaec. Brit. Emp. 51:*181, 1944.
103. Munsick, R. A. "The effect of Neurohypophysial Hormones and Similar Polypeptides on the Uterus and Other Extravascular Smooth Muscle Tissue." In *Neurohypophysial Hormones and Similar Polypeptides,* B. Berde (Ed.), Springer, Heidelberg, 1968, p. 443.
104. Nibbelink, D. W. Paraventricular nuclei, neurohypophysis and parturition. *Amer. J. Physiol. 200:*1299, 1961.
105. Peeters, G., and Coussens, R. The influence of the milking act on the diuresis of the lactating cow. *Arch. Int. Pharmacodyn. 84:*209, 1950.
106. Peeters, G., Debackere, M., Lauryssens, M., and Kühn, E. "Studies on the Release of Oxytocin in Domestic Animals." In *Advances in Oxytocin Research,* J. H. M. Pinkerton (Ed.), Pergamon, Oxford, 1965, p. 75.
107. Pickford, M. "The Release of Oxytocin and Vasopressin." In *Polypeptides Which Affect Smooth Muscles and Blood Vessels,* M. Schachter (Ed.), Pergamon, Oxford, 1960, p. 42.
108. Popenoe, E. A., and du Vigneaud, V. Degradative studies on vasopressin and performic acid-oxidized vasopressin. *J. Biol. Chem. 205:*133, 1953.
109. Poseiro, J. J., and Noriega Guerra, L. "Dose-Response Relationships in Uterine Effects of Oxytocin Infusions." In *Oxytocin,* R. Caldeyro-Barcia and H. Heller (Eds.), Pergamon, Oxford, 1961, p. 158.
110. de Robertis, E. *Histophysiology of Synapses and Neurosecretion,* Pergamon, Oxford, 1964.
111. Roberts, J. S., and Share, L. Oxytocin in plasma of pregnant, lactating and cycling ewes during vaginal stimulation. *Endocrinology 83:*272, 1968.
112. Rudinger, J. Synthetic analogues of oxytocin: an approach to problems of hormone action. *Proc. Roy. Soc.* (*Biol.*) *170:*17, 1968.
113. Rychlik, I. "Inactivation of Oxytocin and Vasopressin by Tissue Enzymes."

In *Proc. 2nd Intern. Pharmacology Meeting,* J. Rudinger (Ed.), Pergamon, London, 1964, p. 153.

114. Ryden, G. Cystine aminopeptidase and oxytocinase activity in pregnancy. *Acta Obstet. Gynec. Scand. 65,* Suppl. *3:*1, 1966.

115. Ryden, G., and Sjöholm, I. Assay of oxytocin by rat mammary gland *in vitro. Brit. J. Pharmacol. 19:*136, 1962.

116. Saameli, K. An indirect method for the estimation of oxytocin blood concentration and half-life in pregnant women near term. *Amer. J. Obstet. Gynec. 85:*186, 1963.

117. Sala, N. The milk-ejecting effect induced by oxytocin and vasopressin during human pregnancy. *Amer. J. Obstet. Gynec. 89:*625, 1964.

118. Sala, N. Milk ejecting effect induced by various octapeptides in human beings. Comparison between the milk ejecting potency of synthetic oxytocin, natural purified oxytocin, natural purified vasopressin and synthetic lysine-8-vasopressin. *Acta Physiol. Lat. Amer. 15:*191, 1965.

119. Sala, N., and Althabe, O. The milk ejecting effect induced by oxytocin during human lactation. *Acta Physiol. Lat. Amer. 18:*88, 1968.

120. Sala, N. L., and Fisch, L. Effect of acetylcholine and atropine upon uterine contractility in pregnant women. *Amer. J. Obstet. Gynec. 91:*1069, 1965.

121. Sala, N. L., Fisch, L., and Schwarcz, R. L. Effect of cervical dilatation upon milk ejection in puerperal women and its relation to oxytocin secretion. *Amer. J. Obstet. Gynec. 91:*1090, 1965.

122. Sawyer, W. H. Inactivation of oxytocin by homogenates of uteri and other tissues from normal and pregnant rats. *Proc. Soc. Exp. Biol. Med. 87:*463, 1954.

123. Schwarcz, R. L., Sala, N. L., Althabe, O., and Fisch, L. "Mecanismos de Producción del Efecto Útero Estimulante de la Dilatación Cervical Artificial en el Embarazo Humano." In *Proc. 2nd Meeting Latin-American Assoc. Res. Human Reprod.* (ALIRH), Viña del Mar, Chile, Nov. 1966, p. 173.

124. Sica-Blanco, Y., Méndez-Bauer, C., Sala, N., Cabot, H., and Caldeyro-Barcia, R. Nuevo método para el estudio de la funcionalidad mamaria en la mujer. *Arch. Ginec. Obstet.* (*Montevideo*) *17:*63, 1959.

125. Sica-Blanco, Y., and Sala, N. L. "Uterine Contractility at the Beginning and End of an Oxytocin Infusion." In *Oxytocin,* R. Caldeyro-Barcia and H. Heller (Eds.), Pergamon, Oxford, 1961, p. 127.

126. Sica-Blanco, Y., Sala, N., and Caldeyro-Barcia, R. Unpublished Data, 1960.

127. Sjöholm, I. Biochemical studies on oxytocin and oxytocinase. *Acta Pharm. Suec. 4:*81, 1967.

128. Smith, M. W. Some properties of rat mammary tissue. *Nature* (London) *190:*541, 1961.

129. Smyth, C. N. "The Oxytocin Sensitivity Test. A Review of Ten Years' Results." In *Advances in Oxytocin Research,* J. H. M. Pinkerton (Ed.), Pergamon, Oxford, 1965, p. 115.

130. STRADA-SAENZ, G., COBO, E., GÓMEZ-ROGERS, C., and SALA, N. Trabajo uterino en parto espontáneo. *III Congr. Uruguayo Ginecotocología 3:*392, 1960.

131. STÜRMER, E. "Bioassay Procedures for Neurohypophysial Hormones and Similar Polypeptides." In *Neurohypophysial Hormones and Similar Polypeptides,* B. Berde (Ed.), Springer, Heidelberg, 1968, p. 130.

132. THEOBALD, G. W. The separate release of oxytocin and ADH. *J. Physiol.* (London) *149:*443, 1959.

133. THEOBALD, G. W. Oxytocin reassessed. *Obstet. Gynec. Survey 23:*109, 1968.

134. TINDAL, J. S., and YOKOYAMA, A. Assay of oxytocin by the milk ejection response on the anaesthetised lactating guinea pig. *Endocrinology 71:*196, 1962.

135. TUPPY, H. The amino-acid sequence in oxytocin. *Biochim. Biophys. Acta 11:*449, 1953.

136. TUPPY, H. "The Influence of Enzymes on Neurohypophysial Hormones and Similar Peptides." In *Neurohypophysial Hormones and Similar Polypeptides,* B. Berde (Ed.), Springer, Heidelberg, 1968, p. 67.

137. TUPPY, H., and NESVADBA, H. Über die Aminopeptidaseaktivität des Schwangerenserums und ihre Beziehung zu dessen Vermögen Oxytocin zu inaktivieren. *Mh. Chem. 88:*977, 1957.

138. VAN DONGEN, C. G., and HAYS, R. L. Oxytocic activity in unextracted blood plasma during calving. *J. Reprod. Fertil. 11:*317, 1966.

139. VAN DONGEN, C. G., and HAYS, R. L. A sensitive *in vitro* assay for oxytocin. *Endocrinology 71:*1, 1966.

140. VAN DONGEN, C. G., and MARSHALL, J. M. Effects of various hormones on the milk ejection response of tissue isolated from the rat mammary gland. *Nature* (London) *213:*632, 1967.

141. VAN DYKE, H. B., ADAMSONS, K., JR., and ENGEL, S. L. Aspects of the biochemistry and physiology of the neurohypophyseal hormones. *Recent Progr. Hormone Res. XI:*1, 1955.

142. VERNEY, E. B. The antidiuretic hormone and the factors which determine its release. *Proc. Roy. Soc. (Biol.) 135:*27, 1947.

143. DU VIGNEAUD, V., LAWLER, H. C., and POPENOE, E. A. Enzymic cleavage of glycinamide from vasopressin and a proposed structure for this pressor-anti-diuretic hormone of the posterior pituitary. *J. Amer. Chem. Soc. 75:*4880, 1953.

144. DU VIGNEAUD, V., RESSLER, C., SWAN, J. M., ROBERTS, C. W., KATSOYANNIS, P. G., and GORDON, S. The synthesis of an octapeptide amide with the hormonal activity of oxytocin. *J. Amer. Chem. Soc. 25:*4879, 1953.

145. DU VIGNEAUD, V., RESSLER, C., and TRIPETT, S. The sequence of amino acids in oxytocin, with a proposal for the structure of oxytocin. *J. Biol. Chem. 205:*949, 1953.

146. WAGNER, G., and FUCHS, A.-R. Effect of ethanol on uterine activity during suckling in post-partum women. *Acta Endocr.* (Kobenhavn) *58:*133, 1968.

147. WALMSLEY, C. F. The concentration of oxytocin in blood in relation to reproduction. Thesis, University of Bristol, 1963.

148. WIDE, L., and PORATH, J. Radioimmunoassay of proteins with the use of Sephadex-coupled antibodies. *Biochim. Biophys. Acta 130:*257, 1966.

149. WIQVIST, N., WIQVIST, I., FIELITZ, C., and CALDEYRO-BARCIA, R. Effects of oxytocin on the uterine response to electrical stimulation. *Acta Endocr.* (Kobenhavn) *41:*161, 1962.

150. ZAMBRANO, D., and DE ROBERTIS, E. The ultrastructural changes in the neurohypophysis after destruction of the paraventricular nuclei in normal and castrated rats. *Z. Zellforsch. 88:*496, 1968.

Chapter Twelve

Uterine Activating Hormones

Anna-Riitta Fuchs

There are many endogenous substances which stimulate the myometrium. They fall into three main categories: neurohormones, tissue hormones, and substances released from inactive precursors in plasma and tissues by enzymatic activity. The last category comprises the kinins and various lipid anions. Of these substances, bradykinin, angiotensin, and prostaglandins have a strong uterotropic activity in pharmacological test preparations. Because of the occurrence of precursors in plasma or in various reproductive organs, they will be mentioned briefly. The neurohormones and tissue hormones which affect uterine smooth muscle include: (1) the posterior pituitary hormones–oxytocin and vasopressin, (2) the adrenal medullary hormones–epinephrine and norepinephrine, and (3) the tissue hormones–serotonin and histamine. The cholinergic and adrenergic chemical transmitter substances may also be considered as neurohormones. Recent studies have shown that their production occurs in structures found in neurones and related cells which are secretory in nature and in many ways homologous to the epinephrine-producing chromaffin cells of the adrenal medulla; therefore, the neurohumors can be included in a generalized concept of neurosecretion.

Contrary to the classical concept of an endocrine gland as an anatomical entity, these substances are produced and stored in complex systems such as the hypothalamo-hypophyseal neurosecretory system or the enterochromaffin cells which are scattered throughout the entire gastrointestinal tract. They are not secreted directly into the circulation but are taken up in special storage granules. Their secretion rate is, therefore, independent of their rate of release which is not regulated by humoral feedback mechanisms but is under the control of the nervous system. This is well established in the case of the neurohormones; the releasing factors affecting tissue hormones, however, are not as well understood. In addition to neural factors, local mechanical (e.g., trauma) and chemical factors seem to be involved in their release.

These substances all elicit a myometrial response when the uterus is under proper steroid-hormonal influence. The threshold to pharmacological stimuli is generally high in the castrate uterus, whereas estrogen treatment lowers the threshold for stimulation and increases the response to all of these substances. Progesterone can modify their action on the estrogen-primed uterus in various ways. It should be emphasized that our knowledge of the regulation of uterine function by ovarian steroids derives mostly from studies in laboratory animals. Their effects on the human uterus are still very poorly understood and results obtained in rodent uteri should only be applied to the human with great caution.

The posterior pituitary hormones are dealt with separately in Chapter Eleven and will not be considered here.

CATECHOLAMINES

The adrenal medullary hormones are chemically characterized as catecholamines, of which two, norepinephrine and epinephrine, are secreted by mammalian tissues. A third, dopamine, which also occurs in the same tissue location, serves as a precursor for the biosynthesis of the two neurohormones. They are synthetized in the brain, in the sympathetic ganglia and nerve endings, as well as in the peripheral chromaffin cells. Most of the chromaffin cells are localized in the adrenal medulla, but such cells are also scattered in other peripheral tissues. In the postsynaptic chromaffin cells of the adrenal medulla both norepinephrine and epinephrine are produced and secreted. At the sympathetic nerve endings, however, only norepinephrine is synthetized and released. Outside the central nervous system most of the catecholamines are located in subcellular particles, the granules or granulated vesicles. The uterus seems to be a major exception to this rule; following ultracentrifugation up to 80 per cent of the catecholamines in uterine homogenates is present in the supernatant and not the vesicular fraction.[105, 115, 116]

A small amount of catecholamine is probably released continuously from the adrenal, but the major portion of the adrenomedullary output is secreted in spurts in response to stimulation of its preganglionic cholinergic fibers or in response to the action of circulatory secretagogues such as insulin or histamine. Stress and exercise stimulate the sympatheticoadrenal system. Under psychic tension and emotional stress only epinephrine seems to be released; whereas, during exercise and physical stress both catecholamines are secreted.

The histochemical fluorescence technique for cellular localization of catecholamines developed by Carlsson, Hillarp, Falck, and Owman[20, 39, 41] has permitted direct determination of the adrenergic innervation of various tissues. The female genital tract of rat,[40] rabbit,[79] cat,[102] and man[78] has been studied, and a system of adrenergic nerves of varying density was demonstrated in all. The nerves were partly associated with the vascular system, but the majority of the nerves could be related to the smooth muscle except in the rat uterus, which lacks muscular adrenergic innervation. The vagina and cervix, and in the human also the area of the internal os, show the richest adrenergic innervation; whereas the uterine nerve supply was less prominent. The transmitter released upon stimulation from hypogastric nerve fibers supplying the uterus of the cat was definitely shown to be norepinephrine by Vogt,[112] but the release of epinephrine could not be excluded.

The catecholamine content of the human uterus[47] and of uteri from other species[77, 103, 105, 116] is low, but it is larger than would correspond to adrenergic perivascular innervation. There is some indication that the uterine norepinephrine content is influenced by the hormonal state;[103] estrogens as well as early pregnancy increase the total content of norepinephrine in the uterus. Others have found the uterine norepinephrine content unaltered by hormonal treatment.[75, 105, 116] During the latter half of pregnancy there is a dramatic decrease in norepinephrine concentration in the uterus, due mainly to the increase in organ weight. By the end of gestation the rabbit uterus is almost completely devoid of norepinephrine-containing nerve fibers.[89] Only norepinephrine is synthetized in the uterus, which lacks the methylating enzyme that converts norepinephrine to epinephrine. The uterus does, however, possess a cellular mechanism for the uptake and the binding of epinephrine.[105, 116] During pregnancy this binding capacity increases. Whether this mechanism functions to inactivate any circulating epinephrine or whether it is stored to be released again by appropriate stimuli is unknown. During parturition the rat uterus discharges about 80 per cent of its epinephrine content in less than six hours.[116]

The catecholamines present in the blood behave like a single metabolic pool, whether they originate from the stimulation of the adrenal medulla or from sympathetic nerves.[7]

Only a very small fraction of the free catecholamines is taken up at the receptor sites of the effector cells, and it is this fraction that is responsible for the tissue response. Most of the released norepinephrine and epinephrine is removed from the blood by uptake into the sympathetic nerve endings, while another part is inactivated by an enzyme, catechol-O-methyl transferase (COMT) which is present in the cytoplasmic fraction of many cells, but is especially concentrated in liver and kidney.[7,52] The nonpregnant uterus contains trace amounts of COMT, but the activity more than doubles during pregnancy.[116]

Only at high rates of sympathetic stimulation does an "overflow" into the circulation occur, and a portion of the released transmitter appears in the venous drainage. As already mentioned, catecholamine release from the uterus during hypogastric stimulation has been demonstrated in both nonpregnant and pregnant cats,[112] but the amounts appearing in uterine venous blood were very small even at supramaximal stimulation rates. A very large blood flow, as in the heart, enhances the overflow and a greater proportion of the transmitter escapes into the general circulation. The sympathetic nerves in the heart are apparently a major source of circulating norepinephrine under normal physiological conditions. It is therefore unlikely that the levels of norepinephrine in peripheral blood reflect the state of uterine sympathetic activity. The plasma catecholamine concentrations have been determined before and during labor in normal parturient women; no significant changes in the plasma norepinephrine levels occurred.[56,58,117] As to epinephrine levels, the results are somewhat variable, but due to the very low concentrations of this hormone in the blood, the results are less reliable. There seems to be a slight increase at the end of labor. The urinary excretion, as determined during 2-hour intervals before and after delivery, did not change significantly during spontaneous or oxytocin-induced delivery.[15]

Tissue Responses

The action of catecholamines on effector cells is independent of the route of access to the cell, whether vascular or neural. The uterine response to hypogastric and splanchnic nerve stimulation is similar to intravenous injections of norepinephrine and epinephrine.[99,101] The response of the myometrium to catecholamines differs in various species,[71,85] and sometimes there is also a difference between in vivo and in vitro effects in the same species. The differential responses to catecholamines are explained by the presence of two different receptor sites on the smooth muscle membranes, called α- and β-receptors, the activation of which leads to the observed mechanical response.[3] Most of the α-receptors are excitatory and most of the β-receptors are inhibitory; notable exceptions are in the intestine and the heart. Norepinephrine has mainly α-effects, although it may have also weak intrinsic β-effects; whereas epinephrine has both α- and β-effects. Isoproterenol, a synthetic sympathomimetic agent, has only β-effects. The resultant mechanical response to each of these substances depends on the relative number and activity of the two receptor sites in each particular effector tissue.

The presence of α- and β-receptors has been demonstrated by means of specific pharmacological blocking agents in the uterus of most mammalian species, including the human.[76] The balance of these receptors in the uterus is regulated by the ovarian hormones. Estrogens seem to enhance mainly the α-activity and progesterone the β-activity. Whether this is due to a de novo formation or unmasking of receptors is not known.[30,76] According to Greiss, uterine blood vessels possess only α- or vasoconstrictor receptors.[54]

In the human the response of the myometrium to epinephrine and norepinephrine differs somewhat in vitro and in vivo. Both norepinephrine and epinephrine are excitatory on the isolated human myometrium from nonpregnant and pregnant uteri throughout gestation.[44,50,92] There is little difference in the response according to the menstrual cycle or the stage of gestation; both hormones elicit a strong tonic contraction followed by a series of smaller rhythmic contractions. These findings agree well with those obtained with norepinephrine in vivo. With epinephrine, however, the in vivo findings are different. Epinephrine, either as a single injection or as an infusion, stimulates the nonpregnant uterus but inhibits the activity of the pregnant uterus, both spontaneous and oxytocin induced. Norepinephrine, on the other hand, elicits contractions in both nonpregnant and pregnant human uteri in vivo.[12,21,49,51,62,82] It is possible that the opposite effects caused by epinephrine in vivo and in vitro are due to some β-receptor blocking substance released from the excised tissues into the bath fluid, as happens with the pregnant cat uterus in vitro.[53,108]

In pregnant women at term, rhythmic contractions were elicited with norepinephrine at infusion rates varying from 2–10 μg/minute.[4,21,62] The induced activity was often uncoordinated, and hypertonus occurred at higher rates. Adaptation of the uterus developed, and in order to maintain activity the infusion rate had to be increased. At the end of the infusion uterine activity returned to preinfusion levels within a few minutes. During epinephrine infusions (5–20 μg/minute) spontaneous or oxytocin-induced activity of the uterus is significantly reduced, but a recovery of the activity starts after a certain period in spite of continued infusion.[82] A rebound phenomenon is often observed when epinephrine infusions are discontinued, resulting in a uterine hypertonus.

Cardiovascular effects are always observed during infusions of either hormone. The effects of both hormones on the cardiovascular system last for a time after plasma concentrations have attained normal levels, whereas uterine effects coincide with plasma levels,[117] indicating a much greater affinity for catecholamines in the heart and vascular tissues than in the uterus. Cardiovascular and other metabolic effects could be observed at infusion rates where uterine activity was not affected (0.06–0.24 μg/minute).[118] Several authors have studied such metabolic effects as the rise in blood sugar and plasma free fatty acids during labor. There seems to be general agreement that an increase in these factors occurs during delivery, but the rise is observed late in labor; it may possibly be related to an increased output of epinephrine from the adrenal medulla during the second stage of labor.[114]

Artificial cervical dilation causes increased uterine activity in the human,[43] and occasionally in the rabbit.[42,45] Ferguson believed that this was due to a reflex release of oxytocin.[42] Fuchs, Olsen, and Petersen did not observe any significant oxytocin release during cervical dilatation in postpartum or parturient rabbits.[45] Fish, Sala, and Schwarcz did not observe a concomitant milk ejection response in pregnant women during artificial cervical dilatation, and presumed therefore that no ocytocin secretion occurred.[43] Atropine did not block the increment in uterine activity.[100] The authors suggest that the increased activity caused by the dilatation might be due to a neurogenic reflex involving norepinephrine release. It is possible that such a reflex is activated also by cervical dilatation during labor.[23] Increased uterine contractions were observed in rabbits during vaginal distension,[26,42,45,] which Cross demonstrated to be entirely neurogenic.[26]

There is no doubt that catecholamines do influence the activity of the uterine muscle under physiological conditions, and that especially the uterine adrenergic innervation does participate in the regulation of uterine function both by regulation of the vasoconstrictor tone and by direct action on the myometrial cell. How important these substances are for the proper functioning of the uterus during pregnancy and at parturition is difficult to estimate. Adrenalectomy is compatible with normal gestation and parturition, provided that cortisone substitution therapy is instituted, indicating that adrenal medullary hormones are not indispensable. Various clinical observations as well as much experimental evidence suggest that the pregnant uterus can fulfill its functions in women and in animals after the nervous communications to the uterus are cut.[19,85,94,106] However, the postsynaptic neuron is independent in the sense that removal of the presynaptic influence does not interfere with the production of the transmitter. The spontaneous release of noradrenaline, although partly dependent on preganglionic nervous impulses, does continue to a certain extent even after denervation.

A complete "denervation" can probably only be achieved through pharmacological blocking agents. Such adrenergic blocking agents have been widely used in vitro, but in relatively few instances in vivo. Deis and Pickford used both ganglionic and peripheral blocking agents in rats and guinea pigs.[29] There was little influence on the contractions of the estrus and late pregnant uterus, whereas in the diestrus as well as midpregnant uterus the contractions invariably increased in size following sympathetic blockade. In the human, dihydroergotamine has been extensively used for clinical purposes. Usually a decrease in uterine tonus and cervical resistance as well as increased contractions were observed after administration of the drug.[93] It is a powerful α-blocking agent, but unfortunately also has some inherent oxytocic action in the human uterus in vivo.[5] Phentolamine, another α-blocker without oxytocic properties, did not inhibit spontaneous contractions in four patients, although it markedly reduced the increment in uterine activity induced by a simultaneous infusion of norepinephrine.[4] Eskes *et al.* infused a β-blocking agent, propranolol, in one case where high spontaneous activity was present without seeing any change in the uterine activity.[37] Barden and Stander recently infused propranolol into 20 pregnant women during spontaneous or oxytocin-induced labor. There was very little influence on the contractions in 9 and a slight increase in 11 of the subjects.[8]

The main influence of catecholamines on uterine function under normal conditions is probably exerted by their action on the uterine vascular bed and possibly on the cervical tonus,[93] but they can, no doubt, temporarily modify the spontaneous or oxytocin-induced uterine contractions that occur independently of the sympathicoadrenal system.

ACETYLCHOLINE

The present knowledge about acetylcholine's role in the uterine function suggests that this neurohumor exerts only a minor modifying action, if any, on uterine activity.

Although adrenergic fibers are associated with the whole of uterine musculature in man[78] cholinergic fibers are concentrated mainly in the region of the cervix and isthmus, where they are particularly related to the cervical blood vessels, glands, and muscle fibers of the isthmus.[24] Acetylcholine-esterase (AChE) containing fibers are also very scarce in rabbit uterus, but the vagina contains a fairly rich plexus of AChE fibers. Nonspecific cholinesterase activity occurs diffusely throughout the uterus in the smooth muscle cells.[79] The acetylcholine content of the uterus is very low, and the earlier findings of Reynolds that estrogens increase the acetylcholine content of the uterus[84] was not confirmed in a later study by Emmens, McIntosh, and Richter.[35] Estrogens have some influence on the serum cholinesterase levels, but the effect is only produced in chronic experiments, under physiological conditions the estrogen action is manifested only as a sex difference in serum cholinesterase levels. No fluctuations occur during the menstrual cycle.[95]

Acetylcholine does elicit contractions in all uterine preparations including the human in vitro, but the necessary concentrations are relatively high (0.001–0.1 mg/ml). At high infusion rates (12–40 mg/minute) acetylcholine elicited rhythmic contraction of the human pregnant uterus at term.[91] However, atropine at a rate of 0.045 mg/minute, which did prevent the increment in uterine activity caused by simultaneous infusion of acetylcholine, did not alter the spontaneous contractions, nor did it inhibit the increment caused by artificial cervical dilatation.[100] Sauter, using external tocography during labor, observed a slight increase in the frequency of contractions and an increase in the uterine tonus following atropine administration.[93] There is, therefore, very little evidence in support of the hypothesis put forward by Sabanah, Toth, and Maugham[90] that uterine motility is entirely controlled by acetylcholine and the adrenergic transmitters, and that the ovarian steroids exert their action on the uterus by influencing the synthesis, metabolism, and receptor sites of these neurohumors.

TISSUE HORMONES

Histamine

Histamine has been available in synthetic form since 1907. It was soon found that it stimulated the pregnant cat uterus as well as the human uterus both in vivo and in vitro.[27] In other species, such as mice and rats, histamine inhibits uterine contractions under all hormonal conditions.[113] It was thought that in these species histamine participates in the maintenance of the uterine quiescence during pregnancy. In rats, however, a sudden, almost complete loss of sensitivity to histamine occurs around the 13th day of gestation with recovery starting on day 18 and the sensitivity slowly returning to normal by 2 days post partum.[113] In species where histamine has an excitatory effect (e.g., guinea pig, rabbit, and man), the doses required to elicit contractions are relatively high; in man the dose required is from 0.3–2 mg as a single intravenous injection.[75] At such dose levels other organs are strongly affected. The uterine response consists of a tonic contraction followed by temporary inhibition of spontaneous activity. During pregnancy or progesterone treatment there is no marked change in uterine sensitivity to histamine. The histamine content of human uterus is much decreased during pregnancy.[55] It is unlikley, therefore, that histamine is of any importance in regulation of myometrial activity in the human or any other species.

Of interest is the finding that profound changes in histamine metabolism take place during pregnancy. This has been thoroughly investigated by Kahlson and his co-workers, and two reviews by Kahlson give all pertinent references in the field.[60,61] In rodents, a striking increase in histamine excretion occurs during the second half of gestation. In the human, a similar although less pronounced increase was observed in about one-half of the cases investigated during the last trimester.[11] This increased excretion is due to a very high rate of histamine formation in the fetus during the period of rapid growth. The high fetal histamine production is very marked in rodents, but there is evidence that the human fetus also produces histamine at a higher rate than adult tissues.[72b] It has been suggested that histamine synthesis is an important factor in cell division and growth, and hence of great importance to the rapidly growing fetus.[60,61]

In many species, including man, a marked increase in plasma histaminase or, more properly, in plasma diamineoxidase activity occurs during gestation. The placenta also has a strong histaminolytic activity and it is shown that the plasma enzyme is derived from the decidual cells.[28] Direct observations indicate that biologically active histamine crosses the placenta in either direction only to a very limited extent, whereas histamine metabolites cross easily.[72a] It is therefore probable that the increased plasma histamine, as well as the placental histaminase, have the function of protecting the maternal organism from the effects of excess histamine produced by the fetus.

It is presently believed that only nascent histamine, formed by the activity of histidine decarboxylase (HDC-ase) in the tissues, is concerned in physiological phenomena.[61,96] HDC-ase is an inducible enzyme, and agents that induce HDC-ase activity cause changes in tone and permeability of terminal blood vessels. On the basis of the correlation between HDC-ase activity and the observed circulatory changes, Schayer has suggested that histamine is an important factor in regulating local circulatory adaptation.[96,97] This would be of great value in the fetus, especially since the placental and umbilical vessels have no nerve supply.

Serotonin

Serotonin occurs mainly in the enterochromaffin system, which is also the most important site of its formation.[36] From 80–95 per cent of total body serotonin is found in the gastrointestinal tract.[104] Serotonin is also produced in the brain where it occurs localized to certain areas, particularly the pineal gland, brain stem, and diencephalic structures. Only trace amounts of free serotonin are found in the blood;[25,104] the main part is bound to platelets which reversibly take up serotonin released into the venous blood from the gastrointestinal tract. In human blood the serotonin content is about 0.1 μg/ml blood. A considerable amount of serotonin is also stored in the mast cells of the skin in the rat and the mouse, but not in the human. Small amounts are found in many tissues, but in most instances it is probably due to the blood contained in these tissues.

Serotonin seems to be of importance in the central nervous system but its physiological function in the brain is not yet fully understood.[14] Besides its effects on the central nervous system, the most important pharmacological characteristic of serotonin is its action on smooth muscle. With few exceptions, all smooth muscles are stimulated by serotonin. The gastrointestinal musculature and certain vascular areas seem to possess a particularly high sensitivity to serotonin. Most notable among the responsive vascular tissues are the pulmonary arterial tree and the blood vessels of the placenta and umbilical cord.

Serotonin has a contractile effect on uterine muscle of all species studied, although the sensitivity may vary from species to species. The rabbit uterus is relatively insensitive,[44] whereas the sensitivity of rat myometrium is high.[46, 87]

We have studied the responses of isolated human myometrium to serotonin and found that nonpregnant strips showed very little response, if any. The strongest responses were observed in early pregnant uterine strips. The intensity of response diminished towards term, although the threshold concentration, usually 0.01 μg/ml, remained more or less the same.

The effect in vivo has been studied in rabbits,[44] dogs,[2] and rats.[10] The response was slight and followed by a period of inhibition; larger doses resulted in no greater response or in inhibition. In rats, much larger doses are required in vivo than in vitro; according to Bisset, ratio of minimum effective dose in vivo to in vitro is 25 to 1.[10] Tachyphylaxis persists after a large dose of serotonin is applied.[13] The sensitivity of other target tissues in vivo (gut, vessels, skin) is much higher than that of the uterus.[48]

The response of the human uterus in situ has not been studied very thoroughly. Serotonin has been given intravenously at term and rhythmic contractions were produced with infusion rates of 10–40 μg/minute.[109] This corresponds to about twice the total estimated production rate of endogenous serotonin. Thus, the experimental evidence does not support the idea that serotonin is of significance in regulation of the uterine contractility during pregnancy and labor.

No significant changes in the metabolism of serotonin seem to occur during pregnancy and labor in normal or toxemic patients. The content of serotonin in the brain and digestive tract has been found to be independent of considerable changes in the endocrine conditions.[83] Placental and uterine contents of serotonin remain very low throughout pregnancy.[66,67] There is no significant change in the number of circulating platelets at the end of pregnancy, and their serotonin content remains constant throughout pregnancy and puerperium.[59,110] The excretion of its main metabolite, 5-hydroxyindoleacetic acid (5HIAA), also remains fairly constant throughout pregnancy and puerperium, although relatively large fluctuations occur from day to day.[59,111] 5HIAA excretion in toxemic patients did not differ significantly from normal.[66]

The placenta has a considerable serotonin-inactivating capacity, which is due to the enzyme monoamine oxidase (MAO-ase) which also inactivates catecholamines.[71] Serotonin injected into the mother does not pass into the fetal circulation.[68,107] This is probably of physiological significance since the umbilical cord is very sensitive to the vasoconstrictive action of serotonin.[6,98] Its concentration in cord blood is much lower than in adult blood; there is no serotonin in amniotic fluid, but relatively large amounts of MAO-ase. Small quantities of 5HIAA could be demonstrated in amniotic fluid, probably derived from fetal metabolic sources.

When injected in large quantities into pregnant rats and mice serotonin induces fetal death.[73] This lethal action has been investigated by Robson and his co-workers who found that it is due to inhibition of placental function brought about by two probably independent effects, namely, reduction of placental blood flow and reduction in the permeability of placental membranes.[57,86] According to a recent report, a monoamine oxidase inhibitor induces abortion in pregnant women when instilled into the amniotic cavity.[69] Apparently placental MAO-ase functions to protect the fetus from the effects of excess maternal serotonin, as well as catecholamines. In patients with carcinoid tumors, who produce large quantities of serotonin, pregnancy is extremely rare. One such case, however, which ended in spontaneous abortion has been reported. The fetus showed no malformations.[70]

PROSTAGLANDINS

Prostaglandins is the name given by von Euler in 1935 to the water and lipid-soluble, smooth-muscle-relaxing and blood-pressure-lowering factor with acidic properties found in human seminal plasma and sheep vesicular glands. It was later isolated and purified and its chemical nature elucidated by Bergström and Samuelsson in Sweden. Recent reviews on their chemistry, occurrence, and biological action are given by von Euler and Eliasson[38] and by Pickles.[81] It was shown that the active principle consisted of several closely related compounds, all called prostaglandins. Fourteen or more have been identified. They are derivatives of an unsaturated nitrogen-free C_{20} acid containing a cyclopentane ring, and either three hydroxy groups in series F or one or two hydroxy groups and a keto group in series E. PGE_1 and PGF_{1a} have one, PGE_2 and PGF_{2a} have two, and PGE_3 has three double bonds.

The biological actions of the prostaglandins vary considerably. Numerous prostaglandins are found in human semen but PGE_1, PGE_2, PGE_3, PGF_{1a}, and PGF_{2a} are the main components; PGE_1 and PGE_2 dominate and account for at least half of the biological activity. Pickles and coworkers showed that human endometrium and menstrual fluid is another source of prostaglandins.[81] It contains predominantly PGF's and the ratio of PGF to PGE increases during the secretory phase and reaches maximum values during menstruation. PGF_{2a} accounts for most of the spasmogenic action of menstrual fluid. The average amount collected during a menstrual period is 5μg PGF_{2a} and about 0.1 μg PGE_2. Since they are absorbed in the vagina they are probably also taken up by the blood vessels in the uterus, and the recovery in menstrual fluid would only reveal the amount escaping absorption. Amniotic fluid and human decidual tissue also contain prostaglandins.[1,63] Recently Karim has found PGF_{2a} in the blood during labor, but was unable to detect it during pregnancy, not even at term.[64]

The responses of the uterus and oviduct to different pure prostaglandins varies in different species. In the human the effects have been studied mainly in isolated myometrial preparations.[16,17,34,80] In a few instances, their effects have also been studied in vivo in nonpregnant[32] and pregnant women.[18,33] In vitro, inhibition or relaxation was the normal response of nonpregnant human myometrium to the seminal fluid prostaglandin or pure PGE's, whereas the usual response of pregnant human myometrium to PGE is one of increased tonus or contractions. The menstrual stimulant group of prostaglandins or the pure PFG's have either no effect or a stimulatory effect on isolated nonpregnant myometrium and always a stimulatory effect on pregnant human myometrium. Human myometrium is most sensitive to the inhibitory effect of PGE's in strips removed around ovulation time. This is probably not the case with the stimulatory effect of PGF's which seems to be greatest just before menstruation and in pregnancy.

In vivo PGF_{2a} had a very strong and long lasting effect during the late secretory phase after instillation of 0.5 μg into the uterine cavity.[32] By intravenous infusion of PGF_{2a}, Karim *et al.* were able to induce labor in 10 women at or near term.[65] There was no elevation of the tonus of the myometrium and the uterus relaxed between contractions. Maternal blood pressure and fetal heart rate was not affected.

PGE in doses of 0.01–0.04 μg/minute/kg was given as an intravenous infusion to two women in early pregnancy and to one woman at term.[18] This caused increased uterine motility and elevated intra-amniotic pressure which occurred with delayed onset and slow disappearance. The pulse rate increased slightly, but there was no change in blood pressure.

The effect of PGE's on nonpregnant human uterus in vivo after intravaginal application has been more difficult to evaluate. It caused decrease in uterine motility in some women, stimulation in some, and no effect in others.[32] The same applies to the studies on the effect of prostaglandins on the motility of the human oviducts.[38]

Prostaglandins seem to interfere somehow with the action of catecholamines in a variety of preparations including rabbit and guinea pig uterus and rat vas deferens.[22] The physiological significance of these findings is not clear, nor is the role of prostaglandins in the organism as a whole well understood. Several proposals have been made; an attractive one is that the PG's in semen both facilitate ejaculation and, after absorption in the vagina, alter the activity of the smooth muscles of the female genital tract in such a way as to facilitate fertilization. Similarly, PG's produced in the endometrium may facilitate the process of menstruation, and those produced in decidual tissue may facilitate the process of labor.

KININS

The kinin hormones form a group of substances of polypeptide nature which act on smooth muscles and either decrease or increase blood pressure. A survey of their occurrence, metabolism, and pharmacological action is given by Rocha e Silva.[88]

Bradykinin and angiotensin have been purified and synthesized. Their precursors are normally present in plasma bound to an α-globulin fraction and released by enzymatic activity, which also is present in plasma.

They have a powerful effect on the circulatory system; angiotensin has a capacity to raise the blood pressure when injected intravenously, whereas bradykinin has a vasodilator action and produces a fall in blood pressure. Bradykinin also decreases capillary permeability, whereas angiotensin does not have an effect on capillaries.

Besides their effect on the vascular system, they have a stimulating effect on other smooth muscles, including the uterus, and they have therefore aroused a certain interest also among uterine physiologists. The isolated rat uterus and guinea pig uterus are about equally sensitive to oxytocin and bradykinin, and only slightly less sensitive to angiotensin.[10] On the other hand, the action of bradykinin on the uterus in situ in several species is weak and irregular, and much larger doses are required to elicit a response in situ than in vitro. In addition, the response of the uterus is only a single contraction while even small amounts of oxytocin have a long lasting effect. In man, Berde and Saameli could not record any effect on human uterus in vitro or in vivo,[9] and their results were confirmed by Eliasson.[31] Both peptides have a marked effect on the blood pressure at lower levels than necessary to stimulate the uterus.[10]

Bradykinin is released from its binding to α-globulins by a complex enzyme system present in plasma. The activation of this enzyme system occurs by the action of various venoms, dilution, or contact with glass, and locally by trauma or heating. Once bradykinin is released it undergoes immediate destruction by another enzyme also present in plasma. So far its physiological role has been related to the phenomena of pain production, increased capillary permeability, and local vasodilatation in an inflamed area. It seems that the uterotropic effect of bradykinin is mainly of pharmacological interest.

In view of the fact that large amounts of renin, the enzyme responsible for release of angiotensin from plasma, are produced in the placenta and the pregnant uterus, it is likely that angiotensin would have some influence upon the uterus. The ephemeral nature of the effect in situ[10] at least in the rat, while producing strong circulatory effects, does not point to an important role for angiotensin in regulating uterine motility.

REFERENCES

1. Abrahams, O. L., and Hawkins, D. F. Lipid-soluble uterine muscle stimulants in human amniotic fluid. *J. Obstet. Gynaec. Brit. Comm. 74:*235, 1967.
2. Abrahams, V. C., and Pickford, M. The effect of 5-hydroxy-tryptamine on the uterus of conscious and anaesthetized dogs. *Brit. J. Pharmacol. 11:*50, 1956.
3. Ahlquist, R. P. A study of the adrenotropic receptors. *Amer. J. Physiol. 153:*586, 1948.
4. Althabe, O., Schwarcz, R. L., Jr., Sala, N. L., and Fish, L. Effect of phentolamine methane sulfonate upon uterine contractility induced by l-norepinephrine in pregnancy. *Amer. J. Obstet. Gynec. 101:*1083, 1968.
5. Altman, S. G., Waltman, R., Lubin, S., and Reynolds, S. R. M. Oxytocic and toxic actions of dihydroergotamine-45. *Amer. J. Obstet. Gynec. 64:*101, 1952.
6. Åström, A., and Samelius, U. The Actions of 5-hydroxytryptamine on the umbilical vessels of the human placenta. *Brit. J. Pharmacol. 12:*410, 1957.
7. Axelrod, J. The metabolism, storage and release of catecholamines. *Rec. Prog. Hormone Res. 21:*597, 1965.
8. Barden, T. P. and Stander, R. W. Myometrial and cardiovascular effects

of an adrenergic blocking drug in human pregnancy. *Amer. J. Obstet. Gynec. 101:*91, 1968.

9. BERDE, B., and SAAMELI, K. Effect of bradykinin on uterine activity. *Nature* (London) *191:*83, 1961.
10. BISSET, G. W., HALDAR, J., and LEWIS, J. E. Actions of oxytocin and other biologically active peptides on the rat uterus. *Mem. Soc. Endocr. 14:*185, 1966.
11. BJURÖ, T., LINDBERG, S., and WESTLING, H. Observations on histamine in pregnancy and the puerperium. *Acta Obstet. Gynec. Scand. 40:*152, 1961.
12. BOURNE, A., and BURN, J. H. The dosage and action of pituitary extract and of the three ergot alkaloids on the uterus in labour with note on action of adrenaline. *J. Obstet. Gynaec. Brit. Emp. 34:*249, 1927.
13. BROCKLEHURST, W. "The Action of 5-Hydroxytryptamine on Smooth Muscle." In *5-Hydroxytryptamine.* G. Lewis (Ed.), Pergamon Press, London, 1958, p. 172.
14. BRODIE, B. B., and COSTA, E. *Monoamines et Systemes Nerveux Central.* Georg & Cie. Geneva, 1962, p. 13.
15. BRUNDIN, J., and ENGSTRÖM, L. Urinary excretion of free catecholamines during spontaneous and oxytocin induced labor. *Obstet. Gynec. 17:*99, 1961.
16. BYGDEMAN, M. The effect of different prostaglandins on human myometrium *in vitro. Acta Physiol. Scand. 63: Suppl.* 242, 1964.
17. BYGDEMAN, M., and ELIASSON, R. The effect of prostaglandin from human seminal fluid on the motility of non-pregnant human myometrium *in vitro. Acta Physiol. Scand. 59:*43, 1963.
18. BYGDEMAN, M., KWON, S., and WIQVIST, N. "The Effect of Prostaglandin E_1 on Human Pregnant Myometrium *in vivo.*" In *Nobel Symposium 2, Prostaglandins,* S. Bergström and B. Samuelsson (Eds.), Almquist and Wiksell, Stockholm, 1967.
19. CARLSON, R. R., and DEFEO, V. J. Role of the pelvic nerve vs. the abdominal sympathetic nerves in the reproductive function of the female rat. *Endocrinology 77:*1014, 1965.
20. CARLSSON, A., FALCK, B., and HILLARP, N.-Å. Cellular localization of brain monoamines. *Acta Physiol. Scand. 56:* Suppl. 196, 1, 1962.
21. CIBILS, L. A., POSE, S. V., and ZUSPAN, F. P. Effect of l-norepinephrine infusion on uterine contractility and cardiovascular system. *Amer. J. Obstet. Gynec. 84:*307, 1962.
22. CLEGG, P. C. The effect of prostaglandins on the response of isolated smooth muscle preparations to sympatomimetic substances. *Mem. Soc. Endocr. 14:*119, 1966.
23. COBO, E. Uterine and milk-ejecting activities during human labor. *J. Appl. Physiol. 24:*317, 1968.
24. COUPLAND, R. E. J. The distribution of cholinesterase positive nerve fibres in the human uterus. *J. Anat. 94:*287.
25. CRAWFORD, N. Plasma free serotonin (5-hydroxytryptamine). *Clin. Chem. Acta 8:*39, 1963.
26. CROSS, B. A. The motility and reactivity of the oestrogenized rabbit uterus

in vivo with comparative observations on milk ejection. *J. Endocr. 16:*237, 1958.

27. Dale, H. H., and Laidlaw, P. P. The physiological action of β-iminazolylethylamine. *J. Physiol.* (London) *41:*1910.
28. Danforth, D. N., and Gorham, F. Placental histaminase. *Amer. J. Physiol. 119:*294, 1937.
29. Deis, R. P., and Pickford, M. The effect of autonomic blocking agents on uterine contractions of the rat and the guinea pig. *J. Physiol.* (London) *173:*215, 1964.
30. Diamond, J., and Brody, T. M. Hormonal alterations in the response of the rat uterus to catecholamines. *Life Sci. 5:*2187, 1966.
31. Eliasson, R. Effect of bradykinin on the human uterus in vitro. *J. Pharmacol. 18:*396, 1966.
32. Eliasson, R., and Posse, N. The effect of prostaglandin on the non-pregnant human uterus *in vivo. Acta. Obstet. Gynec. Scandinav. 39:*12, 1960.
33. Embrey, M. P. The effect of prostaglandins on the human pregnant uterus. *J. Obstet. Gynaec. Brit. Comm. 76:*783, 1969.
34. Embrey, M. P., and Morrison, D. L. The effect of prostaglandins on human pregnant myometrium *in vitro. J. Obstet. Gynaec. Brit. Comm. 75:*829, 1968.
35. Emmens, C. W., McIntosh, F. C., and Richter, D. Oestrogens and acetylcholine. *J. Physiol.* (London) *101:*460, 1943.
36. Erspamer, V., and Asero, B. Identification of Enteramine, the specific hormone of the entero chromaffin cell system as 5-hydroxytryptamine. *Nature* (London) *169:*800, 1952.
37. Eskes, T., Stolte, L., Seelen, J., Moed, H. D., and Vogelsang, C. Epinephrine derivatives and the activity of the human uterus. II. The influence of pronethalol and propranol on the uterine and systemic activity of p-hydroxyphenyl-isopropyl arterenol. *Amer. J. Obstet. Gynec. 92:*871, 1965.
38. von Euler, U. S., and Eliasson, R. *Prostaglandins,* Academic Press, New York, 1967, p. 164.
39. Falck, B. Observations on the possibilities of the cellular localization of monoamines by a fluorescence method. *Acta Physiol. Scand. 56: Suppl. 197:*1, 1962.
40. Falck, B. *cit.* Brundin, J., and Wirsén, C. Adrenergic nerve terminals in the human Fallopian tube examined by fluorescence microscopy. *Acta Physiol. Scand. 61:*585, 1964.
41. Falck, B., and Owman, C. "Histochemistry of Monoaminergic Mechanisms in Peripheral Neurons." In *Mechanisms of Release of Biogenic Amines.* U. S. von Euler, S. Rosell, and B. Uvnäs (Eds.), Pergamon Press, Oxford, 1966, p. 59.
42. Ferguson, J. K. W. A study of the intact uterus at term. *Surg. Gynec. Obstet. 73:*359, 1941.
43. Fish, L., Sala, N. L., and Schwarcz, Jr., R. Effect of cervical dilatation upon uterine contractility in pregnant women and its relation to oxytocin secretion. *Amer. J. Obstet. Gynec. 90:*108, 1964.
44. Fuchs, A.-R. Unpublished observations (1968).

45. Fuchs, A. R., Olsen, P., and Petersen, K. Effect of distension of uterus and vagina on uterine motility and oxytocin release in puerperal rabbits. *Acta Endocr.* (Kobenhavn) *50:*239, 1965.

46. Gaddum, J. H., and Hameed, K. A. Drugs which antagonize 5-hydroxytryptamine. *Brit. J. Pharmacol. 9:*240, 1954.

47. Gaffney, T. E., Burket, R. L., and Woronkow, S. Catecholamine content of the pregnant and non-pregnant human uterus. *Obstet. Gynec. 25:*340, 1965.

48. Garattini, S., and Valzielli, L. *Serotonin,* Elsevier, Amsterdam, 1965.

49. Garrett, W. J. The effects of adrenaline and noradrenaline on the intact human uterus in late pregnancy and labour. *J. Obstet. Gynaec. Brit. Emp. 61:*586, 1954.

50. Garrett, W. J. The effects of adrenaline, noradrenaline, and dihydroergotamine on excised human myometrium. *Brit. J. Pharmacol. 10:*39, 1955.

51. Garrett, W. J. The effects of adrenaline and noradrenaline on the intact nonpregnant human uterus. *J. Obstet. Gynaec. Brit. Emp. 62:*876, 1955.

52. Gillespie, J. Review Lecture: Tissue binding of noradrenaline. *Proc. Roy. Soc. Biol. 166:*1, 1966.

53. Graham, J. D. P., and Gurd, M. K. Effects of adrenaline on the isolated uterus of the cat. *J. Physiol.* (London) *152:*243, 1960.

54. Greiss, F. The uterine vascular bed: Effect of adrenergic stimulation. *Obstet. Gynec. 21:*295, 1963.

55. Gunther, M., and Paton, W. D. M. The histamine content of human uterus. *J. Physiol.* (London) *154:*417, 1960.

56. Hochuli, E., Käser, O., and Burger, M. Adrenalin- und Noradrenalinbestimmungen im Blutplasma unter der Geburt. *Experientia 12:*356, 1956.

57. Honey, D. P., Robson, J. M., and Sullivan, F. M. Mechanism of inhibitory action of 5-hydroxytryptamine on placental function. *Amer. J. Obstet. Gynec. 99:*250, 1967.

58. Israel, S. L., Seligson, H. T., Stroup, P. E., and Seligson, D. I. Epinephrine and norepinephrine in pregnancy and labor. *Obstet. Gynec. 14:*68, 1959.

59. Israel, S. L., Seligson, H. T., Stroup, P. E., and Seligson, D. I. Serotonin in pregnant and parturient women. *Obstet. Gynec. 13:*672, 1959.

60. Kahlson, G. New approaches to the physiology of histamine. *Perspect. Biol. Med. 5:*179, 1962.

61. Kahlson, G. New approaches to the physiology of histamine. *Physiol. Rev. 48:*155, 1968.

62. Kaiser, I. H. The effect of epinephrine and norepinephrine on the contractions of human uterus in labor. *Surg. Gynec. Obstet. 90:*649, 1950.

63. Karim, S. M. M., and Devlin, J. Prostaglandin content of amniotic fluid during pregnancy and labor. *J. Obstet. Gynaec. Brit. Comm. 74:*230, 1967.

64. Karim, S. M. M. Appearance of prostaglandin F_{2a} in human blood during labour. *Brit. Med. J. 4:*618, 1968.

65. Karim, S. M. M., Trussell, R. R., Patel, R. C., and Hillier, K. Response of pregnant human uterus to prostaglandin-F_{2a}-induction of labour. *Brit. Med. J. 4:*621, 1968.

66. Klinge, E., Penttilä, O., and Tissari, A. The content of 5-hydroxytryptamine in human uterine and placental tissue, and their 5-hydroxytryptophan decaboxylase and monoamine oxidase activity in normal and toxaemic pregnancies. *Acta Obstet. Gynec. Scand. 43:*107, 1964.

67. Koren, Z., Pfeiffer, Y., and Sulman, F. G. Serotonin content of human placenta and fetus during pregnancy. *Amer. J. Obstet. Gynec. 93:*411, 1965.

68. Koren, Z., Pfeiffer, Y., and Sulman, F. G. Distribution and placental transfer of C^{14}-5-hydroxytryptamine in pregnant rats. *Amer. J. Obstet. Gynec. 95:*290, 1966.

69. Koren, Z., Pfeiffer, Y., and Sulman, F. G. Induction of legal abortion by intrauterine instillation of pargylene hydrochloride. *J. Reprod. Fertil. 12:*75, 1966.

70. Leeper, S. W., Brown, H., and Rosenberg, H. J. Spontaneous abortion in the carcinoid syndrome. *Amer. J. Obstet. Gynec. 94:*340, 1966.

71. Levy, B., and Ahlquist, R. P. "Adrenergic Drugs." In *Drill's Pharmacology in Medicine,* Ed. 3, J. R. DiPalma (Ed.), McGraw-Hill, New York, 1965, p. 474.

72a. Lindberg, S., Lindell, S.-E., and Westling, H. Metabolism of C^{14}—labelled histamine injected into the umbilical artery. *Acta. Obstet. Gynec. Scand. 42: Suppl. 1:*35, 1963.

72b. Lindberg, S., Lindell, S.-E., and Westling, H. Formation and inactivation of histamine by human foetal tissue *in vitro. Acta Obstet. Gynec. Scand. 42: Suppl. 1* :49, 1963.

73. Lindsay, D., Poulson, E., and Robson, J. M. The effect of 5-hydrotryptamine on pregnancy. *J. Endocr. 26:*85, 1963.

74. Luschinsky, H. L., and Singher, H. O. Identification and assay of monoamine oxidase in the human placenta. *Arch. Biochem. 19:*95, 1948.

75. McElwin, T. W., and Horton, B. T. Response of human uterus to histamine. *Amer. J. Med. Sci. 218:*932, 1949.

76. Miller, J. W. Adrenergic receptors in the myometrium. *Ann. N.Y. Acad. Sci. 139:*788, 1967.

77. Miller, M. D., and Marshall, J. M. Uterine response to nerve simulation, relation to hormonal status and catecholamines. *Amer. J. Physiol. 209:*859, 1965.

78. Owman, C., Rosengren, E., and Sjöberg, N.-O. Adrenergic nerves in the female genital tract of man. *Amer. J. Obstet. Gynec.* To be published. Cit. by Owman, C., and Sjöberg, N.-O., 1966.

79. Owman, C., and Sjöberg, N.-O. Adrenergic nerves in the female genital tract of the rabbit with remarks on cholinesterase containing structures. *Z. Zellforsch. 74:*182, 1966.

80. Pickles, V. R. Myometrial responses to the menstrual plain muscle stimulant. *J. Endoc. 19:*150, 1959.

81. Pickles, V. R. The prostaglandins. *Biol. Rev. 42:*614, 1967.

82. Pose, S. V., Cibils, L. A., and Zuspan, F. P. Effect of l-epinephrine infusion on uterine contractility and cardiovascular system. *Amer. J. Obstet. Gynec. 84:*297, 1962.

83. Resnik, R. H., Smith, G. T., and Gray, S. J. Endocrine influences on tissue serotonin content of the rat. *Amer. J. Physiol. 201:*571, 1961.
84. Reynolds, S. R. M. Acetylcholine-like content of uteri before and after administration of oestrin to ovariectomized rabbits. *J. Physiol.* (London) *95:*258, 1939.
85. Reynolds, S. R. M. *Physiology of the Uterus,* Ed. 2, Hoeber, New York, 1949.
86. Robson, J. M., and Sullivan, F. M. Mechanism of the lethal action of 5-hydroxytryptamine on the foetus. *J. Endocr. 25:*553, 1963.
87. Robson, J. M., Trounce, J. R., and Didcock, K. A. H. Factors affecting the response of the uterus to serotonin. *J. Endocr. 10:*129, 1954.
88. Rocha e Silva, M. "Kinins: Bradykinin, Angiotensin, Substance P." In *Comparative Endocrinology,* Vol. 2, U. S. von Euler and H. Heller (Eds.), Academic Press, New York, 1963, p. 64.
89. Rosengren, E., and Sjöberg, N.-O. Changes in the amount of adrenergic transmitter in the female genital tract of rabbit during pregnancy. *Acta Physiol. Scand. 72:*412, 1968.
90. Sabanah, E. H., Toth, A., and Maughan, G. B. The role of the automatic nervous system in uterine contractility and blood flow. I. The interaction between neurohormones and sex steroids in the intact and isolated uterus. II. The role of the parasympathetic neurohormone acetylcholine in uterine motility and blood flow. *Amer. J. Obstet. Gynec. 89:*841 & 860, 1964.
91. Sala, N. L., and Fish, L. Effect of acetylcholine and atropine upon uterine contractility in pregnant women. *Amer. J. Obstet. Gynec. 91:*1069, 1965.
92. Sandberg, F., Ingelman-Sundberg, A., Lindgren, L., and Rydén, G. *In vitro* studies of the motility of the human uterus. Part III. The effects of adrenaline, noradrenaline, and acetylcholine on the spontaneous motility in different parts of the pregnant and non-pregnant uterus. *J. Obstet. Gynaec. Brit. Emp. 65:*965, 1958.
93. Sauter, H. Beitrag zum Problem der Innervation des Uterus. *Schweiz. Med. Wschr. 10:*221, 1949.
94. Sauter, H. *Die motorische Innervation des menschlichen Uterus.* Karger, Basel, 1954.
95. Sawyer, C. H., and Everett, J. H. The relationship between sex hormones and serum cholinesterase in the rat. *Anat. Rec. 94:*494, 1946.
96. Schayer, R. W. Catabolism of physiological quantities of histamine *in vivo. Physiol. Rev. 39:*116, 1959.
97. Schayer, R. W. "Enzymatic Formation of Histamine from Histidine." In *Handbook of Experimental Pharmacology,* Vol. 18, O. Eicher and A. Farah (Eds.), Springer, Berlin, 1966, p. 688.
98. Schmiermund, H.-J., Rodegra, H., and Soehring, K. Über die Beteiligung von 5-Hydroxytryptamine (Serotonin) beim physiologischem Verschluss der Nabelschnurgefässe post partum. *Arch. Gynaek. 191:*457, 1959.
99. Schofield, B. M. The innervation of cervix and cornu in the rabbit. *J. Physiol.* (London) *117:*317, 1952.

100. Schwarcz, R. W., Jr., Sala, N. L., Althabe, O., and Fish, L. Effect of atropine upon uterine contractility induced by artificial cervical dilation. *Amer. J. Obstet. Gynec. 98:*577, 1959.
101. Setekleiv, J. Uterine motility of the estrogenized rabbit. III. Response to hypogastric and splanchnic nerve stimulation. *Acta Physiol. Scand. 62:*137, 1964.
102. Sjöberg, N.-O. 1966, cit. by Owman and Sjöberg, 1966.
103. Sjöberg, N.-O. Increase in transmitter content of adrenergic nerves in the reproductive tract of female rabbits after estrogen treatment. *Acta Endocr.* (Kobenhavn) *57:*405, 1968.
104. Sjoerdsma, A. Serotonin. *New Eng. J. Med. 261:*131, 1959.
105. Spratto, G., and Miller, J. W. An investigation of the mechanism by which estradiol-17β elevates the epinephrine content of the rat uterus. *J. Pharm. Exp. Ther. 161:*7, 1968.
106. Theobald, G. W. "The Part Played by Nerve Impulses in the Regulation of Uterine Activity in Man." In *Muscle,* W. M. Paul, E. E. Daniel, C. M. Kay, and G. Monkton (Eds.), Pergamon Press, Oxford, 1965, p. 363.
107. Thomsen, K., Schniewind, H., Schultze-Mosgau, H., Kramer, M., and Born, H. Wirkung und Durchtritt vasoaktiver Pharmaka bei künstlich perfundierten Meerschweinchen Placenta. *Arch. Gynaek, 204:*51, 1967.
108. Tsai, T. H., and Fleming, W. W. The adrenotropic receptors of the cat uterus. *J. Pharmacol. 143:*268, 1964.
109. Urban, J. Action of serotonin in uterine inertia. *Ginek. Pol. 36:*1219, 1965.
110. Van den Driesche, R. Biological determination of 5-hydroxytryptamine in blood during pregnancy. *Obstet. Gynec. 55:*34, 1956.
111. Van den Driesche, R., and Delhave, C. A propos de l'élimination urinaire de l'acide 5-hydroxyindole-acetic dans le post-partum immediat. *C. R. Soc. Biol. 156:*416, 1963.
112. Vogt, M. Transmitter released in the cat uterus by stimulation of the hypogastric nerve. *J. Physiol.* (London) *179:*163, 1965.
113. West, G. B. Histamine and the myometrium. *Mem. Soc. Endocr. 14:*199, 1966.
114. Whaley, W. H., Zuspan, F. P., Nelson, G. H., and Ahlquist, R. P. Alterations of plasma free fatty acids and glucose during labor. *Amer. J. Obstet. Gynec. 97:*875, 1967.
115. Wurtman, R. J. *Catecholamines,* Little, Brown, Boston, 1966.
116. Wurtman, R. J., Axelrod, J., and Potter, L. T. The disposition of catecholamines in the rat uterus and the effect of drugs and hormones. *J. Pharm. Exp. Ther. 144:*151, 1965.
117. Zuspan, F. L., Cibils, L. A., and Pose, S. V. Myometrial and cardiovascular responses to alterations in plasma epinephrine. *Amer. J. Obstet. Gynec. 84:*841, 1962.
118. Zuspan, F. L., Nelson, G. H., and Ahlquist, R. P. Epinephrine infusions in normal and toxemic pregnancy. *Amer. J. Obstet. Gynec. 90:*88, 1964.

Chapter Thirteen

Endocrinology of Labor

Fritz Fuchs

It is a unique muscle that grows for a period of nine months, during which time it remains almost completely relaxed, then performs a considerable amount of contractile work during a period of hours, and afterwards shrinks to a fraction of its maximum size and, in preparation for the next reproductive cycle, assumes an essentially resting state, although with considerable contractile activity. It has been proved experimentally, and it is clinically obvious, that the myometrium is capable of contracting at any time during the nine months of gestation just as any other muscle. To prevent contractions—the sustained rhythmic contraction pattern of labor, not the sporadic contractions known as Braxton-Hicks contractions—the existence of a special defense mechanism must be assumed.

Two different types of defense mechanism can be visualized. One involves a change of the physicochemical and biochemical properties of the myometrium by (1) blocking the conduction of impulses from one muscle cell to the other, (2) inhibiting the interaction of the contractile proteins actin and myosin, or (3) inhibiting the enzyme systems involved in the contraction-relaxation process itself or in the metabolic transformations providing energy for the contractile process. The second type of defense mechanism involves the prevention of all stimuli from reaching the target organ, the uterus, by (1) blocking nerve conduction in the central nervous system or in the afferent or efferent pathways of nervous reflexes, (2) preventing the release of humoral factors capable of stimulating the myometrial cells, or (3) inactivating such factors before they reach the target organ. In the first type of defense mechanism, labor may occur when the defense mechanism is withdrawn, thereby permitting contractions to develop. The contractions are due either to the inherent capacity for spontaneous activity of the uterine smooth muscle or to activation by neural or humoral factors which have been present all the time but without a reactive target organ. In the second type of mechanism weakening or withdrawal of the defense mechanism would result in the development or release of activating factors to which the myometrium has been responsive throughout pregnancy.

Since hormones are known to regulate the function of muscle and nerve cells and to be able to influence the function of other endocrine organs, it is reasonable to assume that hormones play an essential role in a defense mechanism and in its withdrawal.[5] In the following discussion the possible endocrine factors will be considered in detail, but it should be borne in mind that other factors may play a role as well.[73]

PROPERTIES OF THE MYOMETRIUM

The human myometrium is composed of long smooth muscle cells in a network of intricately interwoven bundles.[53] The pattern is designed to provide the optimum mechanical conditions for the expulsion of the fetus and the placenta. This pattern need not concern us here, although it should be mentioned that Pinto and co-workers have found certain differences between the various layers with regard to spontaneous activity and reactivity to oxytocic agents.[93] The cell membranes have permeability properties which permit the cells to maintain an internal ionic composition different from that of the extracellular fluid, especially with regard to sodium and potassium, and this establishes a difference in electric potential between the inside and the outside of the membrane. Passive diffusion tends to reduce the potential, but the membrane, under the influence of steroids, is able to counteract the equilibrating tendency by pumping out the sodium ions and allowing potassium ions to enter instead. An activating stimulus produces a rapid change of the membrane potential, and this activates the contractile units, the myofibrils. The same proteins are found in the myofibrils from uterine muscle as in those from skeletal muscle, namely actin, myosin, and tropomysin, but the concentration is much lower and the arrangement is different from that of the striated muscle. In addition, other proteins may be present in uterine muscle.[14]

The myometrium, like other smooth muscles, shows spontaneous activity even in completely denervated preparations or in the presence of nerve-blocking compounds. This inherent property of the myometrial cells is important for the understanding of uterine physiology.[14] The activity of the myometrium originates from a group of cells which acts as a pacemaker, but the cells are not anatomically different from the surrounding cells, as in the cardiac pacemaker. They differ only with regard to excitability, and the areas of highest excitability may change constantly. In normal labor there is evidence to suggest that the pacemaker areas are located in the vicinity of the uterine cornua.

In the myometrium of castrated rabbits and rats, the membrane potential is low and propagated action potentials are absent.[84,85] Estrogen treatment increases the membrane potential to a level where action potentials arise, and the propagation of membrane deplorization is facilitated, resulting in a lower threshold for pharmacological and electrical stimuli. According to Csapo and co-workers, the progesterone-dominated rabbit myometrium has a higher threshold to stimuli and the propagation of depolarization is impaired.[24,25,27,54,85] However, Kao has seriously questioned the interpretations and some of the findings,[66] which do not agree with those of his own or of Saldivar and Melton.[98] To respond to progesterone the myometrium must be estrogen-primed, and the so-called progesterone-dominated myometrium is thus under the influence of both estrogens and progestagens.

It is believed that oxytocic hormones or compounds activate the myometrium by a momentary change in the permeability to sodium, potassium, and calcium, and this gives rise to or increases the number of action potentials. As a result of the increased number of action potentials a contractile response is elicited.[62,66,84] The role of the magnesium ion must also be considered. The effect on the cell membrane is probably brought about through an interaction of the oxytocic compound with membrane-bound calcium. A decrease in the concentration of Ca^{++} in the extracellular fluid will cause depolarization with a decrease of the height and frequency of the action potential and a reduction of the force of contraction. The interaction between ions, steroids, and oxytocic hormones in the human myometrium is not yet known in all details; to a large extent we have to extrapolate from the body of information available from animal experiments. For more detailed reviews see Carsten[14] and Kao.[66]

ENDOCRINE STATUS AT THE ONSET OF LABOR

Placental Hormones

As described in detail in Chapter Three, the excretion of *estrogens* increases markedly with advancing gestation, estriol being the major of the three main estrogens. If serial determinations on individual patients are examined, there is a steady increase and, except in cases of fetal distress or death, no change in the curve to signal the onset of labor, let alone be the cause of it. According to Klopper and Billewicz, those women with the highest excretion values tend to go into labor first, and the average for those as yet undelivered may therefore decrease.[70]

Determination of the blood concentrations and possibly the amniotic fluid concentrations of the three main estrogens would be of more immediate significance in relation to myometrial function than studies of the urinary excretion. However, they are much more difficult, and the number of studies at the end of pregnancy is limited. None of these studies indicate any acute changes in the blood concentrations before the onset of labor.[2,96] After delivery there is, as would be expected, an abrupt fall in the estrogen levels in the blood.

In recent years there has been an interest in abortion or labor induced by intra-amniotic injection of hypertonic solutions. This procedure is followed by a rapid decrease in the urinary excretion of estrogens, as illustrated in Figure 13-1.[111] This drop, which undoubtedly is due to fetal

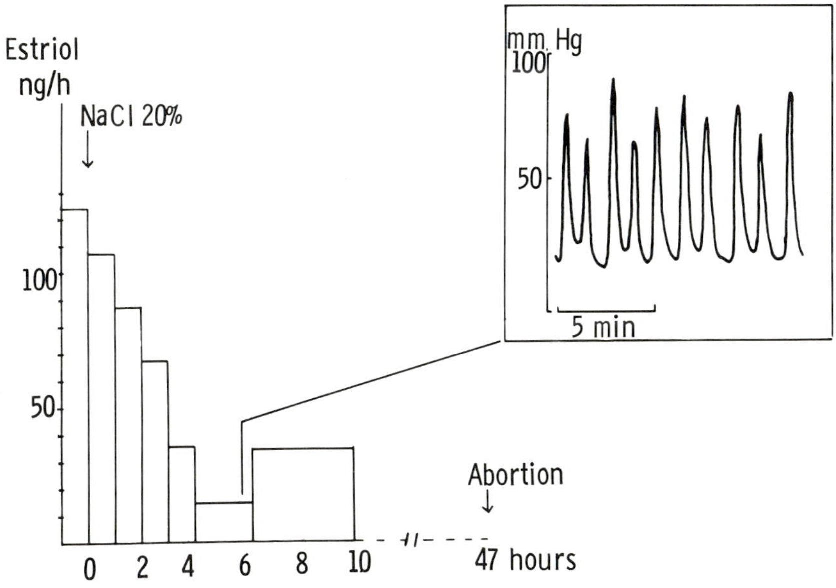

Fig. 13-1. Excretion of estriol during the first 10 hours following intra-amniotic injection of a 20% solution of sodium chloride at 17 weeks of pregnancy. Insert shows an intrauterine pressure recording 5–6 hours after injection. Uterine activity is more than 400 Montevideo Units. (From Wagner, Frandsen, and Stakemann. *Acta Obstet. Gynec. Scand. 42* suppl. *6*:105, 1963.)

death, does not prevent the development of strong uterine contractions. On the other hand, pregnancies with anencephalic fetuses, in which the estriol excretion is very low,[37] usually go past term if not interfered with. Whether this is due to a relative lack of estrogens or to the absence of the fetal pituitary gland is not known.

The three biologically active *progestagens* in the human, progesterone and 20α- and 20β-dihydroprogesterone, are not excreted in the urine in any appreciable amounts. If the excretion of pregnanediol, the most important of the metabolites excreted in the urine, is followed serially, it is found to increase steadily with advancing gestation, gradually leveling off in the last three to four weeks, but with no acute changes before the onset of labor.[72,103]

The progesterone concentration in the maternal blood also increases with advancing gestation, although the rise is not as steep as the rise in estrogen concentrations (Fig. 13-2).[54,104,114,115] There is no evidence for a decrease in the blood level of progesterone before or at the onset of labor, but there is often a moderate fall during the course of labor (Fig. 13-3).[2,76,82,114,115] If pregnancy is interrupted by means of an intra-amniotic injection of hypertonic saline, the pregnanediol excretion decreases about 20 per cent; this decrease is much less than for estrogen,[52,69] which falls by about 80 per cent. Strong uterine contractions develop long before there is any appreciable fall in the peripheral and uterine venous blood levels of progesterone.[49,69,91,104]

It has been suggested that the changes in the *estrogen/progestagen ratio* toward term could be the factor that determines the onset of labor.[5,64] It is certainly true that the ratio changes, since the increase in estrogen production is much greater than that of the progestagen production during gestation. If we look at estriol and pregnanediol in the urine, realizing that these compounds only partially reflect the secretion rates or the blood concentrations, the ratio is roughly 1:100 in the beginning of pregnancy, rising to almost unity at term.[70] There is no acute change just before the onset of labor, and the ratio can show considerable variations from one woman to the other.[70] When hypertonic saline is injected intra-amniotically, the ratio falls before the uterine contractions begin. This fall in the ratio is due to the more rapid decline in the estrogen excretion than in the pregnanediol excretion.[69,111] A rise would fit better with the theory that estrogens stimulate and progestagens inhibit uterine activity. However, there is no question that saline-induced abortion is different from spontaneous labor in many respects.

The pattern of excretion of *chorionic gonadotrophin* (HCG) in the urine is quite different from the excretion patterns of the placental steroids. There is a moderate increase in the excretion during the last

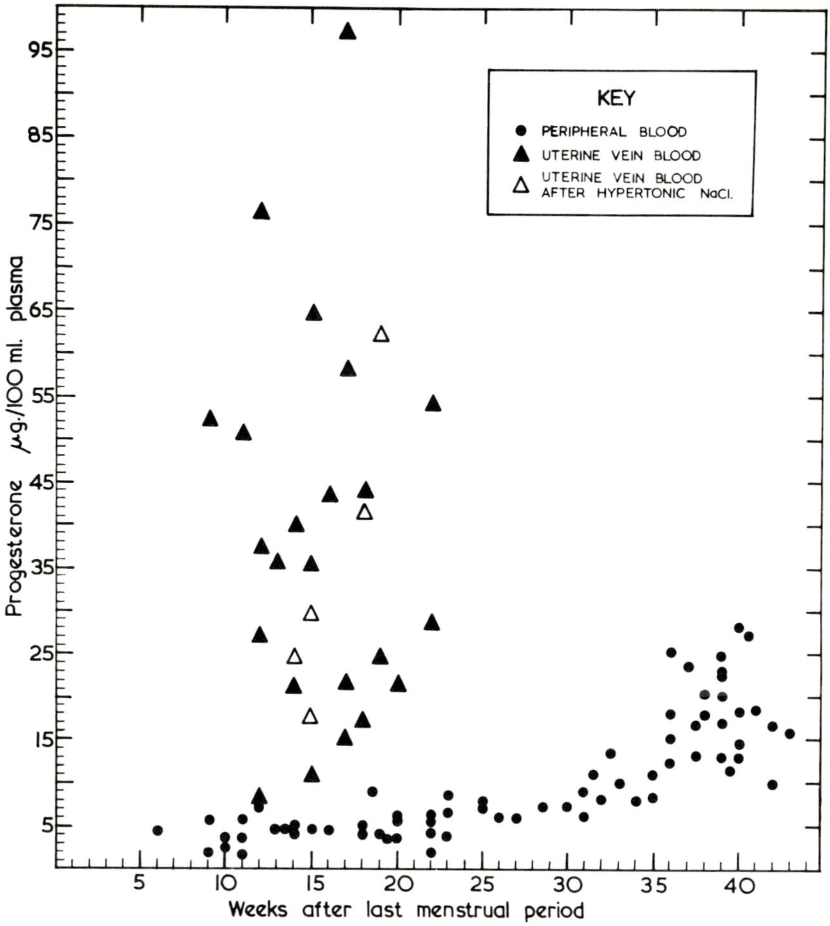

Fig. 13-2. Progesterone concentrations in peripheral venous blood in intact pregnancies and in uterine venous blood before and after intra-amniotic injection of hypertonic saline. (From Short, Wagner, Fuchs, and Fuchs. *Amer. J. Obstet. Gynec. 91*:132, 1965.)

weeks but there are no acute changes to signal the end of pregnancy. Møller and Hamburger in Copenhagen made serial determination of the HCG excretion toward term with the hemagglutination inhibition technique, but found no significant changes at the onset of labor (personal communication). Wide, who developed this technique, studied the excretion in threatened abortions during the second trimester;[113] in those cases where abortion eventually occurred, there was no decrease in the HCG excretion. The blood concentrations of HCG do not appear to have

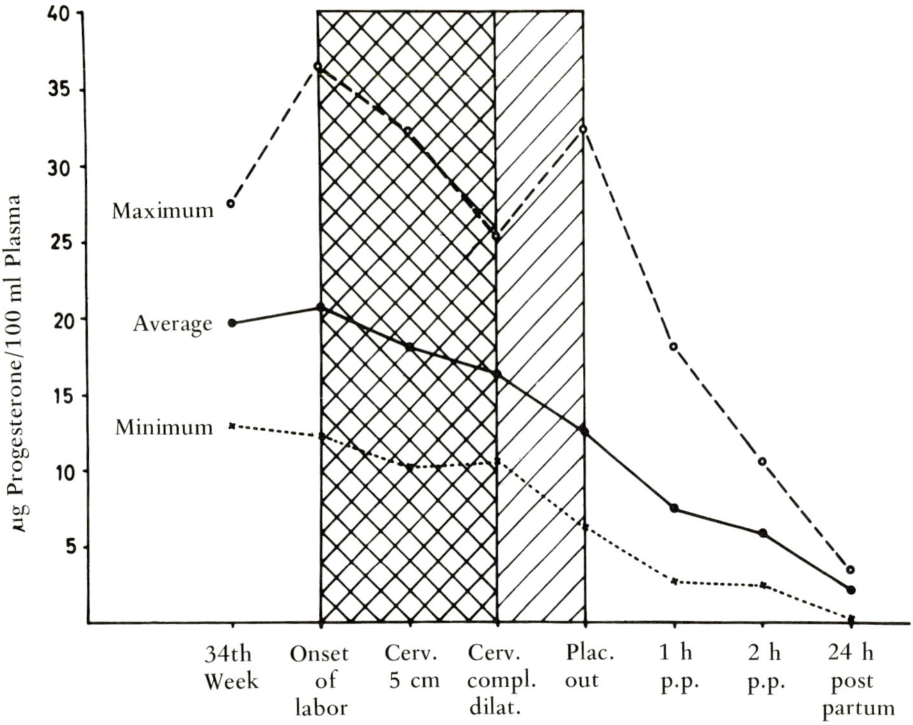

Fig. 13-3. Progesterone concentrations in the peripheral venous blood before, during, and after normal spontaneous labor. Average values and the highest and lowest values found in 13 women. (From Llauro, Runnebaum, and Zander. *Amer. J. Obstet. Gynec. 101*:867, 1968.)

been studied daily at the end of pregnancy, but serial determinations at greater intervals do not indicate any major changes at term.

The concentrations of *placental lactogen* (HPL) in the urine and blood increase with advancing gestation, as described by Josimovich in Chapter Eight. There is no report of any acute changes of the levels at the onset of labor.

Cytohormonal studies of smears from the vagina and the urinary tract have been widely used to evaluate the endocrine balance during pregnancy.[95] Many workers have reported characteristic changes in the vaginal smear during the last few days before the onset of spontaneous labor and maintain that delivery is imminent when such changes can be observed.[65,78,79,116] Other cytologists have looked for such changes but claim that they are seen infrequently and are of limited value to predict the onset of labor.[1,3] Since the staining properties of the exfoliated cells presumably reflect the endocrine balance, especially with regard to the ovarian and placental steriods, this question is of considerable importance. If cytohormonal changes do occur regularly in the last few days before the onset of labor, it must be assumed that they are caused by endocrine changes. Are these changes too subtle to be picked up by our present methods of hormone assays on blood and urine or are they overlooked because of our tendency to consider one hormone at a time instead of trying to get an over-all view of the hormonal balance? Perhaps a computer analysis of the results of serial studies of all the hormones that conceivably could be concerned would provide the answer.

Oxytocic Hormones

The hormones which are able to elicit uterine contractions include oxytocin and vasopressin (ADH), epinephrine and norepinephrine, acetylcholine, serotonin, and histamine. These oxytocic hormones and their possible roles in pregnancy and labor have all been considered in the two previous chapters. As was pointed out, only oxytocin can induce uterine contractions with a pattern which is indistinguishable from that of spontaneous labor, in concentrations that can be considered as physiological.

With the methods presently available, the assay of physiological amounts of *oxytocin* in blood is very difficult. By use of bioassay, Caldeyro-Barcia and his group,[11,12,18] Fitzpatrick and Walmsley,[34,36] and Coutinho[19] have found oxytocin-like activity in the blood during labor. Caldeyro-Barcia's group found oxytocin-equivalent activity in the jugular venous blood corresponding to 300–900 μU of oxytocin per milliliter of plasma during the second stage of labor.[18] The concentrations in the peripheral venous blood, and in the jugular venous blood in the first stage of labor, were much lower, usually between 20 μU/ml, which was the sensitivity limit of the assay, and 200 μU/ml. Coutinho used a less specific assay method;[19] in the peripheral blood during the second stage of labor he found oxytocic activity corresponding to 50–250 μU oxytocin per milliliter blood, going up to 1000–4000 μU/ml during delivery. During pregnancy and the first stage of labor the activity was below 20–40 μU/ml, which is the limit of sensitivity of the assay.

The concentration of *vasopressin* in the maternal blood during labor has been given very little attention, although studies of diuresis and urine osmolality indicate the presence of antidiuretic activity in the blood during parturition. As is the case with oxytoxin, the lack of reliable data is due to the very complicated assay methods presently available. Hoppenstein, Miltenberger, and Moran found very low concentrations of vasopressin in the peripheral venous blood during labor, less than 3

μU ADH per milliliter blood.[60] In the cord blood, on the other hand, the concentration was high, 35 μU/ml on the average, after vaginal delivery. In two infants delivered by cesarean section (one before and one during spontaneous labor), the concentrations were as low as in the maternal blood. Cobo *et al.*, on the other hand, found high levels in maternal blood during labor, except in patients where spinal anesthesia was used to prevent pain.[15] From his studies of the uterine and milk-ejecting activities during labor, Cobo concluded that oxytocin alone cannot account for the uterine activity.[16] It is conceivable that oxytocin and vasopressin both are released during labor and that the uterine activity is due to the combined action of both neurohypophysial hormones, which even may have a synergistic action. The fact that administration of ethanol, which inhibits the release of both hormones from the posterior pituitary gland, can arrest labor during the first stage, is in no way inconsistent with this assumption.[41, 48]

It was shown by Van Dyke and Ames that ethyl alcohol (ethanol) inhibits the release of vasopressin from the posterior pituitary gland.[110] During the last few years, Anna-Riitta Fuchs has demonstrated that this inhibition also holds true for oxytocin.[41, 44, 45] She first showed that the milk ejection reflex can be blocked by prior administration of ethanol, both in the rabbit[45] and in the human.[44] She went on to demonstrate that the onset of labor can be postponed in rabbits by infusion of ethanol.[41] This led to a study of the effect of ethanol on threatened premature labor.[47, 48] In a study which now comprizes 130 cases, it was found that labor could be arrested completely in 91 cases, and the contractions markedly reduced in frequency and amplitude in 38 patients, while only one did not respond at all. Of the 113 patients admitted with intact membranes, delivery was postponed for a minimum of three days and usually several weeks or even months in 65 per cent. If the membranes had ruptured, on the other hand, delivery could not be postponed more than a day or two, although there was an initial effect on the contractions even in these cases. Figure 13-4 shows the external tocographic recording from a patient who had to be treated twice with alcohol intravenously before her threatened premature labor was brought definitely under control. Since ethanol does not inhibit the uterine response to exogenous oxytocin and, in equivalent concentrations, does not inhibit myometrial activity in vitro, it is assumed that the effect of ethanol is due to inhibition of the release of oxytocin from the hypothalamopituitary neurosecretory system. These findings do not exclude the possibility that vasopressin is also involved in the endocrine mechanism of labor, since the release of this hormone is also blocked by ethanol.

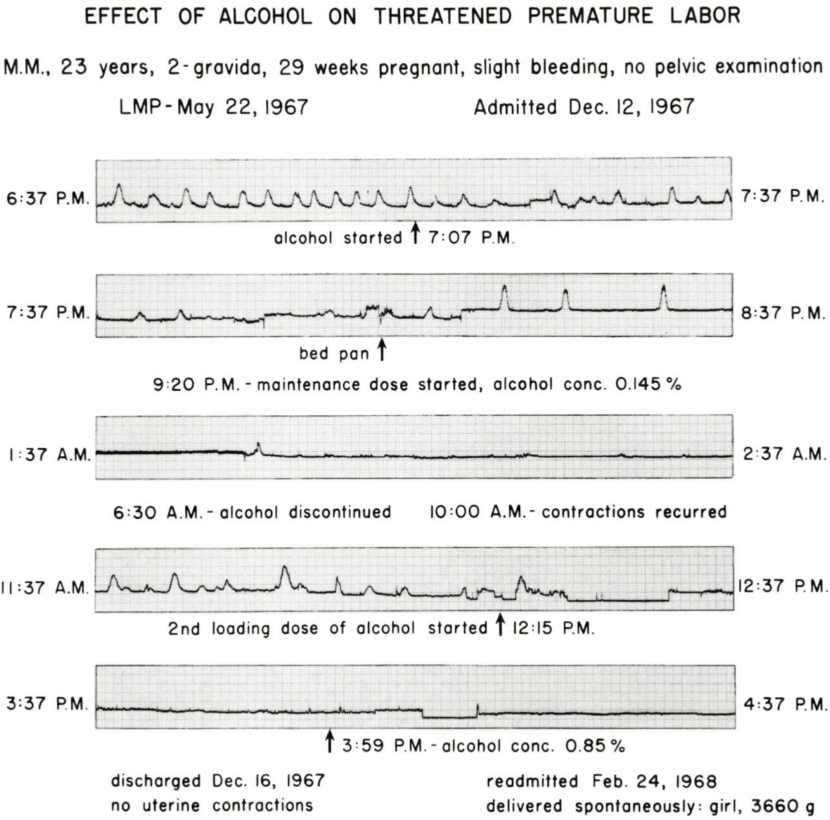

Fig. 13-4. External tocographic record from a patient with threatened premature labor at 29 weeks. After two courses of intravenous alcohol infusion the uterine contractions stopped and the pregnancy continued to term with delivery of a mature infant.

Oxytocinase

The destruction of oxytocin in the blood of pregnant women was discovered by Fekete in 1930.[33] Werle and co-workers established the enzymatic nature of the inactivation reaction and called the responsible compound oxytocinase.[112] This enzyme was later shown not only to inactivate oxytocin but also vasopressin and several other peptides. In spite of this lack of specificity, the term oxytocinase has been retained.[107] In 1957 Tuppy and Nesvadba provided evidence that oxytocinase splits the hormone molecule on the carboxyl side of its amino-terminal hemicystine residue.[108] The enzyme can be demonstrated in the blood very early in pregnancy, and the activity increases with advancing gestation, attaining its highest level during the last month and maintaining it until after delivery.[86, 97, 107]

Several workers claimed that the ability of plasma to inactivate oxytocin diminished towards term and almost disappeared during labor.[30, 59] This would have provided an attractive explanation for the onset of labor, but unfortunately the observations could not be confirmed. The changes in the last weeks before term are small and irregular.[86] During labor the activity usually increases,[56] and after injection or infusion of oxytocin the activity also increases.[51]

There has been much speculation on the physiological significance of the increased oxytocinase activity during pregnancy. Semm[99] and others have advanced the idea that the purpose of the high activity is to shield the uterus from premature stimulation. This effect would be overcome at term by increased release of oxytocin and increased oxytocin sensitivity of the myometrium. However, several factors militate against such a role of oxytocinase. In the circulation, oxytocin is inactivated much faster than can be accounted for by oxytocinase, which could only inactivate about 5 per cent of the oxytocin in the time required for the transport from the posterior pituitary gland to the uterus. And there is no evidence that premature labor occurs predominantly in patients with low oxytocinase levels. In view of the fact that oxytocinase is capable of inactivating also vasopressin and angiotensin, other functions of the enzyme are clearly to be considered, and at present it seems reasonable to conclude that the function of oxytocinase remains obscure.[107]

The situation is further complicated by the fact that another enzyme, which occurs in highest concentrations in the liver and kidneys and reportedly is present in the placenta, can inactivate oxytocin.[9, 107] This "tissue oxytocinase," which is very labile, splits oxytocin in a different place in the molecule; this is evidenced by the fact that it is able to inactivate deamino-oxytocin, which is not split by the plasma oxytocinase.[9] The function of this tissue oxytocinase, which is not specific to pregnancy and which presumably also inactivates vasopressin, is just as obscure as that of the plasma oxytocinase.

UTERINE SENSITIVITY TO OXYTOCIN AND VASOPRESSIN

The myometrial reactivity to oxytocin increases markedly with advancing gestation, as shown by many authors.[13, 57, 89, 105, 109] The sensitivity can be expressed by the threshold dose of oxytocin at various stages of pregnancy or by the uterine activity induced by a standard test dose at various stages. The shape of the curve describing the increasing activity by the latter method depends to some extent on the dose used, which explains some of the disagreement between previous reports (Caldeyro-Barcia, personal communication). The sensitivity increases most markedly shortly before and during labor both in the human and in several other animals.[38, 40, 42, 43, 57, 89, 101, 105] The oxytocin sensitivity has been used to determine when the uterus is "ripe" for induction of labor, first by Smyth[105] and subsequently by many others. Hendricks and Brenner[57] and others found that the sensitivity varied considerably from day to day at the end of pregnancy and did not increase steadily as had been maintained. From clinical experience it is obvious, however, that much less oxytocin is required to induce labor at term than before term.

The oxytocic activity of vasopressin, as measured in the bioassays used for standardization of oxytocic activity, is much less than that of oxytocin. According to Boissonnas *et al.*, the activity is 20 IU/mg for vasopressin and 450 IU/mg for oxytocin when measured on the rat uterus in vitro, and 70 IU/mg for vasopressin and 450 IU/mg for oxytocin when measured by the milk ejection activity in rabbits in vivo.[8] The relative activity thus can vary from one target organ to the other and from one species to another, but may also be influenced by the condition of the organ. Coutinho and Lopes have shown that the nonpregnant human uterus in vivo is much more sensitive to vasopressin than to oxytocin and that the cyclic variations in the sensitivity are much more pronounced for vasopressin than for oxytocin.[20] Embrey found that oxytocin and vasopressin have about equal effect on the human uterus in the first trimester of pregnancy; in the second trimester oxytocin was 2–3 times as potent as vasopressin, in the third trimester it was 5–10 times as potent, and during labor its activity was 10–15 times that of vasopressin.[32] Unfortunately, Embrey used arbitrary units and external recording of uterine activity, and the ratios should therefore be regarded as approximations. A study of the sensitivity of the human uterus to combinations of oxytocin and vasopressin is highly desirable, since a synergistic action of the two neurohypophyseal hormones on the human myometrium cannot be excluded. In the rabbit, however, the two hormones have an antagonistic rather than a synergistic effect.[39]

Placental Steroids and Oxytocin Sensitivity

As previously mentioned, the excitability of the myometrium is influenced by estrogens and progestagens. The estrogens are generally believed to increase the reactivity, while the progestagens are supposed to block the effect on the myometrium.[22-28, 54, 84] In the human, the evidence for this is equivocal, and directly conflicting reports can be found in the literature. Several groups have tried to improve the results of induction of labor with oxytocin by prior or simultaneous administration of estrogens. Pinto *et al.*[93] and Järvinen, Luukkainen, and Väistö[63] have increased the sensitivity to oxytocin by estrogens, while Klopper and Dennis[72] failed to demonstrate any difference in the length of the induction-to-delivery interval in three groups treated with stilbestrol, estriol, and placebo, respectively. Recently, however, Klopper has found a stimulatory effect of estriol sulfate injected into the amniotic cavity at term (personal communication). Mossman and Conrad, on the other hand, found a blocking effect of estradiol sulfate on isolated strips of human myometrium taken at term, although there was some variation in the response.[88] This might be an unspecific effect, since many steroids have an inhibitory effect on myometrial activity in vitro.

A withdrawal of a progesterone block is undoubtedly the cause of the increasing oxytocin sensitivity before the onset of delivery in the rabbit, as shown by Csapo,[22] Bengtsson,[4] Schofield,[100] and Fuchs and Fuchs.[43] In the human, there is very little evidence in support of a simlar relationship. As already mentioned, there is no decrease in the plasma progesterone levels before the onset of labor,[2,76,82,114,115] and oral or intramuscular administration of progesterone or synthetic progestagens has failed to prevent premature or term labor or to reduce the oxytocin sensitivity.[10,50,94,117] Csapo, who still is in favor of the hypothesis that a progesterone "block" must be withdrawn in the human as well as in the rabbit, does not consider the plasma progesterone levels of immediate relevance. He assumes that progesterone diffuses directly from the placenta to the overlying myometrium.[28] However, a relationship between plasma progesterone and oxytocin sensitivity in the human was found recently by Johansson, who examined the progesterone concentration in the blood of 61 term patients to be induced with oxytocin, using the competitive protein-binding technique. In the 23 patients who responded with regular contractions within three hours the average progesterone level was 96 ng/ml, while in the 39 who had a slow or no response the average was 140 ng/ml.[61] The difference between the two groups was highly significant.

As mentioned, administration of progesterone or synthetic progestagens in large doses has failed to delay the onset of spontaneous labor or to arrest threatened premature labor. Several investigators have studied the effect of progestagen treatment on induction of abortion by intra-amniotic injection of hypertonic saline.[7,29,49,52,69,87,90,104,111] Bengtsson and Csapo[7] found that such treatment more than doubled the injection to abortion time, while Møller, Wagner, and Fuchs[87] were unable to find any significant prolongation of the induction to abortion time in 15 cases.

Recently, Gennser, Kullander, and Lundgren reported 48 cases in a double-blind controlled study. They found a slight but statistically not significant increase in the induction to abortion time in the group treated with a progestagen (6-dehydro, 9, 10-retroprogesterone), as compared with the controls.[52] Since other factors than the hormone levels must influence the length of the interval (e.g., the concentration of saline in the amniotic fluid after the injection), these studies do not lead to a final conclusion as to the effect of progestagens on the sensitivity of the pregnant myometrium. It is quite possible that orally or intramuscularly administered progestagens do not reach the myometrium in sufficient quantities to influence the sensitivity, because of their rapid disappearance from the circulation.[104] The inhibitory effect of progestagens injected directly into the myometrium observed by Bengtsson[6] and others would seem to support this explanation.

It is possible that the sensitivity of the myometrium may be influenced by other hormones, but there is very little evidence in support of this. There is no study of the relation between chorionic gonadotrophin or placental lactogen and the oxytocin sensitivity, nor is anything known in the human of the effect of adrenal steroids or of other hormones of maternal origin in this regard. Epinephrine can interfere with the response to oxytocin by making the myometrium temporarily refractory,[39] and this may explain the uncoordinated labor in patients under severe nervous tension, but it is improbable that a withdrawal of epinephrine should trigger the onset of labor. As to hormones that could increase the oxytocin sensitivity, one might speculate about uterus-active substances like serotonin and prostaglandins. In this connection it should be noted that Karim in a recent paper has described elevated concentrations of prostaglandin F_{2a} in the blood just before and during each uterine contraction in spontaneus labor.[67] In a companion paper, Karim *et al.* reported that they had induced labor with normal patterns of contractions by intravenous infusion of prostaglandin F_{2a}.[68]

FETAL HORMONES AND LABOR

One cannot exclude the possibility that hormones of fetal origin play a role in the initiation and maintenance of labor. If the fetal blood contains a substantial amount of vasopressin at birth,[60] as mentioned above, it may also contain high levels of oxytocin; and both could be of fetal origin. The fact that it is possible to arrest threatened premature labor with ethanol[48] does not exclude this possibility, since ethanol moves freely across the placental barrier and equilibrium between the maternal and fetal blood is rapidly established.

Recently, Liggins, Kennedy, and Holm have performed a series of elegant studies of the fetal pituitary function in sheep which support the possibility of fetal factors being important in labor.[81] When they destroyed the fetal pituitary gland by electrocauterization without opening the uterus or the fetal skull, the pregnant ewe did not deliver at the expected time but continued the pregnancy without any signs of impending parturition. Control ewes with sham-operated fetuses with intact pituitary glands delivered at term. The adrenal glands in the hypophysectomized fetuses were found to be much smaller than normal.[79] Drost and Holm then performed adrenalectomy on sheep fetuses, and this also resulted in failure of the pregnant ewes to go into labor.[31] On the other hand, Liggins was able to induce premature labor by infusion of ACTH into the fetuses; the same was seen after infusion of cortisol or dexamethasone, while estradiol-17β did not have any apparent effect (personal communication). With a similar objective, Lanman and Shaffer decapitated fetal lambs in utero; of the three fetuses that survived, two were delivered spontaneously at term, while the third remained in utero and had to be delivered by hysterotomy 24 days past term.[77] The fetal adrenals were much smaller than normal in all three cases. While fetal decapitation thus gives less consistent results than fetal hypophysectomy or adrenalectomy, these studies do point to fetal humoral factors as playing a decisive role in labor in sheep. Whether this holds true for other species remains to be seen, but it should be remembered that dehydroisoandrosterone from the fetal adrenals is the main precursor for estriol in the human.

DISCUSSION

It is evident from the foregoing discussion that our knowledge of the mechanism of labor in the human is deficient. There must be certain factors which activate the uterus, as evidenced by the fact that contractions can be inhibited by alcohol which, in the concentrations used, does not have any significant effect on the myometrium itself. Most of the evidence is in favor of oxytocin as the activating factor, although other oxytocic hormones, either from the mother or the fetus, cannot be excluded. As a smooth muscle the myometrium is capable of autonomous activity, and while such activity does not appear to initiate labor, it may well play a role in its maintenance. The marked lack of sensitivity of the myometrium to oxytocin during most of pregnancy, and the increasing sensitivity toward term, provide support for the assumption of a defense mechanism which keeps the uterus at rest during fetal development. Whether or not progestagens are responsible for such a mechanism in the human, however, remains to be clarified. It is possible that progesterone not only influences the myometrial sensitivity, but also can interfere with the secretion of neurohypophysial hormones.[21,42] This possibility has not been mentioned in the foregoing discussion because it is still hypothetical at the present time. An auxiliary defense mechanism may be provided by the enzymes which inactivate the neurohypophyseal hormones, but there is no evidence that such enzymes are withdrawn to initiate labor.

Just as the newborn provides the stimulus which activates the milk ejection reflex so essential for its survival, it may well be that the fetus provides a stimulus which activates a "child ejection reflex." Whether or not the conjectured stimulus from the fetus is hormonal, as the studies in the sheep would indicate, and whether or not the reflex in the mother is neurohumoral, must remain open for future investigations. A clarification of the endocrine mechanism of human labor would be of enormous clinical significance. After all, premature labor alone is the cause of three-quarters of the perinatal mortality.

REFERENCES

1. Abrams, R. Y., and Abrams, J. Vaginal cytology in the prediction of onset of labor. *Obstet. Gynec. 20:*679, 1962.
2. Aitken, Elsie H., Preedy, J. R. K., Eton, B., and Short, R. V. Oestrogen and progesterone levels in foetal and maternal plasma at parturition. *Lancet 2:*1096, 1958.
3. Barnes, A. C., and Zuspan, F. P. Vaginal cytology as an index of the expected date of confinement. *Amer. J. Obstet. Gynec. 71:*1080, 1956.
4. Bengtsson, L. P. The endocrine control of myometrial contractility in the uterus of the pregnant rabbit. *Amer. J. Obstet. Gynec. 74:*484, 1957.
5. Bengtsson, L. P. Endocrine factors in labour. In Bengtsson, L. P., Diczfalusy, E., and Fuchs, F. Endocrinology of Pregnancy and Labour. *Acta Obstet, Gynec. Scand. 41* suppl. *1:*87, 1962.
6. Bengtsson, L. P. "Some Aspects of the Endocrine Control of Labour." In *Advances in Oxytocin Research,* J. H. M. Pinkerton (Ed.), Pergamon Press, London, 1965, p. 87.
7. Bengtsson, L. P., and Csapo, A. I. Oxytocin response, withdrawal, and reinforcement of defense mechanism of the human uterus in midpregnancy. *Amer. J. Obstet. Gynec. 83:*1083, 1962.
8. Boissonnas, R. A., Guttman, S., Berde, B., and Konzett, H. Relationship between the chemical structure and the biological properties of the posterior pituitary hormones and their synthetic analogues. *Experientia 17:*377, 1961.
9. Branda, L. A., Ferrier, B. M., Archimaut, G., Marchelli, E. A., and

RUCANSKI, B. Deamino-oxytocin: Inactivation by plasma of women in labor. *Science 160:*81, 1968.

10. BRENNER, W. E., and HENDRICKS, C. H. Effect of medroxyprogesterone acetate upon the duration and characteristics of human gestation. *Amer. J. Obstet. Gynec. 83:*1094, 1962.
11. CALDEYRO-BARCIA, R., and POSEIRO, J. J. Oxytocin and contractility of the pregnant human uterus. *Ann. N.Y. Acad. Sci. 75:*813, 1958.
12. CALDEYRO-BARCIA, R., and POSEIRO, J. J. Physiology of the uterine contraction. *Clin. Obstet. Gynec. 3:*386, 1960.
13. CALDEYRO-BARCIA, R., and SERENO, J. A. "The Response of the Human Uterus to Oxytocin Throughout Pregnancy." In *Oxytocin,* R. Caldeyro-Barcia and H. Heller (Eds.), Pergamon Press, Oxford, 1961, p. 177.
14. CARSTEN, MARY E. "Regulation of Myometrial Composition, Growth, and Activity." In *Biology of Gestation,* Vol. 1, N. S. Assali (Ed.), Academic Press, New York, 1968, p. 356.
15. COBO, E., GAITIN, E., MIRZACHI, M., and STRADA, G. Neurohypophyseal hormone release in the human. I. *Amer. J. Obstet. Gynec. 91:*905, 1965.
16. COBO, E. Uterine and milk-ejecting activities during human labor. *J. App. Physiol. 24:*317, 1968.
17. COBO, E. "Inhibicion de la Neurohipofisis Humana, Usando Alcohol y Sobrecarga de Agua." *Summaries Third Reunion Assoc. Latin-Amer. Invest. Human Reprod.* Salvador, Bahia, Brasil, 1968, p. 82.
18. COCH, J. A., BROVETTO, J., CABOT, H. M., FIELITZ, C. A., and CALDEYRO-BARCIA, R. Oxytocin-equivalent activity in the plasma of women in labor and during the puerperium. *Amer. J. Obstet. Gynec. 91:*10, 1965.
19. COUTINHO, E. M. Hormone-induced ionic regulation of labor. *Proc. Second Internat. Congr. Endocr.,* 1964, *Exerpta Med. Congr. Ser. 83:*742, 1965.
20. COUTINHO, E. M., and LOPES, A. C. V. Response of the nonpregnant uterus to vasopressin as an index of ovarian function. *Amer. J. Obstet. Gynec. 102:*479, 1968.
21. CROSS, B. A., and SILVER, I. A. Effect of luteal hormone on the behaviour of hypothalamic neurones in pseudopregnant rats. *J. Endocr. 31:*251, 1965.
22. CSAPO, A. "The Mechanism of Myometrial Function and Its Disorders." In *Modern Trends in Obstetrics and Gynaecology,* Second Series, K. Bowes (Ed.), Butterworth, London, 1955, p. 20.
23. CSAPO, A. I. Progesterone "block." *Amer. J. Anat. 98:*273, 1956.
24. CSAPO, A. I. Function and regulation of the myometrium. *Ann. N.Y. Acad. Sci. 75:*790, 1959.
25. CSAPO, A. I. "The Effect of Oxytocic Substances on the Excitability of the Uterus." In *Oxytocin,* R. Caldeyro-Barcia and H. Heller (Eds.), Pergamon Press, Oxford, 1961, p. 100.
26. CSAPO, A. I. The onset of labour. *Lancet 2:*277, 1961.
27. CSAPO, A. I. Defence mechanism of pregnancy. *Ciba Foundation Study Group No. 9:*3, 1961.
28. CSAPO, A. I. Model experiments and clinical trials in the control of pregnancy and parturition. *Amer. J. Obstet. Gynec. 85:*359, 1963.

29. Csapo, A. I. "The Termination of Pregnancy by the Intra-amniotic Injection of Hypertonic Saline." In *Yearbook of Obstetrics and Gynecology,* J. P. Greenhill (Ed.), 1966–1967, p. 126.
30. Dicker, S. E., and Tyler, C. Inactivation of oxytocin and vasopressin by blood plasma of pregnant women. *J. Obstet. Gynaec. Brit. Emp. 63:*690, 1956.
31. Drost, M., and Holm, L. W. Prolonged gestation in ewes after foetal adrenalectomy. *J. Endocr. 40:*293, 1968.
32. Embrey, M. P. A criterion of oxytocic activity. *J. Obstet. Gynaec. Brit. Emp. 66:*871, 1959.
33. Fekete, K. Beiträge zur Physiologie der Gravidität. *Endokrinologie 7:*364, 1930.
34. Fitzpatrick, R. J. Blood concentration of oxytocin in labour. *J. Endocr. 22:*XIX, 1961.
35. Fitzpatrick, R. J., and Bentley, P. J. "The Assay of Neurohypophysial Hormones in Blood and Other Body Fluids." In *Handbook of Experimental Pharmacology,* Vol. XXIII. Neurohypophysial Hormones and Similar Polypeptides, B. Berde (Ed.), Springer, Heidelberg, 1968, p. 190.
36. Fitzpatrick, R. J., and Walmsley, C. F. "Release of Oxytocin During Parturition." In *Advances in Oxytocin Research,* J. H. M. Pinkerton (Ed.), Pergamon Press, London, 1965, p. 51.
37. Frandsen, V. A., and Stakemann, G. The site of production of oestrogenic hormones in human pregnancy. III. *Acta Endocr.* (Kobenhavn) *47:*265, 1964.
38. Fuchs, A.-R. Oxytocin and the onset of labour in rabbits. *J. Endocr. 30:*217, 1964.
39. Fuchs, A.-R. Effect of adrenaline and vasopressin on the uterine response to oxytocin in conscious rabbits. *Acta Endocr.* (Kobenhavn) *45:*272, 1964.
40. Fuchs, A.-R. The role of oxytocin in the initiation of labour. *Proc. Second Internat. Congr. Endocr.* 1964. *Exerpta Med. Congr. Ser. 83:*753, 1965.
41. Fuchs, A.-R. The inhibitory effect of ethanol on the release of oxytocin during parturition in the rabbit. *J. Endocr. 35:*125, 1966.
42. Fuchs, A.-R. Studies on the control of oxytocin release at parturition in rabbits and rats. *J. Reprod. Fertil. 12:*418, 1966.
43. Fuchs, A.-R., and Fuchs, F. Induction and inhibition of labour in the rabbit. *Acta Endocr.* (Kobenhavn) *29:*615, 1958.
44. Fuchs, A.-R., and Wagner, G. Effect of alcohol on release of oxytocin. *Nature* (London) *198:*92, 1963.
45. Fuchs, A.-R., and Wagner, G. The effect of ethyl alcohol in the release of oxytocin in rabbits. *Acta Endocr.* (Kobenhavn) *44:*593, 1963.
46. Fuchs, F. Endocrine factors in the maintenance of pregnancy. In Bengtsson, L. P., Diczfalusy, E., and Fuchs, F. Endocrinology of Pregnancy and Labour. *Acta Obstet. Gynec. Scand. 41 suppl. 1:*7, 1962.
47. Fuchs, F. Treatment of threatened premature labour with alcohol. *J. Obstet. Gynaec. Brit. Comm. 72:*1011, 1965.
48. Fuchs, F., Fuchs, A.-R., Poblete, V. F., Jr., and Risk, A. Effect of alcohol

on threatened premature labor. *Amer. J. Obstet. Gynec. 99:*627, 1967. *Ugeskr. Laeger 130:*399, 1968.

49. Fuchs, F., Fuchs, A.-R., Short, R. V., and Wagner, G. Uterine motility and concentrations of progesterone in uterine venous blood after intra-amniotic injection of hypertonic saline. *Acta Obstet. Gynec. Scand. 44:*63, 1965.
50. Fuchs, F., and Stakemann, G. Treatment of threatened premature labor with large doses of progesterone. *Amer. J. Obstet. Gynec. 79:*172, 1960.
51. Fylling, P. Serum and plasma oxytocinase activity during induction of labour. *Acta Obstet. Gynec. Scand. 42:*227, 1963.
52. Gennser, G., Kullander, S., and Lundgren, N. Studies of therapeutic abortion induced by hypertonic saline. *J. Obstet. Gynaec. Brit. Comm. 75:*1058, 1968.
53. Goerttler, K. Die Architektur der Muskelwand des menschlichen Uterus und ihre funktionelle Bedeutung. *Gegenbaurs Morph. Jahrb. 65:*45, 1931.
54. Goto, M., and Csapo, A. I. The effect of the ovarian steroids on the membrane potential of uterine muscle. *J. Gen. Physiol. 43:*455, 1960.
55. Greig, Marion, Coyle, Mary G., Cooper, W., and Walker, J. Plasma progesterone in mother and foetus in the second half of human pregnancy. *J. Obstet. Gynaec. Brit. Comm. 69:*772, 1962.
56. Hashimoto, T. Studies on l-cystine-aminopeptidase. II. *J. Jap. Obstet. Gynec. Soc. 8:*96, 1961.
57. Hendricks, C. H., and Brenner, W. E. Patterns of increasing uterine activity in late pregnancy and the development of uterine responsiveness to oxytocin. *Amer. J. Obstet. Gynec. 90:*485, 1964.
58. Heusghem, C. *Contribution a l'étude analytique et biochimique des Œstrogènes naturals.* Masson, Paris, 1957.
59. Hilton, J. G., and Johnson, R. F. Changes in blood oxytocinase during parturition. *Amer. J. Obstet. Gynec. 78:*479, 1959.
60. Hoppenstein, J. M., Miltenberger, F. W., and Moran, W. H. The increase in blood levels of vasopressin in infants during birth and surgical procedures. *Surg Gynec. Obstet. 127:*1, 1968.
61. Johansson, E. D. B. Progesterone level and response to oxytocin at term. *Lancet 2:*570, 1968.
62. Jung, H. "The Effect of Oxytocin on the Mechanism of Uterine Excitation." In *Oxytocin,* R. Caldeyro-Barcia and H. Heller (Eds.), Pergamon Press, Oxford, 1961 p. 87.
63. Järvinen, P. A., Luukkainen, T., and Väistö, L. The effect of oestrogen treatment on myometrial activity in late pregnancy. *Acta Obstet. Gynec. Scand. 44:*258, 1965.
64. Kaiser, R. Ueber die Aenderung des Oestrogen/Pregnandiol-Quotienten im Verlauf der Graviditaet. *Arch. Gynäk. 192:*428, 1960.
65. Kamnitzer, M. B. Vaginal cytology at the end of pregnancy. *Acta Cytol. 3:*255, 1959.
66. Kao, C. Y. "Ionic Basis of Electrical Activity in Uterine Smooth Muscle." In *Cellular Biology of the Uterus,* R. Wynn (Ed.), Appleton-Century-Crofts, New York, 1967, p. 386.

67. Karim, S. M. M. Appearance of prostaglandin F_{2a} in human blood during labour. *Brit. Med. J. 4*:618, 1968.

68. Karim, S. M. M., Trussell, R. R., Patel, R. C., and Hillier, K. Response of pregnant human uterus to prostaglandin-F_{2a}-induction of labour. *Brit. Med. J. 4*:621, 1968.

69. Kerr, M. G., Roy, Eveline, Harkness, R. A., Short, R. V., and Baird, D. T. Studies of the mode of action of intra-amniotic injection of hypertonic solutions in the induction of labour. *Amer. J. Obstet. Gynec. 94*:214, 1966.

70. Klopper, A., and Billewicz, W. Urinary excretion of oestriol and pregnanediol during normal pregnancy. *J. Obstet. Gynaec. Brit. Comm. 70*:1024, 1963.

71. Klopper, A., and Dennis, K. J. Effect of oestrogens on myometrial contractions. *Brit. Med. J. 2*:1157, 1962.

72. Klopper, A., Macnaughton, M. C., and Michie, E. A. Oestriol and pregnanediol excretion during pregnancy and at the onset of labour. *J. Endocr. 22*:XIV, 1961.

73. Knaus, H. H. Der Eintritt der Geburt. *Zbl. Gynäk. 90*:7 & 49, 1968.

74. Kumar, D. "Hormonal Regulation of Myometrial Activity: Clinical Implications." In *Cellular Biology of the Uterus,* R. Wynn (Ed.), Appleton-Century-Crofts, New York, 1967, p. 449.

75. Kumar, D., Wagatsuma, T., Sullivan, W. J., and Barnes, A. C. Studies on the mechanism of action of progesterone on the human myometrium. II. *Amer. J. Obstet. Gynec. 90*:1355, 1964.

76. Kumar, D., Ward, Elisabeth D., and Barnes, A. C. Serial plasma progesterone levels and onset of labor. *Amer. J. Obstet. Gynec. 90*:1360, 1964.

77. Lanman, J. T., and Schaffer, A. Gestational effects of fetal decapitation in sheep. *Fertil. Steril. 19*:598, 1968.

78. Lemberg-Siegfried, S., Stamm, O., and de Watteville, H. Le frottis vaginal aux différents stades de la grossesse normale et pathologique. *Presse Med. 63*:1558, 1955.

79. Lichtfus, C. P. Vaginal cytology at the end of pregnancy. *Acta Cytol. 3*:247, 1959.

80. Liggins, G. C., and Kennedy, P. C. Effects of electrocoagulation of the foetal lamb hypophysis on growth and development. *J. Endocr. 40*:371, 1968.

81. Liggins, G. C., Kennedy, P. C., and Holm, L. W. Failure of initiation of parturition after electrocoagulation of the pituitary of the fetal lamb. *Amer. J. Obstet. Gynec. 98*:1080, 1967.

82. Llauro, J. L., Runnebaum, B., and Zander, J. Progesterone in human peripheral blood before, during, and after labor. *Amer. J. Obstet. Gynec. 101*:867, 1968.

83. Marshall, J. M. *Initiation of Labor.* U.S. Department of Health, Education and Welfare, Public Health Service Publ. No. 1390, 1965.

84. Marshall, J. M. Relation between the ionic environment and the action of drugs on the myometrium. *Fed. Proc. 27*:115, 1968.

85. Marshall, J. M., and Csapo, A. I. Hormonal and ionic influences on the membrane activity of uterine smooth muscle cells. *Endocrinology 68:*1026, 1961.

86. Melander, S. Plasma oxytocinase activity. *Acta Endocr.* (Kobenhavn) *48:* suppl. 96, 1965.

87. Møller, K. J. A., Wagner, G., and Fuchs, F. Inability of progestagens to delay abortions induced by hypertonic saline. *Amer. J. Obstet. Gynec. 90:*694, 1964.

88. Mossman, R. G., and Conrad, J. T. *In vitro* blocking and oxytocic effects of water-soluble estrogens on pregnant human, mouse, and rat uteri. *Amer. J. Obstet. Gynec. 99:*539, 1967.

89. Munsick, R. A. "The Effect of Neurohypophysial Hormones and Similar Polypeptides on the Uterus and Other Extravascular Smooth Muscle Tissue." In *Handbook of Experimental Pharmacology.* XXIII. Neurohypophysial Hormones and Similar Polypeptides, B. Berde (Ed.), Springer, Heidelberg, 1968, p. 443.

90. Osborn, R. H., Goplerud, C. P., and Yannone, M. E. Response of peripheral plasma progesterone concentration to intra-amniotic hypertonic saline. *Amer. J. Obstet. Gynec. 101:*1073, 1968.

91. Øvlisen, B., and Iversen, J. Treatment of threatened premature labor with 6α-methyl-17α-acetoprogesterone. *Amer. J. Obstet. Gynec. 86:*291, 1963.

92. Pinto, R. M., Lerner, U., and Pontelli, H. The effect of progesterone on oxytocin-induced contraction of the three separate layers of human gestational myometrium in the uterine body and lower segment. *Amer. J. Obstet. Gynec. 98:*547, 1967.

93. Pinto, R. M., Leon, C., Mazzocco, N., and Scasserra, V. Action of estradiol-17-β at term and at the onset of labor. *Amer. J. Obstet. Gynec. 98:*540, 1967.

94. Pose, S. V., and Fielitz, C. "The Effects of Progesterone on the Response of the Pregnant Human Uterus to Oxytocin." In *Oxytocin,* R. Caldeyro-Barcia and H. Heller (Eds.), Pergamon Press, Oxford, 1961, p. 229.

95. Pundel, J. P., and Van Meensel, F. *Gestation et Cytologie Vaginale.* Masson, Paris, 1951.

96. Roy, E., and Mackay, R. The concentration of oestrogens in blood during pregnancy. *J. Obstet. Gynec. Brit. Comm. 69:*13, 1962.

97. Ryden, G. Cystine aminopeptidase and oxytocinase activity in pregnancy. *Acta Obstet. Gynec. Scand. 45:*suppl. 3, 1966.

98. Saldivar, J. T., Jr., and Melton, C. E., Jr. Effects *in vivo* and *in vitro* of sex steroids on rat myometrium. *Amer. J. Physiol. 211:*835, 1966.

99. Semm, K. Das Wehenproblem mit besonderer Berücksichtigung des Oxytocin-Oxytocinasehaushaltes. *Z. Geburtsh. Gynäk.* (Suppl.) *154:*1, 1960.

100. Schofield, B. M. The hormonal control of myometrial function during pregnancy, *J. Physiol. 138:*1, 1957.

101. Schofield, B. M. "The Physiology of the Myometrium." In *Recent Advances in Physiology,* R. Crease (Ed.), Churchill, London, 1963, p. 222.

102. Schofield, B. M. "Parturition." In *Advances in Reproductive Physiology,* A. McLaren (Ed.), Logos Press, London, 1968, p. 9.

103. Shearman, R. P. Some aspects of the urinary excretion of pregnanediol in pregnancy. *J. Obstet. Gynaec. Brit. Emp. 66:*1, 1959.

104. Short, R. V., Fuchs, A.-R., Fuchs, F., and Wagner, G. Progesterone concentrations in uterine venous blood after intra-amniotic injection of hypertonic saline in midpregnancy. *Amer. J. Obstet. Gynec. 91*:132, 1965.

105. Smyth, C. N. Uterine irritability. *Lancet 1*:237, 1958.

106. Taubert, H. D., and Haskins, A. L. Intravenous infusion of progesterone in human females: blood levels obtained and effect on labor. *Obstet. Gynec. 22*:405, 1963.

107. Tuppy, H. "The Influence of Enzymes on Neurohypophysial Hormones and Similar Peptides." In *Handbook of Experimental Pharmacology.* XXXIII. Neurohypophysial Hormones and Similar Polypeptides, B. Berde (Ed.), Springer, Heidelberg, 1968, p. 67.

108. Tuppy, H., and Nesvadba, H. Ueber die Aminopeptidaseaktivität des Schwangerenserum. *Mh. Chem. 88*:977, 1957.

109. Turnbull, A. C., and Anderson, A. B. M. Uterine contractility and oxytocin sensitivity during human pregnancy in relation to the onset of labour. *J. Obstet. Gynaec. Brit. Comm. 75:*278, 1968.

110. Van Dyke, H. B., and Ames, R. Alcohol diuresis. *Acta Endocr.* (Kobenhavn) *7:*110, 1951.

111. Wagner, G., Frandsen, V. Aa., and Stakemann, G. Oestriol excretion during induced abortion. *Acta Obstet. Gynec. Scand. 42:*suppl. 6:105, 1963.

112. Werle, E., Hevelke, A., and Buthmann, K. Zur Kenntniss des oxytocinabbauenden Prinzips des Blutes. *Biochem. Z. 309*:270, 1941.

113. Wide, L. An immunological method for the assay of human chorionic gonadotrophin. *Acta Endocr.* (Kobenhavn) Suppl. *70,* 1962.

114. Woolever, C. A. Progesterone and progesterone therapy in pregnancy. *Clin. Obstet. Gynec. 8*:565, 1965.

115. Yannone, M. E., McCurdy, J. R., and Goldfien, A. Plasma progesterone levels in normal pregnancy, labor and the puerperium. *Amer. J. Obstet. Gynec. 101:*1058, 1968.

116. Zidovsky, J. Significance of parabasal ('postnatal') cells in the vaginal smear in prolonged pregnancy. *Acta Cytol. 5*:393, 1961.

Chapter Fourteen

Endocrine Factors in Abortion and Premature Labor

Arnold Klopper

Much research has been devoted to the study of abortion and premature labor, and a great volume of writings on the subject has accumulated. However, our understanding of the processes involved has expanded little in the last few decades and our ability to control them has not expanded at all. There are many reasons for this, not the least of which is the fact that much of the study, of necessity, has had to be conducted within the context of clinical medicine. The scientific principles of exact definition of material and of controls have largely been ignored. The institution of controls in abortion studies is a difficult and controversial matter, but the lack of design and the failure of categorization which has characterized most studies in this field is inexcusable. It is all the more deplorable when one realizes that widely accepted definitions of threatened abortion, inevitable abortion, missed abortion, recurrent abortion, and premature labor have existed for decades. These categories should be rigidly separated and, in writings on the subject, the criteria for preventing findings pertaining to inevitable or missed abortion from obtruding on data in the other categories should be stated; the experi-

This work was done under a grant to the author by the Medical Research Council of Britain.

mental design should be such as to permit maximum discrimination between these entities.

In clinical practice, threatened abortion is a very heterogeneous group containing diverse causal elements, and even under circumstances of the most careful clinical categorization the group will contain a considerable admixture of *post hoc* established fetoplacental damage rendering the material unsuitable for causal endocrine study. For this reason we shall direct our attention in this chapter mainly to prospective studies of recurrent abortion. The term habitual abortion has unfortunate connotations of volition, making it, in a sense, on a par with drug taking or other bad habits. The term habitual abortion will therefore be eschewed. The definition of recurrent abortion as three or more consecutive abortions arises from a misconceived view on the incidence of abortion in subsequent pregnancies, and recurrent abortion will be used, therefore, to signify two or more previous abortions. Primary recurrent aborters who have never carried a pregnancy beyond 28 weeks are on *prima facie* grounds likely to constitute the most homogeneous group, but secondary aborters, who had had a term pregnancy followed by two or more consecutive abortions, are too numerous to be ignored, provided the data on these can be separated from the primary group.

It is a matter of common clinical impression (perhaps not sufficiently critically examined) that an abortion at 12–14 weeks is an essentially dissimilar process from the miniature labor which may happen at 22–24 weeks. The view that the causation of the latter may have much in common with the onset of normal labor has much to recommend it. In this chapter, in order to keep these two dissimilar processes separate, the event which occurs at 5–20 weeks will be called an abortion, and the event which occurs at 20–36 weeks will be called a premature labor. It is likely that in the 16–20 week group there is a considerable overlap of these categories.

One further point needs to be made concerning the selection and definition of abortion material. In nearly all studies on recurrent abortion, the women have not come under observation until the pregnancy was at least 10–12 weeks in duration. A recent study has directed attention to the fact that in recurrent abortion more than half of the women who are going to abort have done so by the twelfth week.[38] Any study in which a substantial proportion of the patients were 12 weeks or more pregnant when they came under surveillance has been done, therefore, on a population which is *ipso facto* heavily biased in favor of fetal salvage. It is essential to specify at which stage of pregnancy study was begun, and it is of prime importance that observations should commence early in pregnancy.

This chapter will deal only with the endocrine factors in abortion; other elements such as genetic faults will be mentioned only in passing. Although many hormones play a role in the endocrinology of pregnancy, the paucity of experimental evidence concerning other compounds obliges us to limit consideration to three types of compounds: chorionic gonadotrophin, progestagens, and the estrogens. As far as abortion is concerned, two aspects will be surveyed: (1) the excretion of hormone metabolites by women liable to abort, and (2) the therapy of abortion with hormones. Premature labor will be examined in terms of hormone-related changes in the uterus and cervix. For reasons of space, it is not possible to attempt to review the voluminous literature of even this restricted field. The chapter outlines a personal view of the development of thought in the last two decades and occasionally supports possibly idiosyncratic views by data from our experimental work.

STUDIES ON HORMONE LEVELS IN ABORTION

These studies can conveniently be grouped into those where the initial hormone levels were determined as a means of prognosis and those in which serial studies were made as a means of studying the changes in hormone level associated with the process of abortion.

Initial Hormone Levels

Chorionic Gonadotrophin

Assays of chorionic gonadotrophin as an index of the likelihood of abortion have a long history, much of it reflecting technical developments in assay methods rather than advances in our knowledge of the genesis of abortion. It is the only one of the hormones to be considered which has been measured in blood, rather than as a urinary excretion product, with any satisfactory degree of accuracy, and therefore it is the only one to be examined in terms of serum rather than urinary levels. Until the 1960's the only method available for the measurement of chorionic grandotrophin was to observe its secondary effects on the gonads or secondary sex organs of small animals, the end points being such phenomena as ovarian hyperemia, increase in uterine weight, or the release of sperms. In spite of a good deal of sophistication in the statistics of this approach,[6] this early era contributed nothing of lasting value to our understanding of abortion.

A general consensus about the pregnancy curve for HCG was arrived at which has not yet been seriously challenged. This shows a rapidly increasing serum concentration rising to a peak 60 days from the last menstrual period and then falling to a midpregnancy low of one-fourth to one-third peak value. Many series also show a second much smaller rise at term, although this is not often remarked upon.[3,54] Almost no studies were done on day to day variation in the same person, and even normal person to person variation was seldom described in acceptable statistical terms.

The combination of this paucity of information about the normal universe, the gross inaccuracy and imprecision of biological assay, and the fact that measurements had to be made at a time when levels were changing rapidly defeats any possibility of discriminating judgment today. However, many studies purporting to show a high liability to abort in subjects with low initial chorionic gonadotrophin levels have appeared. There is little doubt that chorionic gonadotrophin levels fall once the chorionic tissue which is producing the hormone is severely damaged. What must be regarded as an entirely open question is whether a fall in gonadotrophin level precedes the damage to the placenta or is in any way a primary cause of the abortion. These studies may be entirely transformed by the new immunological techniques for the assay of chorionic gonadotrophin produced within a short while of one another by Wide[53] and by Brody and Carlström.[8] Brody and Carlström have certainly gone on to show that the prognosis in those patients with threatened abortion, in whom the ultimate diagnosis cannot be made clinically on admission, is closely correlated with their initial serum gonadotrophin level.[9] This, of course, still leaves unanswered the question of whether the fall in gonadotrophin is causal. It is a matter of some interest that a few of their patients showed normal levels but went on to abort in midpregnancy; this is another straw in the wind showing that early and late abortions are essentially dissimilar processes.

Progesterone

Although adequate methods for the estimation of progesterone in blood have been devised, the information on changes in blood progesterone concentration in pathological pregnancy is fragmentary. The normal pregnancy values show a large scatter.[50,57] There are, in fact, few data on the variation from subject to subject or from day to day in the same subject. Without these data it is impossible to evaluate changes in pathological states. Blood progesterone levels are poorly correlated with what are presumed to be progesterone-conditioned physiological events, and show hardly any correlation with corresponding urinary pregnanediol levels. This may be due, at least in part, to the fact that progesterone is very rapidly removed from the circulation. The amount of hormone found in the peripheral circulation is only a small part of that produced by the feto-placental unit; a substantial proportion is metabolized in its passage through the maternal liver. We are obliged to adopt the unsatisfactory expedient of evaluating the changes in progesterone production which may accompany abortion largely in terms of urinary pregnanediol. Although methods for the assay of pregnanediol in blood have been published,[43, 52] they are inadequate to examine the changes associated with abortion and no reliable evidence on the changes in blood pregnanediol exists. Changes of progesterone concentration in the retroplacental blood associated with the therapeutic induction of abortion have cast an interesting light on the role of this hormone in the onset of normal labor; these changes are discussed in Chapter Thirteen.

Investigations of the value of initial pregnanediol excretion in forecasting the outcome of the pregnancy by women liable to abort now date back nearly 30 years. Perhaps the most authoritative early study was done by Guterman.[23] In a study of threatened abortion he found that 90 per cent of those patients who had a low pregnanediol excretion eventually aborted while only 14 per cent of those with normal levels aborted.

In recurrent abortion, the results were less dramatic; 93 per cent of the patients with normal levels carried the pregnancy to term while only 43 per cent of those with low levels went to term. In a flash of insight which was to be ignored for the next decade, he pointed out that he was unable to confirm the therapeutic effect of progesterone and that the incidence of recurrent abortion in his series was not nearly as high as had been predicted on previous statistical calculations.[39] Guterman's view that initial pregnanediol levels indicated the likely outcome of the pregnancy was confirmed by an authoritative European publication,[7] and each year has produced a fresh crop of publications in which similar findings have been noted. The distinction between cause and consequence has become increasingly blurred. In many quarters the causal role of progesterone deficiency is now regarded as self evident and the obvious therapeutic deduction is drawn with enthusiasm.[46]

A contrary wind has started to blow in recent years. Shearman and Garrett,[49] Goldzieher[21] and Klopper and Macnaughton[35] have all failed to find any significant difference in pregnanediol excretion between patients who were going to abort and those who would carry their pregnancy to term. In a group of 33 primary recurrent aborters studied by Klopper and Macnaughton, those who carried their pregnancy beyond 30 weeks had an average initial excretion rate of pregnanediol of 8.77 mg/24 hours; whereas those who aborted before 30 weeks had an initial rate of 7.57 mg/24 hours. All these patients had pregnanediol assays done before they were 10 weeks pregnant. A larger mixed series of 74 primary and secondary recurrent aborters had similar values. Many of the earlier studies were done by assay methods which would be quite unacceptable today, but it is hard to see how this could give rise to apparent differences between aborters and non-aborters. On the other hand, many earlier series included a high proportion of women more than 8–10 weeks advanced in pregnancy, and it is difficult to escape the conclusion that these data were biased by the inclusion of many patients who already had serious placental injury by the time the first measurements were made.

At most it is an open question whether progesterone deficiency is ever *propter hoc* rather than *post hoc.* The evidence on grounds other than pregnanediol assays strongly supports the thesis that a primary feto-placental defect is a far more common cause of abortion.

Estrogens

Methods for the estimation of estrogens in blood are as yet in their infancy. The role of estrogens in abortion will therefore be discussed in terms of the excretion of a major estrogen metabolite, estriol, in the urine. Although estriol measurements have been widely applied to the study of placental function later in pregnancy, surprisingly few papers have been published on estriol excretion in relation to abortion.[17] Attention has been concentrated on pregnanediol measurements in the mistaken belief that these were examining a causal factor. In normal pregnancy, pregnanediol excretion rises slowly between 5 and 10 weeks and it is possible to group together initial excretion value over this whole period without bias even if the proportion of 5 or 10 week pregnancies is unduly low or high. Estriol excretion, however, rises much more rapidly over this time, and the 9–10 week gestation group would raise unduly the average value for the 5–8 week group if the groups were taken together. For this reason, the 5–8 week and 9–10 week groups have been considered separately in Table 14-1.

The higher average initial estriol excretion of those who will carry their pregnancy through 30 weeks as compared to those who are going to abort is interesting and worth a closer look. Figure 14-1 shows the standard deviation about these mean values.

TABLE 14-1
INITIAL ESTRIOL EXCRETION IN PRIMARY RECURRENT ABORTION*

Stage of pregnancy at initial assay	Pregnancy carried beyond 30 weeks	Pregnancy aborted before 30 weeks
5– 8 weeks	100 μg/24 hr	84 μg/24 hr
9–10 weeks	319 μg/24 hr	113 μg/24 hr

* From Klopper and Macnaughton. *J. Obstet. Gynaec. Brit. Comm. 72:*1022, 1965.

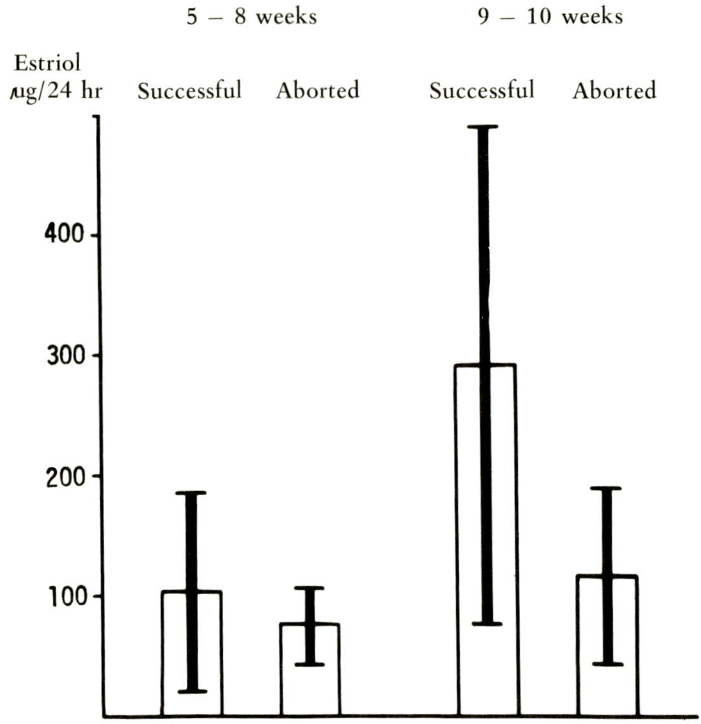

Fig. 14-1. Average and standard deviation of estriol output in patients who aborted compared with the excretion of those who carried the pregnancy beyond 30 weeks. Figures for the 5–8 week group and the 9–10 week group at initial assay are given separately. (From Klopper and Macnaughton. *J. Obstet. Gynaec. Brit. Comm. 72:*1022, 1965.)

There is a considerable overlap, at both stages of gestation, between the lower values among the successful pregnancies and the highest values among the aborters. Therefore, one cannot predict with any degree of assurance in the individual case what the outcome of the pregnancy will be on the basis of the initial estriol value. The large scatter about the mean in all groups makes the differences between the means not significant. It is nevertheless interesting that, in the same group of patients, the mean difference in estriol values between successful pregnancies and abortions is much greater proportionally than the mean difference in pregnanediol values.

Serial Studies

Serial studies of hormone excretion have been widely advocated. They certainly have formidable advantages over single estimations. The element of uncertainty introduced by the large day-to-day variation in normal hormone excretion is largely eliminated, and it is possible to see whether the output is rising or falling with time. It is helpful to know that the excretion of a hormone metabolite is falling at a time when it should be increasing, and it is possible by serial studies to demarcate zones of increasing danger with some assurance. It is the causal interpretation of serial studies which should be viewed with caution. Because a successive fall in pregnanediol or estriol can often be shown to precede an abortion it does not mean that a failure in the production of the parent hormone is the cause of the abortion or that the process can be reversed by suitable steroid therapy. The available evidence supports more strongly the view that the changes in steroid output are themselves engendered by the primary cause of the abortion. The falling steroid values reflect the increasing damage to feto-placental function which may go on to fetal death and abortion.

This view of the secondary role of the endocrine changes is to some extent borne out by the data displayed in Figure 14-2.

This figure is taken from a group of 74 primary and secondary recurrent aborters studied by Klopper and Macnaughton.[35] It shows the mean value week-by-week of the pregnanediol excretion of patients who aborted as contrasted with the excretion of those who carried the pregnancy beyond 30 weeks. These values were derived somewhat differently from those of previous studies. The estimations were started early in pregnancy and no values from a patient who aborted were included in the abortion mean if the urine was collected within a week of the onset of symptoms of the abortion. It was hoped in this way to reduce the number of values derived from patients who were already suffering from inevitable or missed abortion. It can be seen that no real difference between aborters and non-aborters becomes apparent until after 12 weeks gestation. By the time the lines deviate clearly the number of patients contributing to the mean of the aborting group is falling sharply as those who have aborted or will do so within a week are, of course, removed from the group.

The mean estriol excretion of aborters contrasted with non-aborters, shows a somewhat different picture. (Fig. 14-3). Here the mean value of the aborters deviates much earlier in pregnancy and the difference between the two groups is relatively much greater. This may be taken to argue a causal role for the estrogens, but at least one other explanation is also feasible. This concerns the somewhat different meanings of pregnanediol and estriol in the mother's urine. It can be assumed that pregnanediol is a simple function representing the amount of active trophoblastic tissue while estriol is more complex, its level in urine being the outcome of both fetal and placental activity. If, therefore, the abor-

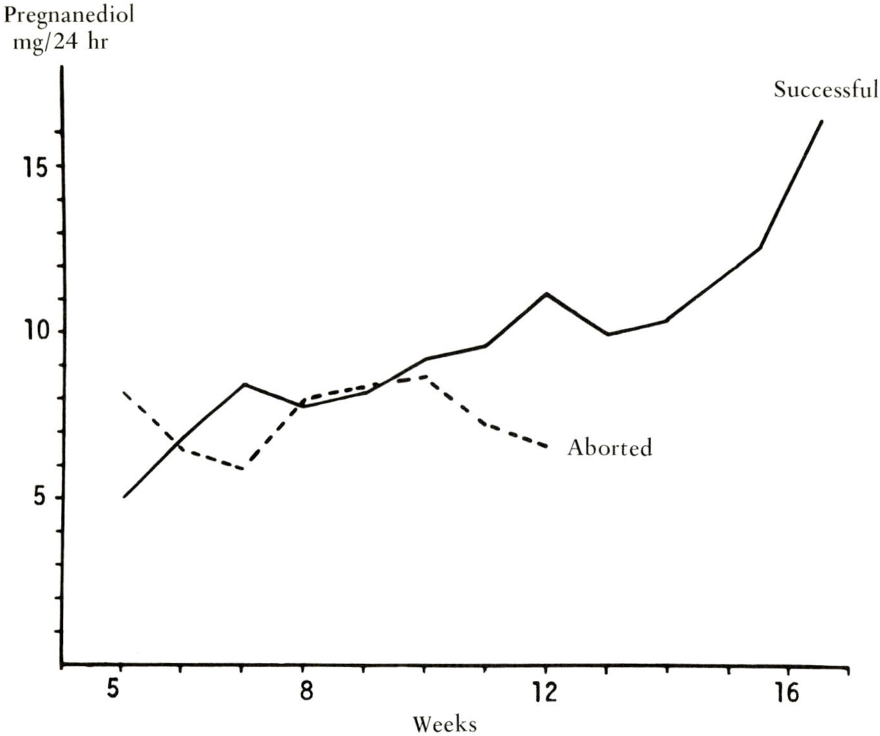

Fig. 14-2. Average weekly pregnanediol excretion of patients who aborted compared with that of patients who carried the pregnancy beyond 30 weeks. No results from patients who were within a week before aborting are included in the mean values. (From Klopper and Macnaughton. *J. Obstet. Gynaec. Brit. Comm. 72:*1022, 1965.)

tion is preceded by devitalisation and death of the fetus, the estriol output will be greatly depressed by the loss of the fetal role. Pregnanediol levels, on the other hand, may remain nearly normal as long as trophoblastic activity is maintained by the maternal circulation in the intervillous spaces.

The differential role of estriol and of pregnanediol is illustrated in Figure 14-4. This patient was not a recurrent aborter but a primigravida excluded from the normal pregnancy series of Klopper and Billewicz[33] because she produced a macerated fetus at 23–24 weeks. Evidently fetal death took place slowly because, although estriol levels showed an alarming deviation early in pregnancy, the uterine growth continued and pregnanediol levels remained normal. Presumably, placental function survived relatively intact until nearly 20 weeks when the pregnanediol

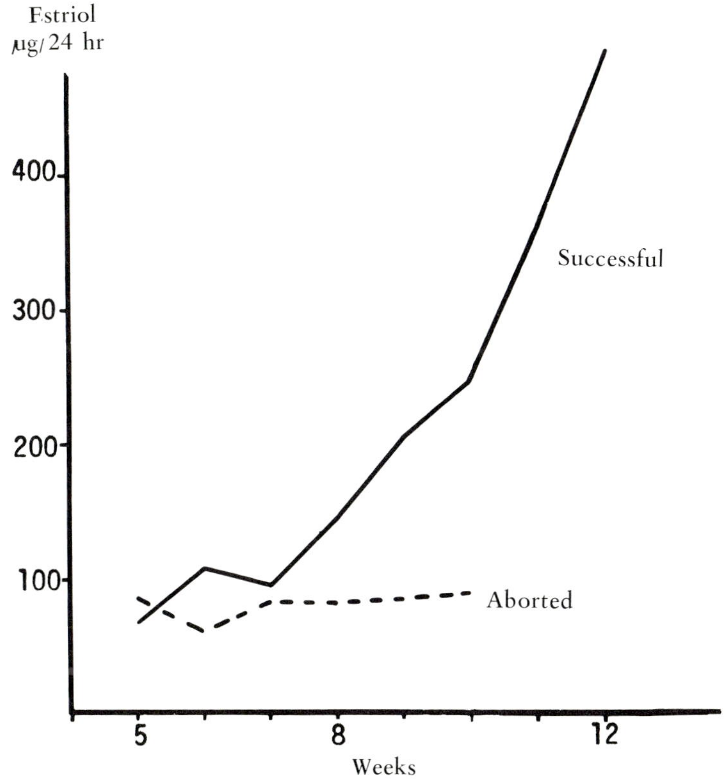

Fig. 14-3. Average weekly estriol excretion of patients who aborted compared with that of patients who carried the pregnancy beyond 30 weeks. No results from patients who were within a week of aborting are included in the mean values. (From Klopper and Macnaughton. *J. Obstet. Gynaec. Brit. Comm.* *72*:1022, 1965.)

output suddenly fell precipitously. It is of interest that in this patient other metabolic changes of pregnancy, such as fluid retention and the laying down of fat which have been associated with estrogens and progesterone, respectively, by Hytten and Leitch,[32] followed the pattern which might be expected if estrogen production were low and progesterone normal.

HORMONE THERAPY OF ABORTION

Some information on the role of hormones in abortion may be deduced from the results of hormone therapy. Unfortunately, the true state of affairs regarding therapy has long been obscured by two fundamental misconceptions. The first, that a substantial proportion of

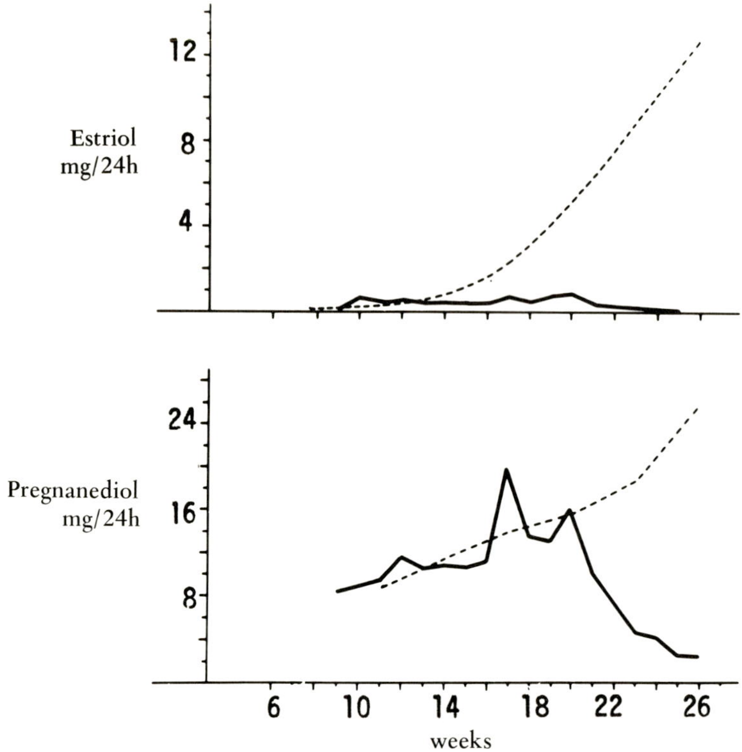

Fig. 14-4. Serial assays of estriol and pregnanediol excretion in a primigravida before and after intrauterine death of the fetus. Macerated fetus delivered at 23–24 weeks. Dashed lines represent normal values, solid lines represent patient. (From Hytten and Leitch. Blackwell, Oxford, 1964.)

abortions is caused by primary hormone deficiency, has already been examined. The second arises from a mistaken belief that the incidence of abortion increases with the number of previous abortions. Malpas is primarily responsible for the view that a woman who has aborted on several occasions has an increased chance of abortion in subsequent pregnancies.[39] Indeed, according to his calculations, a woman who has had four successive abortions has nearly a 100 per cent chance of aborting in a subsequent pregnancy. This view was further elaborated by Eastman, and came to be universally adopted in the obstetrical world. Thereafter, it was only necessary for an investigator to show that the administration of a particular compound was followed by a fetal salvage rate notably greater than would be expected by the Malplas calculation in order to demonstrate the effectiveness of the compound. By these means many investigators claimed that various progestagens were beneficial in abortions.

This subject will not be discussed here since it has been ably reviewed by Goldzieher and Benigno.[22] It was presumed that the abortion-preventing capacity of progestagens had been amply demonstrated, and it was thought that the causative role of progesterone deficiency had, by the same token, been substantiated. Goldzieher and Benigno questioned the Malpas calculation and showed that the predicted high incidence of abortion following four or more abortions did not occur, whatever the therapy. It slowly became evident that in recurrent abortion a salvage rate of about 70 per cent could be expected from any form of intensive care, without specific therapy.

A more sophisticated version of this approach has also been applied to demonstrate the efficacy of synthetic progestational compounds in habitual abortion.[47] In this work, the patient is used "to act as her own control;" that is, the previous fetal loss rate of a group of aborters is used to judge whether the compound used in the present pregnancy was effective. There is, in fact, no evidence that the conclusions thus derived are any more valid than those of the earlier blind trial, testing the progestational compound against a placebo in the same population. By this means it was shown that a variety of synthetic progestational compounds did not significantly improve fetal salvage in abortion. The failure of progestational compounds to affect the process of abortion does not prove that progesterone deficiency plays no role in the causation of abortion, but it weakens somewhat arguments which are based upon the presumed therapeutic effect of progesterone.

Attempts to evaluate the use of estrogens in the therapy of abortion have not been notably successful. Upon occasion, stilbestrol in particular has had enthusiastic advocates, but the figures for fetal salvage are not convincing in the light of present criteria. Goldzieher and Benigno reviewed five series in which stilbestrol was used and found an average abortion rate of 35 per cent, much the same as could be expected in any untreated group.[22] Although, in abortion, the fall in estriol levels occurs earlier and is more marked than is the case with pregnanediol, the results of estrogen therapy do not substantiate the role of estrogen deficiency in the etiology of abortion.

The results both of assays of endogenous hormone production and of treatment with hormones do not support the hypothesis that primary hormone deficiency plays a considerable role in abortion. This does not mean that no such cases do occur. They may constitute too small a proportion of the total number of abortions to be detected by either of these means. The result of hormone therapy in particular is a very blunt weapon in this context. The nonspecific cure rate in recurrent abortion is high, and it would require a large number of patients to demonstrate even a modest improvement. It has, in fact, been calculated that it would require a double blind trial of 1078 recurrent aborters to demonstrate even a 10 per cent improvement in fetal salvage.[21] Improved means of measuring the endocrine *mileau interieur* have a better chance of evaluating the role of hormones in abortion. To do so, however, requires considerable improvements in the techniques for the assay of hormones in blood and urine. In addition, much more attention must be paid to statistical principles in the design of trials, and there must be a rigorous clinical control of patients starting earlier in pregnancy.

ENDOCRINE FACTORS IN PREMATURE LABOR

It has already been pointed out that abortion and premature labor appear to be essentially dissimilar in nature, and that we shall call the event occurring between 20 and 36 weeks a premature labor. There will obviously be some overlap between the two groups at the earlier stage but such a chronological distinction is otherwise a convenient means of categorization which does discriminate between different processes.

The traumatic and sociological components in the etiology of premature labor have received much attention in recent years. Obstetrical interest has centered particularly on the role of previous cervical trauma in causing an anatomical defect which detracts from complete uterine closure. This interest in a relatively minor component in the causation of premature labor has diverted attention from the more important physiological changes in the cervix which are an essential part of pregnancy. The balance has been somewhat restored by the work of Wood *et al.*[55] Each week, from 24 weeks until delivery, they assessed the cervical and myometrial activity of a group of women. They found that either premature dilation of the cervix or excessive uterine activity by themselves did not very often give rise to premature labor, but the two factors in combination were very likely to do so. Attention has been drawn to a third element by Armenia.[1] He pointed out that under normal circumstances the chorion is firmly attached to the decidua. If the cervix dilates the membranes will not prolapse until they are sheared from the lower uterine segment. Three factors may be operative in such shearing: (1) uterine contractions, (2) bleeding (e.g., from a marginal sinus), and (3) inadequacy in the formation of the decidua vera and capsularis. Very much more is known about cervical changes and about alterations in myometrial contractility than about the loosening of the membranes from the decidua; therefore, only the role which hormones might play in the physiology of the cervix and myometrium will be discussed here.

Cervical Changes

Three related aspects of the changes induced by pregnancy in the cervix have been studied. They are changes in the chemical composition of the cervix, changes in its microscopic architecture, and changes in its mechanical properties. Much of the pioneer work in this field was done by Harkness and his colleagues at University College Hospital in London.[24–31] They studied rats and found that during pregnancy the total amount of collagen in the uterus increased greatly, nearly as much proportionally as the total uterine wet weight. A similar but smaller increase took place in the total collagen content of the cervix. Some 24–48 hours after delivery, the cervical collagen content fell very rapidly as the protein was reabsorbed. The collagen content of the membranes rose to a peak on the 17th day of pregnancy and thereafter fell off. The tensile strength of the fetal membranes appeared to be related to their collagen content, the maximum strength being reached the day after the peak concentration of collagen in the membranes and then, like the latter, falling off rapidly as term approached.

Harkness found that these changes in the chemical composition of the rat's cervix during pregnancy went *pari passu* with changes in its physical properties. He measured the extensibility of the cervix at various stages of pregnancy and found that there was a great increase in extensibility. It was concluded that the changes in the cervix were related to the ease with which collagen fibrils could slip upon one another, as though there had been a change in molecular links between collagen fibrils and in the viscosity of the ground substance binding them together. A study of the time relationships of these changes in the mechanical properties of the cervix showed that, although some continuous change could be detected from early pregnancy, the dramatic alterations took place in the 24 hours before birth.

Similar studies were made on the rat cervix by Zarrow and Yochim.[58] They emphasized the increasing water content of the cervix in pregnancy so that the collagen fibers become spread further apart and the collagen concentration in terms of cervical wet weight actually decreases while the total content increases. The changes in chemical composition and mechanical properties are reflections of changes in the microscopic architecture of the cervix. Changes in the microscopic build of the cervix were elucidated by Danforth and his colleagues.[12-14] They pioneered the application of these studies to the human female and thus alerted obstetricians to the possible bearing of cervical changes on premature labor. In the nonpregnant cervix the collagen is a dense tightly woven felt. During pregnancy there is some dissociation of collagen bundles into fibrillar constituents. There is a loosening of the collagen with an increase of interfibrillar ground substance but, as in the rat, dramatic changes only take place shortly before the onset of labor. The ground substance mass increases during pregnancy, but the hexosamine, which is one of the principal constituents of the mucopolysaccharides of the ground substance, stays more or less constant in concentration. The primary change may therefore be in the ground substance of the cervix which becomes increasingly hydrated and whose properties determine the solubility of collagen.

Attempts to correlate cervical changes with the onset of premature labor have not been uniformly successful. Buckingham, Buethe, and Danforth were able to show a marked change in the collagen:muscle ratio of the incompetent cervix,[12] and it is tempting to suppose that many instances of premature labor can be accounted for by the premature onset of the rapid changes which occur in the cervix just before term labor.

Although it seems probable that premature labor and cervical changes are connected and that these cervical changes are under hormonal influence, studies designed to explore which hormones do what, are yet in their infancy. A few scattered findings show interesting pointers along the way. In rats, the pregnancy changes in cervical collagen can be imitated in kind but not in degree by the simultaneous administration of estrogen, progesterone, and relaxin, and it may be surmised that the combination has a stimulatory effect upon collagenase, the enzyme which hydrolyzes collagen. It has already been suggested that the primary change is more likely to be related to the ground substance than to the collagen. It is therefore of interest to examine the effect of various hormones on the mucopolysaccharides of the genital tract. Much of the definitive work in this field has been done by Zachariae, who showed that under the influence of estrogen large amounts of short-lived acid mucopolysaccharides are produced in the uterus.[56] Progesterone blocks this estrogen-induced production of mucopolysaccharides. It must be noted, however, that in the experiments of Zachariae the chief effect of estrogens was upon the ground substance of the endometrium, the sulphomucopolysaccharides of the cervix being relatively resistant to estrogen. The effect of estrogens on mucopolysaccharides was further explored by Kvarstein, Nordbo, and Schultz-Haudt who showed that estrogen treatment lowered the chondroitin sulfate B content of rat skin.[37] It seems likely, therefore, that estrogens can effect both the amount and composition of the ground substance of the cervix.

A further aspect of the relationship between estrogens and changes in cervical composition deserves attention. The belief that estriol, rather than being a relatively inert metabolite of other more active estrogens, is a hormone in its own right with specific effects on the cervix, has been gaining ground in the last few years. The evidence in favor of this view has been reviewed by Merrill.[40] It has long been known that estriol is produced in large quantities during human pregnancy. This disproportionate secretion of estriol in particular appears to be peculiar to the human. The role of estriol in pregnancy may not be general to all mammals, but it is just possible that, in the human, estriol levels play a determinant part in the development of cervical change. One may surmise that the reason a connection between estriol and cervical change has not been demonstrated before is that biologists have been looking at the wrong hormone in the wrong species.

Changes in Myometrial Activity

In general, the changes in myometrial activity associated with the onset of premature labor resemble those which occur with labor at term. The onset of normal labor has been discussed in the previous chapter. Here we will take only a passing glance at some aspects of endocrine function pertinent to the problem of premature labor.

The part played by estrogens in premature labor will not be understood until their role in normal pregnancy is elucidated. A few facts, however, about the changes caused by estrogens in the myometrial cell are clearly established. The work of Mueller has shown that the primary effect of estradiol is on the protein metabolism of the uterus, probably through its effect in promoting the synthesis of nucleoprotein.[42] Specifically, it has been shown that the incorporation of formate, glycine, and serine into the nucleic acid purines, adenine and guanine, is greatly stimulated. Over-all protein synthesis, as measured by incorporation of amino acids like serine or tryptophan, is stimulated. The end result of this process can be detected as a hypertrophy and hyperplasia of the myometrial cells.[11] Possibly these processes are germane to growth changes in the pregnant uterus rather than to myometrial contractility, but it is very likely that the effects of estrogens on uterine carbohydrates,[10] water,[5] and electrolytes[15] are all pertinent to myometrial activity. Indeed, estrogens have been shown to have profound effects on the type of contractions which can be induced in the myometrium of a rabbit in late pregnancy.[48] Estrogens cause an expansion of the intracellular compartment relative to the extracellular space in the uterus together with a shift of sodium into, and of potassium out of, the cells.

Until now estrogen assays have not shown any consistent change in estrogen levels associated with the onset of labor, although a statistical correlation between urinary estriol excretion at 36 weeks and the stage of gestation at which labor eventually begins was claimed by Klopper and Billewicz.[33] Premature labor is occasionally preceded by particular types of placental damage, such as retroplacental hemorrhage, which may quite obscure the true nature of the change in estrogens levels which takes place at this time. The evidence concerning the effect of estrogen administration on myometrial contractility is equally confusing. Bayer[2] and Pinto, Fisch, and Schwarcz[45] have claimed that hexestrol and estradiol, respectively, will greatly enhance myometrial contractility. Klopper and Dennis, however, found no effect from estriol or stilbestrol on the induction-delivery interval following artificial rupture of the membranes.[34] The situation can best be summarized by saying that it is likely that estrogens alone or in combination with other hormones do have an effect on the onset of normal or premature labor, but just how the estrogens are involved is not known.

The role of progesterone in the onset of premature labor may be bound up with its effect in reducing the potential across the myometrial cell. The results of treatment of threatened premature labor with progesterone have been disappointing.[20] Nor have the more potent synthetic compounds like 17α-hydroxyprogesterone caproate[16] or 6α-methyl-17α-acetoxyprogesterone[44] yielded better results, although the latter compound had been shown by Fuchs and Koch to be capable of stopping oxytocin-induced premature labor in the rabbit much more efficiently than progesterone.[19] These findings do not prove that a fall in progesterone production or an alteration in its metabolism is not a cause of premature labor. Such an alteration in progesterone levels may be evident only in the blood of the retroplacental space. It has been claimed by Bengtsson and Csapo that a fall in placental progesterone production is responsible for the premature labor which results when hypertonic saline is injected into the uterus.[4] On the other hand, Klopper, Turnbull, and Anderson found no significant change in urinary pregnanediol before the onset of labor in these patients,[36] and Short *et al.* were unable to detect any fall in the progesterone concentration of the uterine venous blood.[51] Like the estrogens, progesterone probably plays a part in premature labor, but key factors in the process have not yet been elucidated.

In contrast to the early abortions, endocrine factors may play a causative role in premature labor. It can be surmised that what occurs in premature labor is similar in nature to what happens in the onset of normal labor, and that premature labor very often represents an endocrine-induced dysjunction in time of the integrated physiological processes of pregnancy rather than a specific pathology. Of interest in this connection is the fact that in most of the cases of threatened premature labor in which labor was arrested with intravenous administration of ethyl alcohol the uterus remained inactive after discontinuation of the alcohol.[18] Labor did not recur until after an interval of days, weeks, or even months. Whatever the triggering factor is in these cases of premature labor, it does not appear to be any permanent change in the endocrine milieu, but rather a reversible, temporary stimulus, which, under normal conditions is released at a time characteristic for the species in question when endocrine factors have made the uterus optimally sensitive.

REFERENCES

1. ARMENIA, C. S. The "incompetent internal os" as a cause of late abortion and premature labor. *Obstet. Gynec. 21*:349, 1963.
2. BAYER, R. Labor induction and the determination of the termination of labor with water-soluble estrogens in obstetrics outside the hospital. *Zbl. Gynak. 84*:1841, 1962.
3. BEHRMAN, S. J., and NIEMANN, P. Serum gonadotrophins in normal and abnormal pregnancy; quantitative and qualitative analysis. *Fertil. Steril. 6*:236, 1955.
4. BENGTSSON, L. P., and CSAPO, A. Oxytocin response, withdrawal and reinforcement of the defence mechanism in the human uterus at midpregnancy. *Amer. J. Obstet. Gynec. 83*:1083, 1962.
5. BITMAN, J., CECIL, H. C., HAWK, H. W., and SYKES, J. F. Effect of estrogen and progesterone on water and electrolyte content of rabbit uteri. *Amer. J. Physiol. 197*:93, 1959.
6. BORTH, R. L'importance de la biométrie en médicine en biologie et en biochimie. *Internat. Ztschr. Vitaminforsch. 22*:226, 1950.
7. BORTH, R., and DE WATTEVILLE, H. Hormone assays in obstetrics and gynecology. *Vitamins Hormones* (*N. Y.*) *10*:141, 1952.
8. BRODY, S., and CARLSTRÖM, G. Immunoassay of human chorionic gonadotrophin in normal and pathologic pregnancy. *J. Clin. Endocr.* 22:564, 1962.
9. BRODY, S., and CARLSTRÖM, G. Human chorionic gonadotrophin in abnormal pregnancy. Serum and urinary findings using various immunoassay techniques. *Acta Obstet. Gynec. Scand. 44*:32, 1965.
10. BRODY, S., and WESTMAN, A. Effects of oestradiol and progesterone on the glycogen content of the rabbit uterus. *Acta Endocr.* (Kobenhavn) *28:*39, 1958.
11. BRODY, S., and WIQUIST, N. Ovarian hormones and uterine growth: effects of estradiol, progesterone and relaxin on cell growth and cell division in the rat uterus. *Endocrinology 68*:971, 1961.
12. BUCKINGHAM, J. C., BUETHE, R. A., and DANFORTH, D. N. Collagen-muscle ratio in clinically normal and clinically incompetent cervices. *Amer. J. Obstet. Gynec. 91:*232, 1965.
13. BUCKINGHAM, J. C., SELDON, R., and DANFORTH, D. N. Connective tissue changes in the cervix during pregnancy and labor. *Ann. N.Y. Acad. Sci. 97*:733, 1962.

14. Danforth, D. N., Buckingham, J. C., and Roddick, J. W. Connective tissue changes incident to cervical effacement. *Amer. J. Obstet. Gynec. 80*:939, 1960.

15. Daniel, E., and Daniel, B. Effects of ovarian hormones on the content and distribution of cation in intact and extracted rabbit and cat uterus. *Canad. J. Biochem. 35*:1205, 1957.

16. Eichner, E. Clinical use of 17α-hydroxyprogesterone caporate in the prevention of premature labor and its effect upon fetal salvage. *Ann. N.Y. Acad. Sci. 71*:789, 1958.

17. Frandsen, V. A., and Stakemann, G. The urinary excretion of estriol during the early months of pregnancy. *Acta Endocr.* (Kobenhavn) *44*:196, 1963.

18. Fuchs, F., Fuchs, A.-R., Poblete, V. F., Jr., and Risk, A. Effect of alcohol on threatened premature labor. *Amer. J. Obstet. Gynec. 99*:627, 1967.

19. Fuchs, F., and Koch, F. Inhibition of oxytocin-induced labor in rabbits with various gestagens. *Acta Endocr.* (Kobenhavn) *42*:403, 1963.

20. Fuchs, F., and Stakemann, G. Treatment of threatened premature labor with large doses of progesterone. *Amer. J. Obstet. Gynec. 79*:172, 1960.

21. Goldzieher, J. W. Double-blind trial of a progestin in habitual abortion. *J.A.M.A. 188*:651.

22. Goldzieher, J. W., and Benigno, B. B. The treatment of threatened and recurrent abortion: A critical review. *Amer. J. Obstet. Gynec. 75*:1202, 1958.

23. Guterman, H. S. Physiologic basis for clinical applications of progesterone. *J. Clin. Endocr. 10*:641, 1950.

24. Harkness, M. L., and Harkness, R. D. Further observations on collagen in regenerating liver of rat. *J. Physiol. 123*:482, 1954.

25. Harkness, M. L., and Harkness, R. D. Growth of collagen in foetus, placenta and foetal membranes of rat. *J. Physiol. 128*:225, 1955.

26. Harkness, M. L., and Harkness, R. D. Changes in physical properties and in collagen and hexosamine contents of foetal membranes during pregnancy in rat. *J. Physiol. 132*:482, 1956.

27. Harkness, M. L., and Harkness, R. D. Changes in the distensibility on the uterine cervix of the rat after parturition. *J. Physiol. 141*:34P, 1958.

28. Harkness, M. L., and Harkness, R. D. Changes in the physical properties of the uterine cervix of the rat during pregnancy. *J. Physiol. 148*:524, 1959.

29. Harkness, M. L., and Harkness, R. D. Effect of enzymes on the mechanical properties of tissues. *Nature* (London) *183*:1821, 1959.

30. Harkness, M. L., and Harkness, R. D. The mechanical properties of the rat uterine cervix during involution after parturition. *J. Physiol. 156*:112, 1961.

31. Harkness, R. D., and Moralee, B. E. Time-course and route of loss of collagen from rat's uterus during postpartum involution. *J. Physiol. 132*:502, 1956.

32. Hytten, F. E., and Leitch, I. *The Physiology of Human Pregnancy.* Blackwell, Oxford, 1964.

33. Klopper, A., and Billewicz, W. Urinary excretion of oestriol and pregnanediol during normal pregnancy. *J. Obstet. Gynaec. Brit. Comm. 70*:1024, 1963.
34. Klopper, A. I., and Dennis, K. J. Effect of oestrogens on myometrial contractions. *Brit. Med. J. 2*:1157, 1962.
35. Klopper, A., and Macnaughton, M. Hormones in recurrent abortion. *J. Obstet. Gynaec. Brit. Comm. 72*:1022, 1965.
36. Klopper, A. I., Turnbull, A. C., and Anderson, A. B. Changes in steroid hormone excretion during abortion in midpregnancy by the intra-amniotic injection of hypertonic saline. *J. Obstet. Gynaec. Brit. Comm. 73*:390, 1966.
37. Kvarstein, B., Nordbo, H., and Schultz-Haudt, S. An effect of estrogen on the chondroitin sulphate of rat skin connective tissue. *Acta Endocr.* (Kobenhavn) *44*:209, 1963.
38. Macnaughton, M. C. The probability of recurrent abortion. *J. Obstet. Gynaec. Brit. Comm. 71*:784, 1964.
39. Malpas, P. A study of abortion sequences. *J. Obstet. Gynaec. Brit. Emp. 45*:932, 1938.
40. Merrill, R. C. Estriol: A review. *Physiol. Rev. 38*:463, 1958.
41. Møller, K. J. A., and Fuchs, F. Double-blind controlled trial of 6-methyl, 17-acetoxyprogesterone in threatened abortion. *J. Obstet. Gynaec. Brit. Comm. 72*:1042, 1965.
42. Mueller, G. C. Some biochemical studies on the mechanism of action of estrogens. *Cancer 10*:716, 1957.
43. Oertel, G. W., Bechmann, I. N., and Eik-Nes, K. B. The measurement of pregnane-3α, 20α-diol and its isomers in human plasma. *Arch. Biochem. 86*:148, 1960.
44. Øvlisen, B., and Iversen, J. Treatment of threatened premature labor with 6α-methyl-17α-acetoxyprogesterone. *Amer. J. Obstet. Gynec. 86*:291, 1963.
45. Pinto, R. M., Fisch, L., and Schwarcz, R. Action of estradiol 17β upon uterine contractility and the milk-ejecting effect in the pregnant woman. *Amer. J. Obstet. Gynec. 90*:99, 1964.
46. Rawlings, W. J., and Krieger, V. I. Studies in the prevention of recurrent abortion due to corpus luteum deficiency. *Med. J. Aust. 45*:561, 1958.
47. Reifenstein, E. C. Clinical use of 17α-hydroxy progesterone caproate in habitual abortion. *Ann. N.Y. Acad. Sci. 71*:762, 1958.
48. Schofield, B. M. The effect of injected oestrogen on pregnancy in the rabbit. *J. Endocr. 25*:95, 1962.
49. Shearman, R., and Garrett, W. Double-blind study of effect of 17-hydroxyprogesterone caproate on abortion rate. *Brit. Med. J. 1*:292, 1963.
50. Short, R. V. Progesterone in blood. The chemical determination of progesterone in peripheral blood. *J. Endocr. 16*:415, 1958.
51. Short, R. V., Wagner, G., Fuchs, A.-R., and Fuchs, F. Progesterone concentrations in uterine venous blood after intra-amniotic injection of hypertonic saline in mid-pregnancy. *Amer. J. Obstet. Gynec. 91*:132, 1965.
52. Sommerville, I. F., and Deshpande, G. N. The quantitative determination

of progesterone and pregnanediol in human plasma. *J. Clin. Endocr.* *18:*1223, 1958.

53. Wide, L. An immunological method for the assay of human chorionic gonadotrophin. *Acta Endocr.* (Kobenhavn) *88:* Suppl. 70, 1962.
54. Wilson, R. B., Albert, A., and Randall, L. M. Quantitative studies on production, destruction and elimination of chorionic gonadotrophin in normal pregnancy. *Amer. J. Obstet. Gynec.* *58*:960, 1949.
55. Wood, C., Bannerman, R. H., Booth, R. I., and Pinkerton, J. H. The prediction of premature labor by observation of the cervix and external tocography. *Amer. J. Obstet. Gynec.* *91*:396, 1965.
56. Zachariae, F. Autoradiographic (S35) and histochemical studies of sulphomucopolysaccharides in the rabbit uterus, oviducts and vagina; variations under hormonal influence. *Acta Endocr.* (Kobenhavn) *29*:118, 1958.
57. Zander, J. Progesteron in menschlichem Blut und Geweben: Progesteron im peripheren venösen Blut der Frau. *Klin. Wschr.* *33*:697, 1955.
58. Zarrow, M. X., and Vochim, J. Dilatation of the uterine cervix of the rat and accompanying changes during the estrous cycle, pregnancy and following treatment with estradiol, progesterone and relaxin. *Endocrinology* *69*:292, 1961.

Index

70 71 72 73 10 9 8 7 6 5 4 3 2 1